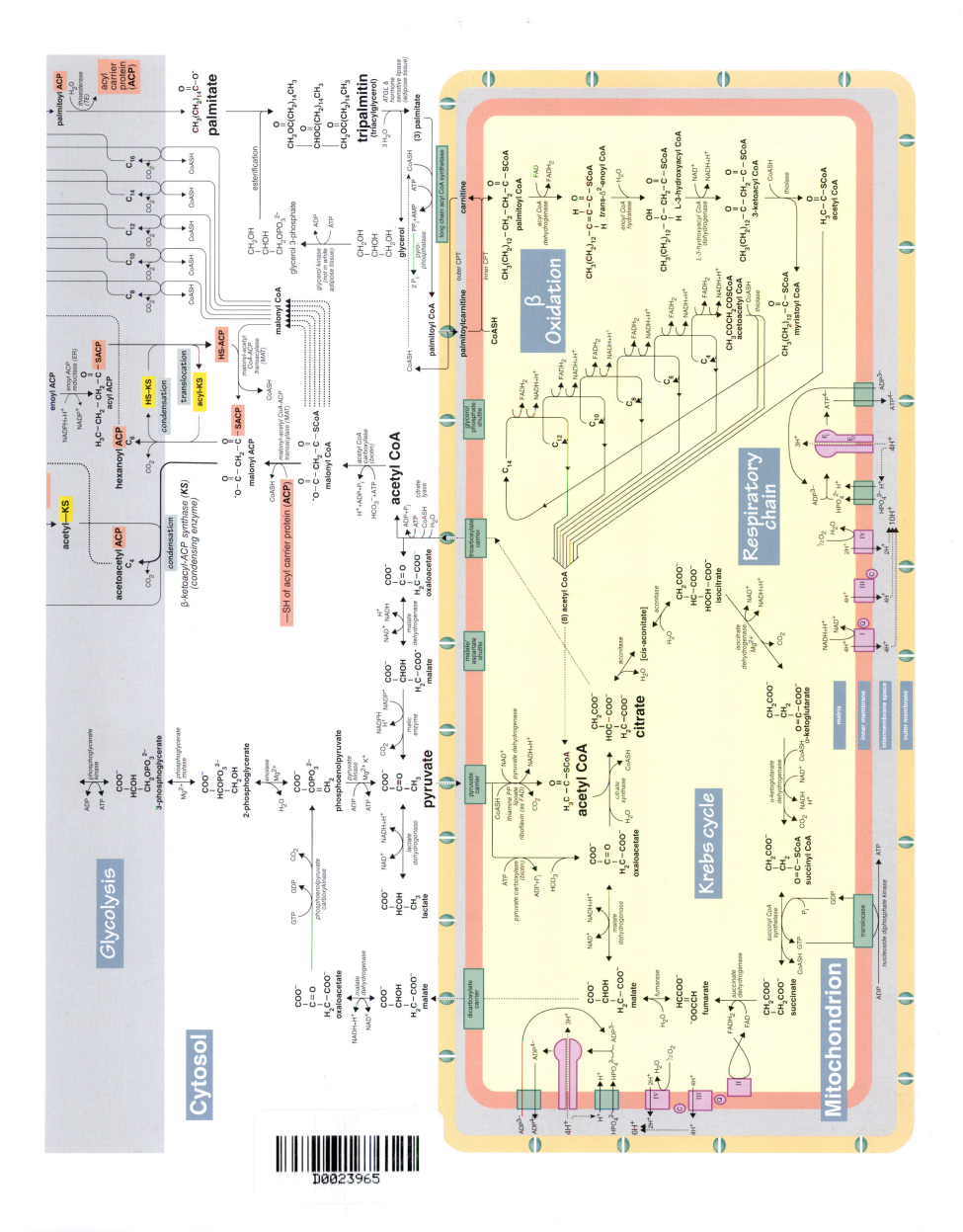

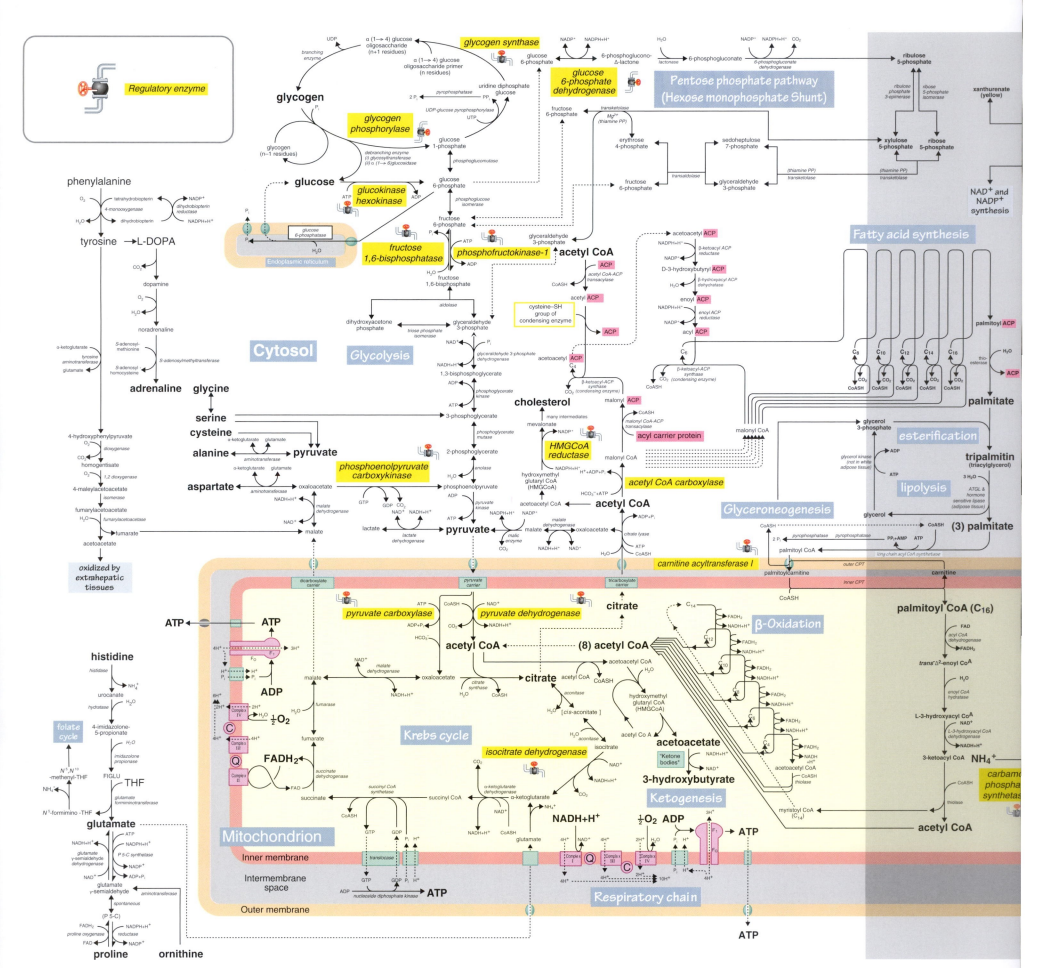

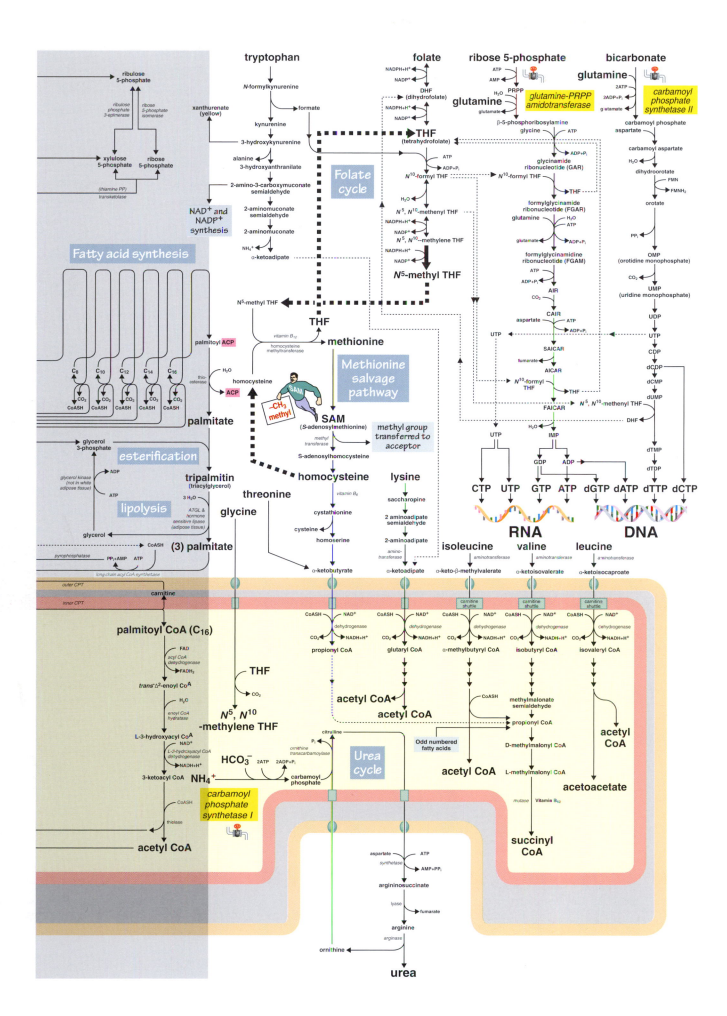

To the memory of Richard W. Hanson (1935–2014), Case Western Reserve University, Ohio, USA

Metabolism at a Glance

J. G. Salway
University of Surrey
Guildford, UK

FOURTH EDITION

WILEY Blackwell

This edition first published 2017 © 2017 by John Wiley & Sons Ltd
First published 1994
First Japanese edition 1994
First Complex Chinese edition 1996
First German edition 1997
Second edition 1999
Second Japanese edition 2000
Second German edition 2000
Spanish edition 2002
Third edition 2004
Korean edition 2006
Brazilian edition 2009
Portuguese edition 2009
Turkish edition 2012

Registered Office
John Wiley & Sons Ltd, The Atrium, Southern Gate, Chichester, West Sussex, PO19 8SQ, UK

Editorial Offices
9600 Garsington Road, Oxford, OX4 2DQ, UK
The Atrium, Southern Gate, Chichester, West Sussex, PO19 8SQ, UK
111 River Street, Hoboken, NJ 07030-5774, USA

For details of our global editorial offices, for customer services and for information about how to apply for permission to reuse the copyright material in this book please see our website at www.wiley.com/wiley-blackwell

The right of the author to be identified as the author of this work has been asserted in accordance with the UK Copyright, Designs and Patents Act 1988.

Library of Congress Cataloging-in-Publication Data

Names: Salway, J. G., author.
Title: Metabolism at a glance / J.G. Salway.
Other titles: At a glance series (Oxford, England)
Description: Fourth edition. | Chichester, West Sussex ; Hoboken, NJ : John
    Wiley & Sons Inc., 2017. | Series: At a glance series | Includes
    bibliographical references and index.
Identifiers: LCCN 2016007782| ISBN 9780470674710 (pbk.) | ISBN 9781119277781
    (Adobe PDF)
Subjects: | MESH: Metabolism | Metabolic Diseases | Handbooks
Classification: LCC QP171 | NLM QU 39 | DDC 616.3/9–dc23 LC record available at
    http://lccn.loc.gov/2016007782

A catalogue record for this book is available from the British Library.

Wiley also publishes its books in a variety of electronic formats. Some content that appears in print may not be available in electronic books.

Cover image: © Caroline Mardon 2016

Set in 9.25/12.5pt Minion by SPi Global, Pondicherry, India
Printed and bound in Malaysia by Vivar Printing Sdn Bhd

1 2017

Contents

Preface   ix
Acknowledgements   x

 Part 1 **Energy metabolism**

1   Introduction to metabolic pathways   2

2   Biosynthesis of ATP I: ATP, the molecule that powers metabolism   4

3   Biosynthesis of ATP II: mitochondrial respiratory chain   6

4   Oxidation of cytosolic NADH: the malate/aspartate shuttle and glycerol phosphate shuttle   8

5   Metabolism of glucose to provide energy   10

6   Metabolism of one molecule of glucose yields 31 (or should it be 38?) molecules of ATP   12

7   Anaerobic metabolism of glucose and glycogen to yield energy as ATP   14

8   2,3-Bisphosphoglycerate (2,3-BPG) and the red blood cell   16

9   Metabolism of triacylglycerol to provide energy as ATP   18

Part 2 **Carbohydrate metabolism**

10   Metabolism of glucose to glycogen   20

11   Glycogen metabolism I   22

12   Glycogen metabolism II   24

13   Glycogen metabolism III: regulation of glycogen breakdown (glycogenolysis)   26

14   Glycogen metabolism IV: regulation of glycogen synthesis (glycogenesis)   28

15   Pentose phosphate pathway: the production of NADPH and reduced glutathione   30

16   Regulation of glycolysis: overview exemplified by glycolysis in cardiac muscle   32

17   Glycolysis in skeletal muscle: biochemistry of sport and exercise   34

18   Regulation of gluconeogenesis   36

19   Regulation of Krebs cycle   38

20   Mammals cannot synthesize glucose from fatty acids   40

21   Supermouse: overexpression of cytosolic PEPCK in skeletal muscle causes super-athletic performance   42

22   Sorbitol, galactitol, glucuronate and xylitol   44

23   Fructose metabolism   46

24   Ethanol metabolism   48

Part 3 **Fat metabolism**

25   Pyruvate/malate cycle and the production of NADPH   50

26   Metabolism of glucose to fat (triacylglycerol)   52

27   Metabolism of glucose to fatty acids and triacylglycerol   54

28   Glycolysis and the pentose phosphate pathway collaborate in liver to make fat   56

29   Esterification of fatty acids to triacylglycerol in liver and white adipose tissue   58

30   Mobilization of fatty acids from adipose tissue I: regulation of lipolysis   60

31   Mobilization of fatty acids from adipose tissue II: triacylglycerol/fatty acid cycle   62

32   Glyceroneogenesis   64

33   Metabolism of protein to fat after feeding   66

34   Elongation and desaturation of fatty acids   68

35   Fatty acid oxidation and the carnitine shuttle   70

36   Ketone bodies   72

37 Ketone body utilization   74

38 β-Oxidation of unsaturated fatty acids   76

39 Peroxisomal β-oxidation   78

40 α- and β-oxidation   80

41 ω-Oxidation   82

Part 4 Steroid metabolism

42 Cholesterol   84

43 Steroid hormones and bile salts   86

Part 5 Amino acid metabolism

44 Biosynthesis of the non-essential amino acids   88

45 Catabolism of amino acids I   90

46 Catabolism of amino acids II   92

47 Metabolism of amino acids to glucose in starvation and during the period immediately after refeeding   94

48 Disorders of amino acid metabolism   96

49 Phenylalanine and tyrosine metabolism   98

50 Tryptophan metabolism: the biosynthesis of NAD$^+$, serotonin and melatonin   100

51 Ornithine cycle for the production of urea: the 'urea cycle'   102

Part 6 Metabolic channelling

52 Metabolic channelling I: enzymes are organized to enable channelling of metabolic intermediates   104

53 Metabolic channelling II: fatty acid synthase   106

Part 7 Purines, pyrimidines and porphyrins

54 Amino acid metabolism, folate metabolism and the '1-carbon pool' I: purine biosynthesis   108

55 Amino acid metabolism, folate metabolism and the '1-carbon pool' II: pyrimidine biosynthesis   110

56 Krebs uric acid cycle for the disposal of nitrogenous waste   112

57 Porphyrin metabolism, haem and the bile pigments   114

Part 8 Integration of metabolic pathways and diabetes

58 Metabolic pathways in fasting liver and their disorder in Reye's syndrome   116

59 Diabetes I: metabolic changes in diabetes   118

60 Diabetes II: types I and II diabetes, MODY and pancreatic β-cell metabolism   120

61 Diabetes III: type 2 diabetes and dysfunctional liver metabolism   122

Index   125

Preface

The 'At a Glance' format of two-page spreads for each topic imposes on the author the discipline of brevity. This fourth edition includes a general updating of new concepts in metabolism plus extensive revision of the chapters on carbohydrate and fatty acid/triacylglycerol metabolism to include glyceroneogenesis. The biosynthesis of cholesterol in health and disease has been extensively revised, and the topic of sports science is extended by reference to the hyper-athletic performance of the 'super-mouse'. Although there is an excellent monograph on substrate chanelling by Agius and Sherratt (see Chapter 52), this chronically neglected subject has received further emphasis by including a new chapter on the extraordinary molecular production-line process of fatty acid synthesis. When I was a young biochemist I was invited by a paediatrician at one hour's notice to provide a review at a clinical meeting on the subject of phytanic acid metabolism to precede his report on a patient with Refsum's disease. I was unfamiliar with the topic and bamboozled by the complexity of phytanic acid metabolism. To my shame I invented an excuse to decline the invitation. I am pleased to say this edition includes chapters on the α- and ω-oxidation of branched chain fatty acids which will help others faced with this challenge. Sir Hans Krebs is well known for his work on the citric acid cycle and the urea cycle, and is less well known for his contribution to the glyoxylate cycle. However, there is a fourth Krebs cycle that has been almost completely neglected by text books. This is the Krebs uric acid cycle for the disposal of nitrogenous waste in uricotelic animals and is featured in a new chapter in this edition.

The format allows the book to be used by students of medicine, veterinary science and the biomedical sciences. It will also serve postgraduates, researchers and practising specialists in the fields of diabetes, metabolic disorders, chemical pathology and sports science. However, readers new to biochemistry will need to cherry-pick the information appropriate to their level of study with guidance from their course notes. I have also written a companion book in this series, *Medical Biochemistry at a Glance*, which provides a basic introduction to metabolism and biochemistry that might be more accessible to readers unfamiliar with this subject. Finally, to those who say that metabolism is hopelessly complicated: the important thing is not to be overwhelmed by information but to treat metabolic maps just as you would any road map or plan of the underground rail network and simply select the information needed for your specific purpose.

J. G. Salway
j.salway@btinternet.com

Further reading

Frayn K.N. (2010) *Metabolic Regulation: A Human Perspective*, 3rd edn. Wiley-Blackwell Publishing, Oxford.

Acknowledgements

The late Professor Richard Hanson, who was dubbed 'the maestro of metabolism', has been a constant source of support and encouragement. He reminded me of the importance of 'glyceroneogenesis', a neglected aspect of metabolism featured in this edition, alas too late for Richard to see it.

I am very grateful to the many readers who have sent encouraging emails, frequently followed by a qualifying comment drawing my attention to an error or omission. This is so very helpful and much appreciated. I have also had invaluable help, expert advice and guidance from Loranne Agius, Stan Brown, Keith Frayn, Anna Gloyn, Jean Harker, Gail E. Herman and Ron Hubbard.

This is the fifth occasion over nearly 20 years I have worked with Elaine Leggett of Oxford Design and Illustrators. Elaine's patience has been challenged on occasions but once again she has endured to produce wonderful artwork which reviewers of other editions have described as 'awesome'.

This complicated book has been a challenge for the staff at Wiley-Blackwell and has been overseen by a quartet of editors in succession: Martin Davies, Fiona Goodgame, Magenta Styles and James Watson. However, throughout I am especially grateful for the continuity of wise advice and calm counsel of Karen Moore. Karen has worked on all four editions of *Metabolism at a Glance* and both editions of *Medical Biochemistry at a Glance* over a period spanning almost 25 years. This new edition involved a change of font which produced unexpected 'computer errors' in the numerous structural formulae in the artwork. I was very fortunate when Sarah Bate agreed to rise to the challenge and her patient attention to detail in spotting thousands of errors and omissions in the metabolic charts has been a source of reassurance. Once again my thanks to Rosemary James who has read the proofs with her eagle-eyed enthusiasm for accuracy and knack for identifying mistakes. I am also very grateful to Francesca Giovannetti, production editor, Loan Nguyen and lastly to Jane Andrew for her patient attention to detail and helpful suggestions in the final copy-editing process.

Introduction to metabolic pathways

1

Metabolic charts

The metabolic map opposite will, at first sight, appear to most readers to be a confusing, incomprehensible jumble of chemical formulae. There can be no doubt that metabolic charts **are** complex, and many biochemists remember their own first introduction to metabolism as a somewhat bewildering experience.

The first important thing to remember is that the chart is no more than a form of map. In many respects it is similar to a map of the London Underground, which is also very complicated (Diagram 1.1). With the latter, however, we have learned to suppress the overwhelming detail in order to concentrate on those aspects relevant to a particular journey. For example, if asked 'How would you get from **Archway** to **Queensway**?' the reply is likely to be: 'Take the Northern Line travelling south to **Tottenham Court Road**, then change to the Central Line travelling west to **Queensway**'. An equally valid answer would be: 'Enter Archway station, buy a ticket at the kiosk, pass through the ticket inspector's barrier and proceed to the platform. When a train arrives, enter and remain seated as it passes through Tuffnell Park, Kentish Town, Camden Town, Euston, Warren Street and Goodge Street. When it reaches Tottenham Court Road, stand up and leave the train, transfer to platform 1, etc.' Each of these details, although essential for completion of the journey, is not necessary to an **overall** understanding of the journey.

A similar approach should be used when studying the metabolic chart. The details of individual enzyme reactions are very complex and very important. Many biochemists, including some of the world's most famous, have been researching individual enzymes such as **phosphofructokinase-1**, **pyruvate dehydrogenase** and **glucokinase** for many years. The detailed properties of these important enzymes and the mechanism of their reactions are superbly summarized in several standard biochemistry textbooks. However, these details should not be allowed to confuse the mind of the reader when asked the question: 'How is glucose metabolized to fat?' When faced with such a problem, the student should learn to recall sufficient detail relevant to an overall understanding of the pathways involved, while maintaining an awareness of the detailed background information and mechanisms.

Chart 1.1: subcellular distribution of metabolic pathways

The metabolic chart opposite shows how certain pathways are located in the **cytosol** of the cell, whereas others are located in the **mitochondrion**. Certain other enzymes are associated with subcellular structures such as the **endoplasmic reticulum**, for example **glucose 6-phosphatase**. Others are associated with organelles such as the nucleus and peroxisomes which, for simplicity, are not shown in the chart.

The enzymes required to catalyse the reactions in the various metabolic pathways are organized among the different subcellular compartments within the cell. For example, the enzymes involved in **fatty acid synthesis**, the **pentose phosphate pathway** and **glycolysis** are nearly all located in the **cytosol**. As we can see, most of the reactions involved in harnessing energy for the cell, **Krebs cycle**, **β-oxidation** and **respiratory chain**, are located in the **mitochondrion**, which is frequently called 'the power house of the cell'.

Mitochondrion (plural, mitochondria)

Most animal and plant cells contain mitochondria. An important exception in most animal species is the mature red blood cell. Mitochondria are usually sausage-shaped organelles. They are surrounded by a double system of membranes conveniently described as the **outer membrane** and the **inner membrane**, which separate an **intermembrane space**. Interestingly, they contain ribosomes for protein synthesis plus some of their own genes, and reproduce by binary fission. In short, they are largely autonomous and biologists have suggested that they were originally bacterial cells that evolved a symbiotic relationship with a larger cell. They have therefore been described as 'cells within a cell'.

The outer membrane of the mitochondrion is fairly typical of most cell membranes, being composed of 50% protein and 50% lipids. It contains a channel-forming protein called **porin**, which renders it permeable to molecules of less than 10 kDa. This is in contrast to the inner membrane, which forms one of the most impermeable barriers within the cell. This inner membrane contains 80% protein and 20% lipid, and is folded inwards to form cristae (not shown), which project into the matrix. It is, however, permeable to water and gases such as oxygen. Also, certain metabolites can cross the inner membrane, but only when assisted by carrier systems such as the **dicarboxylate carrier**.

When sections of the inner membrane are stained for electron microscopy, mushroom-like projections, the F_O/F_1 **particles** appear. These are respiratory particles that are thought to be embedded in the membrane *in vivo*, but following oxidation project into the matrix. These particles are involved in **adenosine triphosphate** (ATP) synthesis by oxidative phosphorylation, and are functionally associated with the respiratory chain.

The **matrix** of the mitochondrion contains the enzymes of the **β-oxidation** pathway and also most of the enzymes needed for **Krebs cycle**. An important exception is **succinate dehydrogenase**, which is linked to the **respiratory chain** in the inner membrane. Certain mitochondria have special enzymes, for example, liver mitochondria contain the enzymes necessary for ketogenesis (see Chapter 36) and urea synthesis (see Chapter 51).

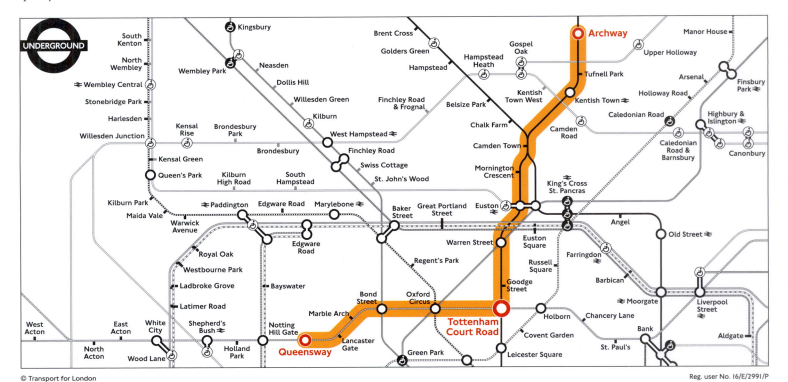

Diagram 1.1 Map of the London Underground. Reproduced with permission of Pulse Creative Limited. LRT Registered User No. 16/E/2991/P.

© Transport for London

Reg. user No. 16/E/2991/P

Metabolism at a Glance, Fourth Edition. J. G. Salway. © 2017 John Wiley & Sons Ltd. Published 2017 by John Wiley & Sons Ltd.

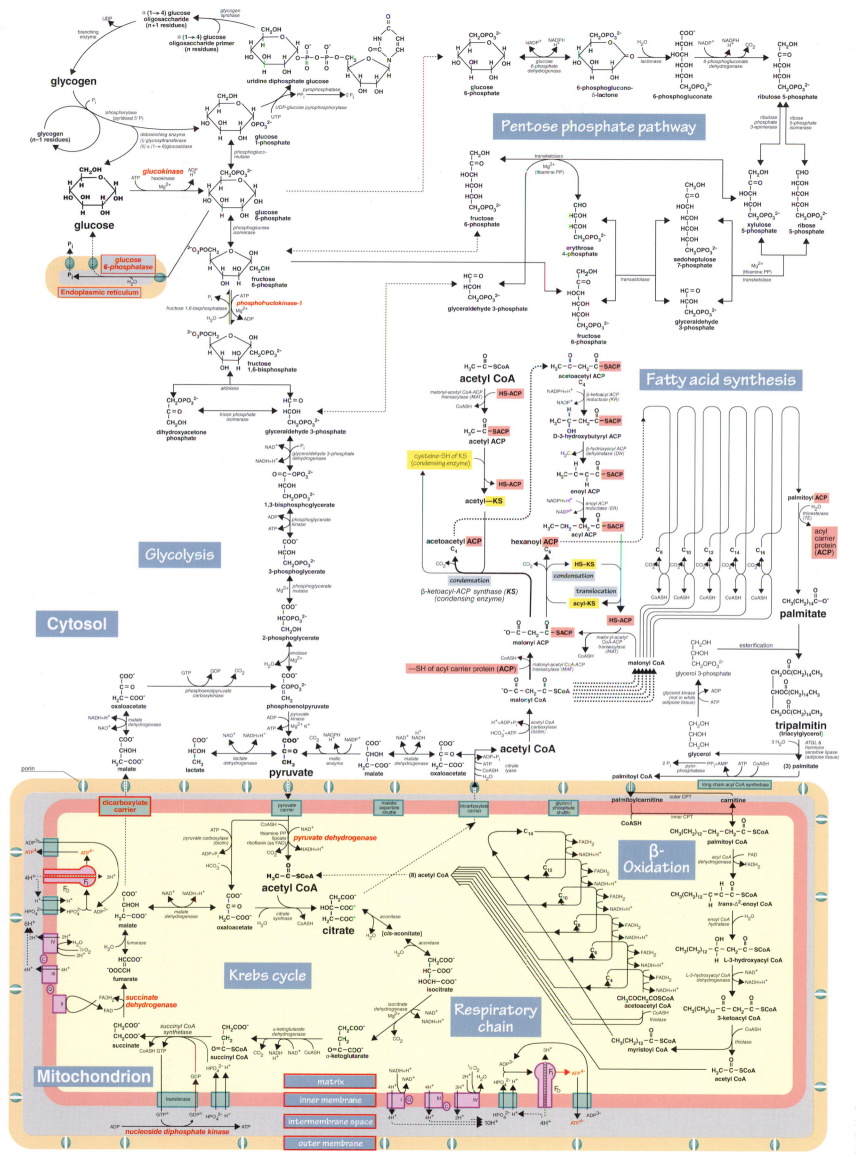

Chart 1.1 Map of the main pathways of intermediary metabolism.

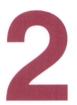

Biosynthesis of ATP I: ATP, the molecule that powers metabolism

How living cells conserve energy in a biologically useful form

A lump of coal can be burned in a power station to generate electricity, which is a very useful and versatile form of energy. Apart from coal, several other fuels, such as oil, peat and even public refuse, can be used to generate electricity. This electrical energy can then be used to power innumerable industrial machines and domestic appliances, which are essential to our modern way of life.

Living cells have a similarly versatile energy resource in the molecule, **adenosine triphosphate (ATP)**. ATP can be generated by oxidizing several metabolic fuels, although carbohydrates and fats are especially important. ATP is used in innumerable vital metabolic reactions and physiological functions, not only in humans, but in all forms of life. The primary objective of intermediary metabolism is to maintain a steady supply of ATP so that living cells can grow, reproduce and respond to the stresses and strains imposed by starvation, exercise, overeating, etc.

Chart 2.1: biosynthesis of ATP

We will see later (Chapter 5) how glucose is oxidized and energy is conserved as ATP. ATP can be synthesized by phosphorylation of adenosine diphosphate (ADP) by two types of process. One does not need oxygen and is known as **substrate-level phosphorylation**. The other requires oxygen and is known as **oxidative phosphorylation**.

Substrate-level phosphorylation

Examination of the chart opposite shows that two reactions in glycolysis, namely the **phosphoglycerate kinase** and **pyruvate kinase** reactions, produce ATP by direct phosphorylation of ADP. This is **substrate-level phosphorylation** and is especially important for generating ATP if the tissues are inadequately supplied with oxygen.

ATP can also be made anaerobically from the phosphagen **phosphocreatine** (see Chapter 17).

Another example of substrate-level phosphorylation occurs in Krebs cycle. The reaction (Diagram 2.1), catalysed by **succinyl CoA synthetase**, produces guanosine triphosphate (GTP), which is structurally similar to ATP. The enzyme **nucleoside diphosphate kinase** catalyses the conversion of GTP to ATP in the intermembrane space. **NB:** One proton (H^+) is needed to transport one phosphate anion into the matrix in a process coupled to the import of guanosine diphosphate (GDP) (Diagram 2.1).

Oxidative phosphorylation

In the presence of oxygen, oxidative phosphorylation is by far the most important mechanism for synthesizing ATP. This process is coupled to the oxidation of the reduced 'hydrogen carriers' **NADH** and **$FADH_2$** via the respiratory chain.

'Hydrogen carriers' NAD⁺ and FAD

NAD⁺ (nicotinamide adenine dinucleotide)

NAD^+ is a hydrogen carrier derived from the vitamin niacin. It is a coenzyme involved in several oxidation/reduction reactions catalysed by dehydrogenases. In the example opposite, taken from Krebs cycle, **malate dehydrogenase** catalyses the oxidation of malate to oxaloacetate. During this reaction, NAD^+ is reduced to form NADH, which is oxidized by the respiratory chain and 2.5 molecules of ATP are formed (see Chapter 6).

FAD (flavin adenine dinucleotide)

FAD is a hydrogen carrier derived from the vitamin riboflavin. It differs from NAD^+ in that it is covalently bound to its dehydrogenase enzyme, and is therefore known as a prosthetic group. In the example opposite, the **succinate dehydrogenase** reaction is shown with FAD being reduced to $FADH_2$. Succinate dehydrogenase is bound to the inner membrane of the mitochondrion and is an integral part of the respiratory chain. When $FADH_2$ is oxidized by this process, a total of 1.5 ATP molecules are formed (see Chapter 6).

ATP/ADP translocase

The inner membrane of the mitochondrion is impermeable to ATP. A protein complex known as the ATP/ADP translocase is needed for the export of ATP in return for the import of ADP and phosphate anion.

The ATP molecule has two phosphoanhydride bonds that provide the energy for life

The ATP molecule has two phosphoanhydride bonds (Diagram 2.2). When hydrolysed at physiological pH, 1 mole of ATP releases 7.3 kcal (30.66 kJ) as energy, which can be used for metabolic purposes. These two phosphoanhydride bonds were referred to by Lipmann in 1941 as 'high-energy' bonds. However, this term is a misleading concept that (apologies apart) has been banished from the textbooks. In fact, these phosphoanhydride bonds are no different from any other covalent bonds.

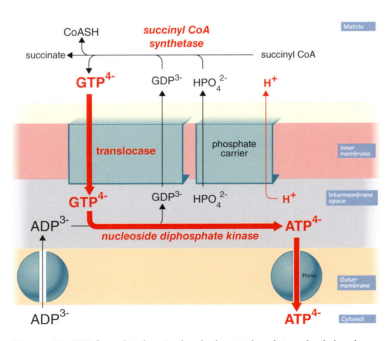

Diagram 2.1 GTP formed in the mitochondrial matrix by substrate-level phosphorylation is used to form ATP in the intermembrane space for export to the cytosol.

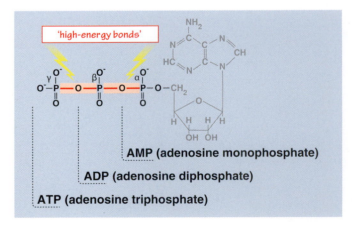

Diagram 2.2 Adenosine triphosphate.

References

Carusi E.A. (1992) It's time we replaced 'high-energy phosphate group' with 'phosphoryl group'. *Biochem Ed*, **20**, 145–7.

For a description of the function and structure of NAD^+ and FAD see:

Salway J.G. (2012) *Medical Biochemistry at a Glance*, 3rd edn. Wiley-Blackwell, Oxford.

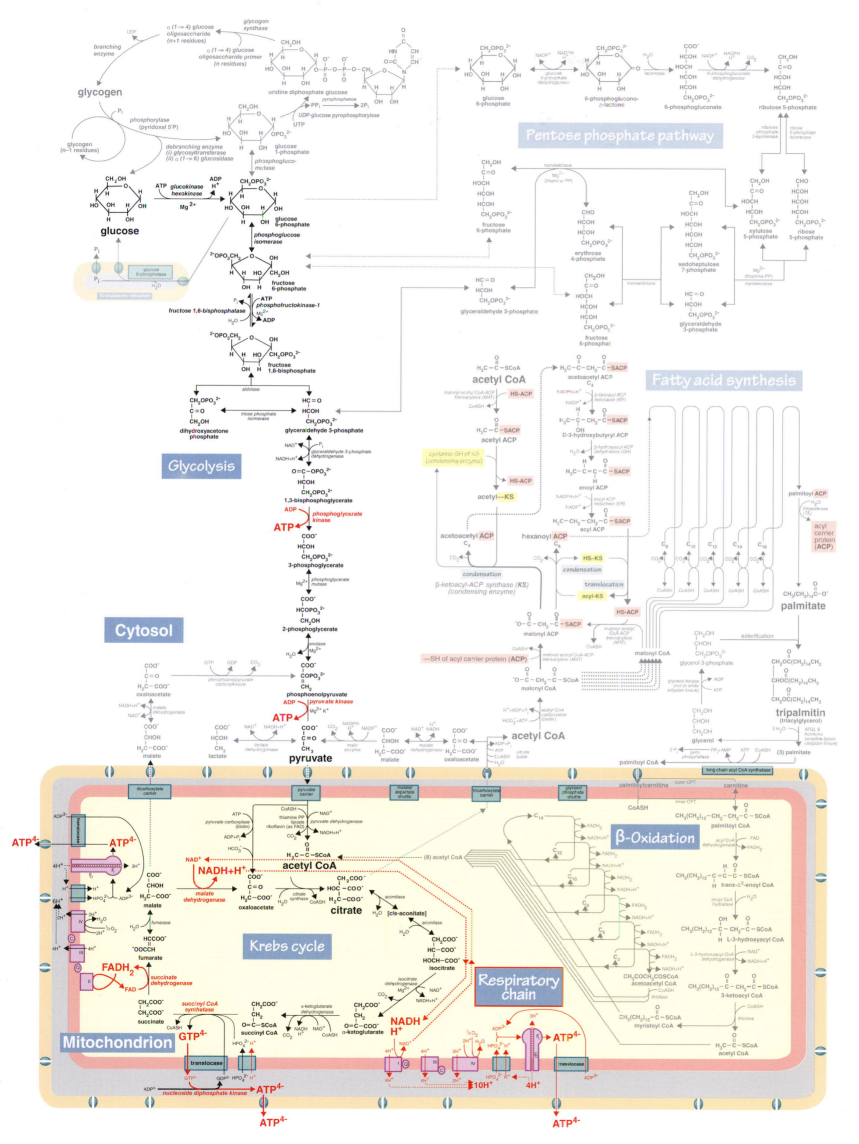

Chart 2.1
Biosynthesis of ATP.

Biosynthesis of ATP II: mitochondrial respiratory chain

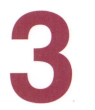

Diagram 3.1a Electron transport.
The respiratory chain showing the flow of electrons from NADH and FADH$_2$ to oxygen with the formation of water. NB: Ascorbate (vitamin C) and TMPD are **experimental** donors/acceptors that are used in studies of mitochondria *in vitro*.

Don't panic! At a first reading, students should use the simplified Diagrams 3.1a and 3.1b. Diagram 3.2 provides a more detailed summary for advanced students, or see the companion book *Medical Biochemistry at a Glance* (Salway 2012).

The mitochondrial respiratory chain (Diagram 3.1) comprises a series of reduction/oxidation reactions within complexes I, II, III and IV. These are linked by ubiquinone (Q) and cytochrome c (cytc). Ubiquinone, which accepts electrons and protons (H$^+$) as it is reduced to ubiquinol (QH$_2$), shuttles from both complexes I and II, to complex III. Similarly, cytochrome c shuttles electrons from complex III to complex IV. The synthesis of ATP via the respiratory chain is the result of two coupled processes: (i) **electron transport**; and (ii) **oxidative phosphorylation**.

1 **Electron transport** (Diagram 3.1a). This involves the oxidation (i.e. the removal of electrons) from NADH, or FADH$_2$, with transport of the electrons through a chain of oxidation/reduction reactions involving cytochromes until they are donated to molecular oxygen, which is consequently reduced to water.

2 **Oxidative phosphorylation and proton transport** (Diagram 3.1b). According to Mitchell's chemiosmotic theory, the electron transport drives proton pumps in complexes I, III and IV. Positively charged protons are pumped out of the mitochondrial matrix but **not** with any associated negatively charged anions. Consequently, as a result of this **charge separation**, the matrix side of the membrane becomes negatively charged, whilst the extruded protons ensure that its opposite side becomes positively charged. The difference in electrochemical potential across the membrane, which is 8 nm thick, is about 150–250 mV. This may seem unremarkable but is equivalent to 250 000 V/cm! It is this potential difference that provides the energy for ATP synthesis when the protons return to the matrix through the F$_o$ proton channel, thereby driving the F$_1$ ATP synthetase.

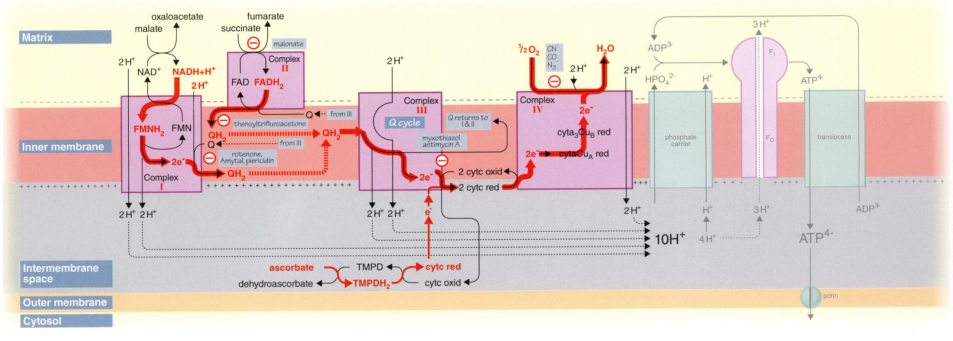

Diagram 3.1b Proton flow. The respiratory chain showing the extrusion of protons by complexes I, III and IV creating an electrochemical gradient. As the protons return through the ATP synthetase complex, ADP is phosphorylated to ATP.

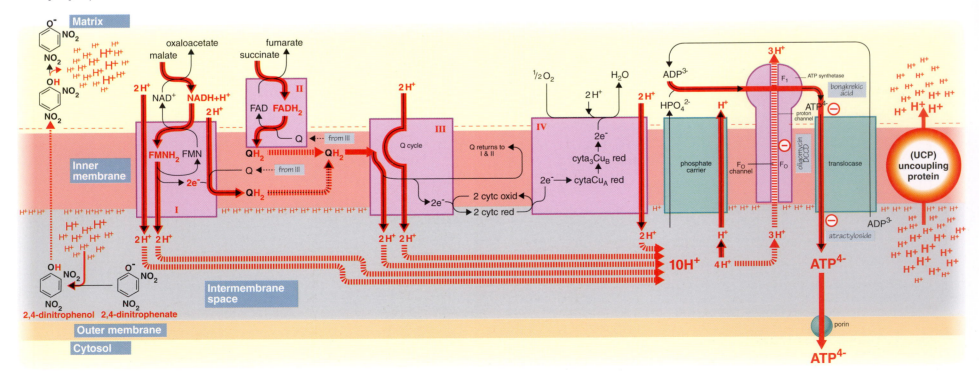

Metabolism at a Glance, Fourth Edition. J. G. Salway. © 2017 John Wiley & Sons Ltd. Published 2017 by John Wiley & Sons Ltd.

Proton extrusion

The **transport of two electrons** enables complexes I and III each to extrude $4 H^+$, while complex IV pumps $2 H^+$, that is a total of **10 protons**.

Stoichiometry of ATP synthesis

Current consensus opinion is that $3 H^+$ are needed to form 1 ATP, and an additional H^+ is needed to translocate it to the cytosol, i.e. a total of $4 H^+$ per ATP synthesized.

P/O ratios: 'traditional' integer and 'modern' non-integer values

The number of molecules of ATP synthesized per molecule of oxygen consumed has traditionally been accepted as integer (i.e. whole number) values, i.e. **three** for NADH, and **two** for $FADH_2$. However, current opinion challenges this assumption. Diagram 3.1b shows that when NADH is oxidized, a total of $10 H^+$ are extruded. Since $4 H^+$ are needed to make 1 ATP, oxidation of NADH yields the equivalent of **2.5** ATP molecules (i.e. the P/O ratio is the non-integer value 2.5). Similarly, for $FADH_2$, the P/O ratio is 1.5 (see Chapter 6).

Inhibitors of the respiratory chain

Compounds that inhibit or interact with Keilin's respiratory chain (pronounced 'Kaylin') have contributed to our understanding of this process. These compounds (Diagram 3.1) can be organized into three groups: those that inhibit the flow of electrons, those that interfere with the flow of protons and miscellaneous compounds.

Diagram 3.1a: interference with the flow of electrons

1 **Rotenone, piericidin and amytal.** Ubiquinone is reduced to ubiquinol, which shuttles between complexes I and III, and, in so doing, transports electrons from complex I to complex III. Rotenone, piericidin and amytal prevent the transfer of electrons from complex I to ubiquinone.

2 **Malonate.** Malonate, being structurally similar to succinate, is a competitive inhibitor of succinate dehydrogenase, which is a component of complex II.

3 **Thenoyltrifluoroacetone.** Ubiquinone can also shuttle electrons from complex II to complex III. This is inhibited by thenoyltrifluoroacetone, which prevents the transfer of electrons from complex II to ubiquinone.

4 **Antimycin A, stigmatellin and myxothiazol.** Antimycin A, stigmatellin and myxothiazol block the flow of electrons from ubiquinol to the iron/sulphur Rieske protein. This passes electrons to cytochrome c, which is loosely associated with the outer face of the inner membrane and shuttles electrons from complex III to complex IV.

5 **Cyanide, carbon monoxide and azide.** Electrons are transferred from complex IV (also known as cytochrome c oxidase) to molecular oxygen. This process is inhibited by cyanide, carbon monoxide and azide.

Diagram 3.1b: interference with the flow of protons (H⁺)

1 **Oligomycin and dicyclohexylcarbodiimide (DCCD).** These compounds block the proton channel of the F_o segment of ATP synthetase. Consequently the flux of protons needed for ATP synthesis by the enzyme is prevented.

2 **2,4-Dinitrophenol (DNP) and carbonylcyanide-p-trifluoromethoxy-phenylhydrazone (FCCP).** DNP (ditto FCCP) is a weak acid. Its base 2,4-dinitrophenate accepts H^+ producing the undissociated acid form, DNP, which is lipophilic and diffuses across the inner mitochondrial membrane. This leakage of H^+ diverts the flux of H^+ from the ATP synthetase thus bypassing ATP synthesis. However, the flow of electrons is unrestricted by DNP and its effect is described as 'uncoupling ATP synthesis from electron transport'.

3 **Uncoupling protein (UCP).** This is found in the inner mitochondrial membrane of brown adipose tissue and is involved in non-shivering thermogenesis. Like DNP and FCCP, it lowers the electrochemical gradient by allowing leakage of protons so that energy is dissipated as heat instead of being used for ATP synthesis.

Some other compounds that affect the respiratory chain

1 **Tetramethyl-p-phenyldiamine (TMPD).** TMPD is an artificial electron donor that can transfer electrons to cytochrome c. Since ascorbate can reduce TMPD, these compounds can be used experimentally to study the respiratory chain (Diagram 3.1a).

2 **Bongkrekic acid and atractyloside.** Bongkrekic acid (a toxic contaminant of bongkrek, which is a food prepared from coconuts) and atractyloside, both inhibit the ATP/ADP translocase preventing the export of ATP and the import of ADP. Whereas bongkrekic acid binds to the inner aspect of the adenine nucleotide carrier, atractyloside binds to its outer aspect.

Reference

Salway J.G. (2012) *Medical Biochemistry at a Glance*, 3rd edn. Wiley-Blackwell, Oxford.

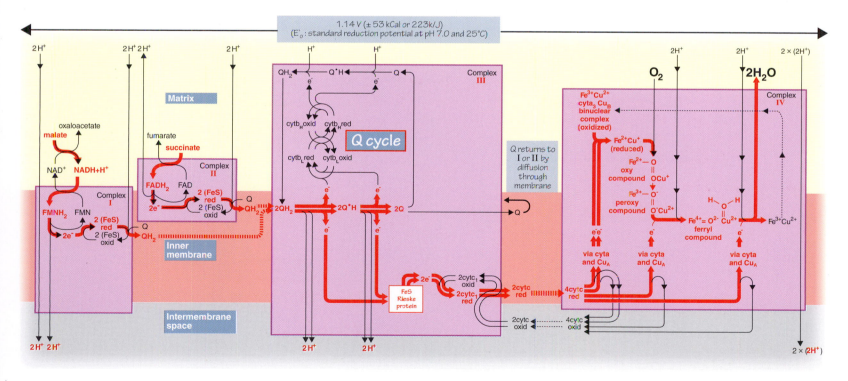

Diagram 3.2 Complexes I, II, III and IV in detail. Complex I: protons and electrons from NADH are passed to a flavin mononucleotide (FMN). The electrons pass to the iron/sulphur complex then to ubiqinone (Q), which also gains $2 H^+$ and is reduced to ubiquinol (QH_2). **Complex II**: electrons are passed from $FADH_2$ via the iron/sulphur complex to ubiquinone and are joined by protons to form ubiquinol. **Complex III**: here ubiquinol delivers the protons that are extruded into the intermembrane space. Meanwhile, electrons are passed via the iron/sulphur Rieske protein and membrane-bound cytochrome c_1 before leaving the complex by reducing the cytosolic cytochrome c.

The 'Q cycle' is a device for regenerating ubiquinone from ubiquinone semiquinone Q·H involving two cytochrome b. **Complex IV**: cytochrome c donates two electrons (indirectly via Cu_A and cytochrome a) to the oxidized binuclear complex $cyta_3Cu_B$. The resulting reduced complex binds O_2 to form the oxy species that rearranges to the peroxy form. Protonation and addition of a third electron, followed by oxygen–oxygen bond splitting, produce the ferryl compound. A fourth electron and further protonation produce intermediates (not shown) that form water and regenerate the oxidized complex, completing the cycle.

Oxidation of cytosolic NADH: the malate/aspartate shuttle and glycerol phosphate shuttle

Oxidation of cytosolic NADH

The **glyceraldehyde 3-phosphate dehydrogenase** reaction occurs in the cytosol and forms NADH, which can be oxidized by the respiratory chain in the mitochondrion to produce ATP. However, molecules of NADH are unable to cross the inner membrane of the mitochondrion. This paradox is overcome by two mechanisms that enable 'reducing equivalents' to be transferred from the cytosol to the mitochondrion. They are the **malate/aspartate shuttle** and the **glycerol phosphate shuttle**.

Glycerol phosphate shuttle

This shuttle (Chart 4.1), which is particularly important in the flight muscle of insects, uses cytosolic NADH in the presence of **glycerol 3-phosphate dehydrogenase** to reduce **dihydroxyacetone phosphate** to form **glycerol 3-phosphate**. The latter diffuses into the intermembrane space of the mitochondrion. Here it is oxidized by the mitochondrial glycerol 3-phosphate dehydrogenase isoenzyme, which is associated with the outer surface of the inner membrane. The products of the reaction are dihydroxyacetone phosphate (which diffuses back into the cytosol) and FADH$_2$. This FADH$_2$ can be oxidized by the respiratory chain but, since it donates its electrons to **ubiquinone (Q)**, there is enough energy to pump only 6 H$^+$. These can synthesize the equivalent of 1.5 molecules of ATP (see Chapter 3).

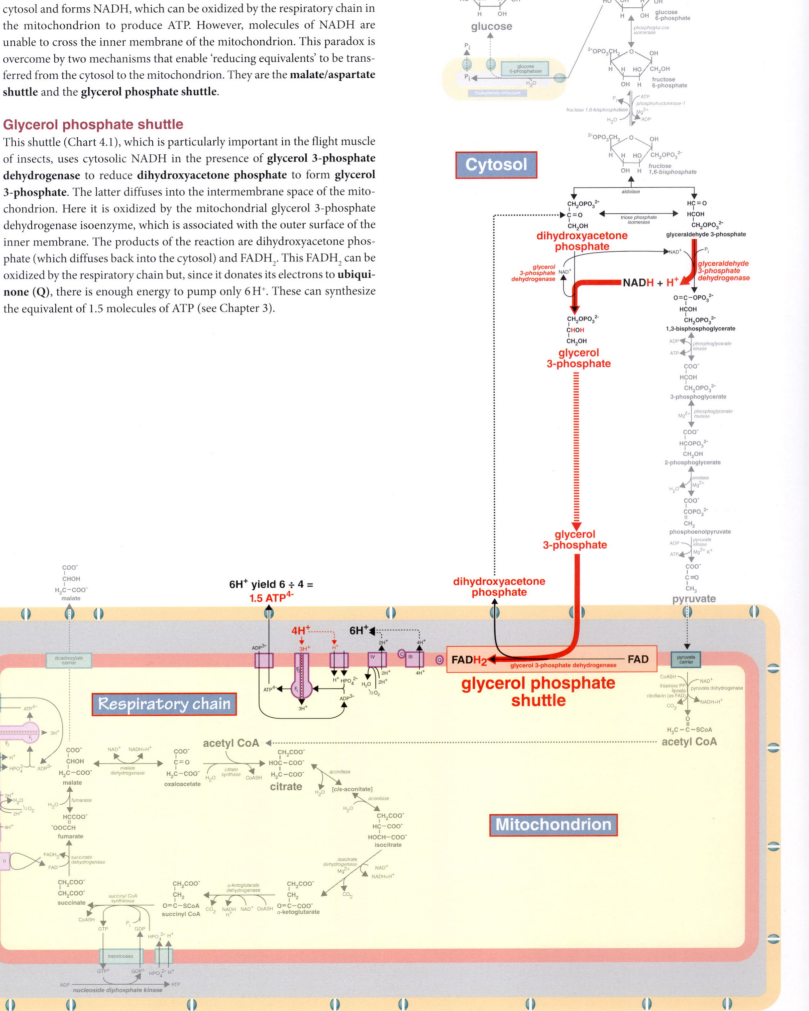

Chart 4.1 Glycerol phosphate shuttle.

Metabolism at a Glance, Fourth Edition. J. G. Salway. © 2017 John Wiley & Sons Ltd. Published 2017 by John Wiley & Sons Ltd.

Malate/aspartate shuttle

This shuttle (Chart 4.2) starts with cytosolic **oxaloacetate**. First, cytosolic **malate dehydrogenase** uses the NADH to reduce oxaloacetate to malate. The latter is transported into the mitochondrial matrix in exchange for α-ketoglutarate. Here it is oxidized by malate dehydrogenase back to oxaloacetate, and the NADH released is available for oxidative phosphorylation by the respiratory chain, producing ATP.

The oxaloacetate must now be returned to the cytosol. The problem is that it too is unable to cross the inner mitochondrial membrane. Accordingly, it is transformed to **aspartate** in a reaction catalysed by aspartate aminotransferase. Aspartate leaves the mitochondrion via the glutamate/aspartate carrier in exchange for the import of glutamate and a proton. Once in the cytosol, aspartate is transaminated by aspartate aminotransferase, and thus oxaloacetate is restored to the cytosol, thereby completing the cycle.

NB: Oxidation of each mitochondrial NADH in the respiratory chain provides energy to pump **10 H**[+]. However, since **1 H**[+] is needed for the glutamate/aspartate carrier, a total of **9 H**[+] are available to synthesize the equivalent of 2.25 molecules of ATP.

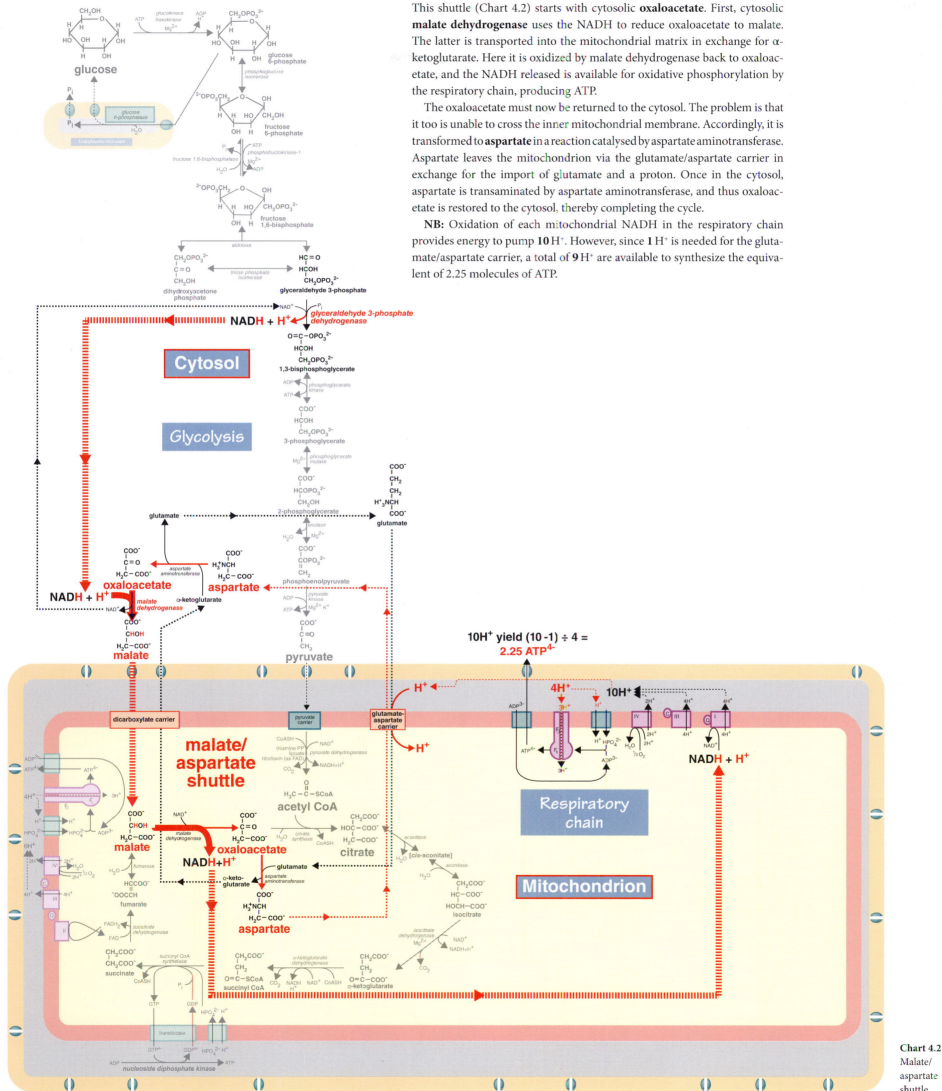

Chart 4.2
Malate/
aspartate
shuttle.

Metabolism of glucose to provide energy

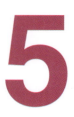

The glucose molecule, which is a rich store of chemical energy, burns vigorously in air to form carbon dioxide and water and, in the process, energy escapes as heat. This can be represented by the following equation:

$$C_6H_{12}O_6 + 6\,O_2 \rightarrow 6\,CO_2 + 6\,H_2O + \text{energy as heat}$$
glucose　　oxygen　　carbon　　water
　　　　　　　　　　　dioxide

Carbohydrate-containing foods such as starch are digested to glucose, which is then absorbed into the blood, and it is well known that 'glucose gives you energy'. Bearing in mind that the laws of thermodynamics apply to both animate and inanimate systems, we must now consider how living cells can release energy from a glucose molecule in a controlled way, so that the cell neither bursts into flames nor explodes in the process.

Once a glucose molecule has passed from the bloodstream into a cell, it is gradually transformed and dismantled in a controlled sequence of some two dozen biochemical steps, in a manner analogous to a production line in a factory. The several biochemical transformations are assisted by enzymes, some of which need cofactors derived from vitamins to function properly. Such a series of biochemical reactions is known as a metabolic pathway.

Chart 5.1: glucose metabolism

The chart shows that, in order to conserve the energy from glucose as ATP, three metabolic pathways are involved. First, glucose is oxidized through the pathway known as **glycolysis**. The end product of glycolysis, two molecules of **pyruvate**, are then fed into **Krebs cycle**, where they are completely oxidized to form six molecules of carbon dioxide. In the process, the hydrogen carriers **NAD+** and **FAD**, which are compounds derived from the vitamins niacin and riboflavin respectively, become reduced to **NADH** and **FADH$_2$** and carry hydrogen to the **respiratory chain**. Here, energy is conserved in **ATP** molecules, while the hydrogen is eventually used to reduce oxygen to water (see Chapter 3).

The energy released from ATP on hydrolysis can then be used for biological work such as muscle contraction, protein synthesis and conduction of nerve impulses.

Several vitamins provide cofactors for the enzymes involved in these metabolic pathways. For example, the pyruvate dehydrogenase reaction needs cofactors derived from niacin, thiamine, riboflavin, lipoic acid and pantothenic acid. A deficiency of any of these could cause malfunctioning of a metabolic pathway at the particular enzymic reaction(s) where the cofactor is involved.

The overall reaction for the oxidation of glucose by living cells is therefore:

$$C_6H_{12}O_6 + 6\,O_2 \rightarrow 6\,CO_2 + 6\,H_2O + \text{energy as ATP}$$
glucose　　oxygen　　carbon　　water
　　　　　　　　　　　dioxide

Importance of insulin in glucose transport

Insulin is a hormone secreted into the blood by the β-cells of the pancreas in response to increased blood glucose concentrations such as might follow a carbohydrate meal. Because of the large mass of muscle and fat tissue in the human body, the ability of insulin to control the uptake and metabolism of glucose in these cells plays a major part in regulating the blood glucose concentration (Diagram 5.1). In diabetes mellitus, where there is inadequate insulin action, glucose cannot enter muscle and fat cells and consequently the blood glucose concentration rises (hyperglycaemia). This situation has inspired the aphorism describing diabetes as 'starvation in the midst of plenty'.

If there is an inappropriate excess of insulin relative to the available glucose, then a low blood glucose concentration (hypoglycaemia) results. This might arise if a diabetic patient receives too much insulin in proportion to the carbohydrate supply – or in other words, fails to achieve the balance essential to diabetic control. A rare example of excessive insulin secretion occurs in patients with an insulin-secreting tumour (insulinoma) where the β-cells are overactive. In both cases, the resulting hypoglycaemia is dangerous because the brain, which is largely dependent on glucose for fuel, is deprived of its energy supply, and coma may follow.

Insulin is a very important hormone. It has a controlling influence on the metabolism of fats and proteins as well as a direct involvement with glucose metabolism. Its many metabolic actions are mentioned throughout this book.

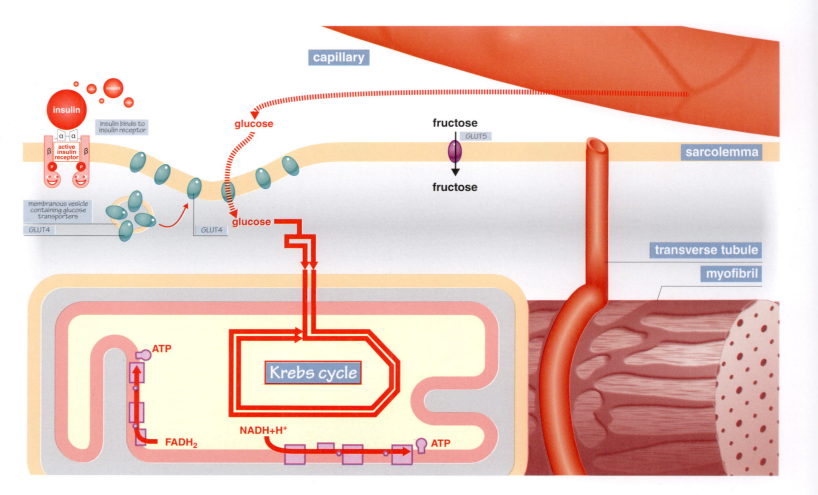

Diagram 5.1 Insulin and the transport of glucose into muscle cells. Glucose is carried by the blood arterial system to the capillaries, which supply the various body tissues. Glucose penetrates the gaps in the capillary wall to form an aqueous fluid, called the interstitial fluid, which bathes the cells. In the case of erythrocytes, liver cells and brain cells, glucose is transported through the outer membrane into the cytosol via a family of insulin-independent facilitative glucose transporters known respectively as GLUT1, GLUT2 and GLUT3. However, in the case of skeletal muscle (not shown to scale) and fat cells, the **insulin-dependent glucose transporter GLUT4** is involved. Here, insulin is needed to recruit GLUT4 from a latent intracellular location. Insulin causes a vesicle containing the GLUT4 to fuse with the sarcolemma, thereby stimulating glucose transport into the sarcoplasm, where it is oxidized and ATP is formed. Also in the sarcolemma are **GLUT5** transporters, which preferentially transport **fructose**.

Metabolism at a Glance, Fourth Edition. J. G. Salway. © 2017 John Wiley & Sons Ltd. Published 2017 by John Wiley & Sons Ltd.

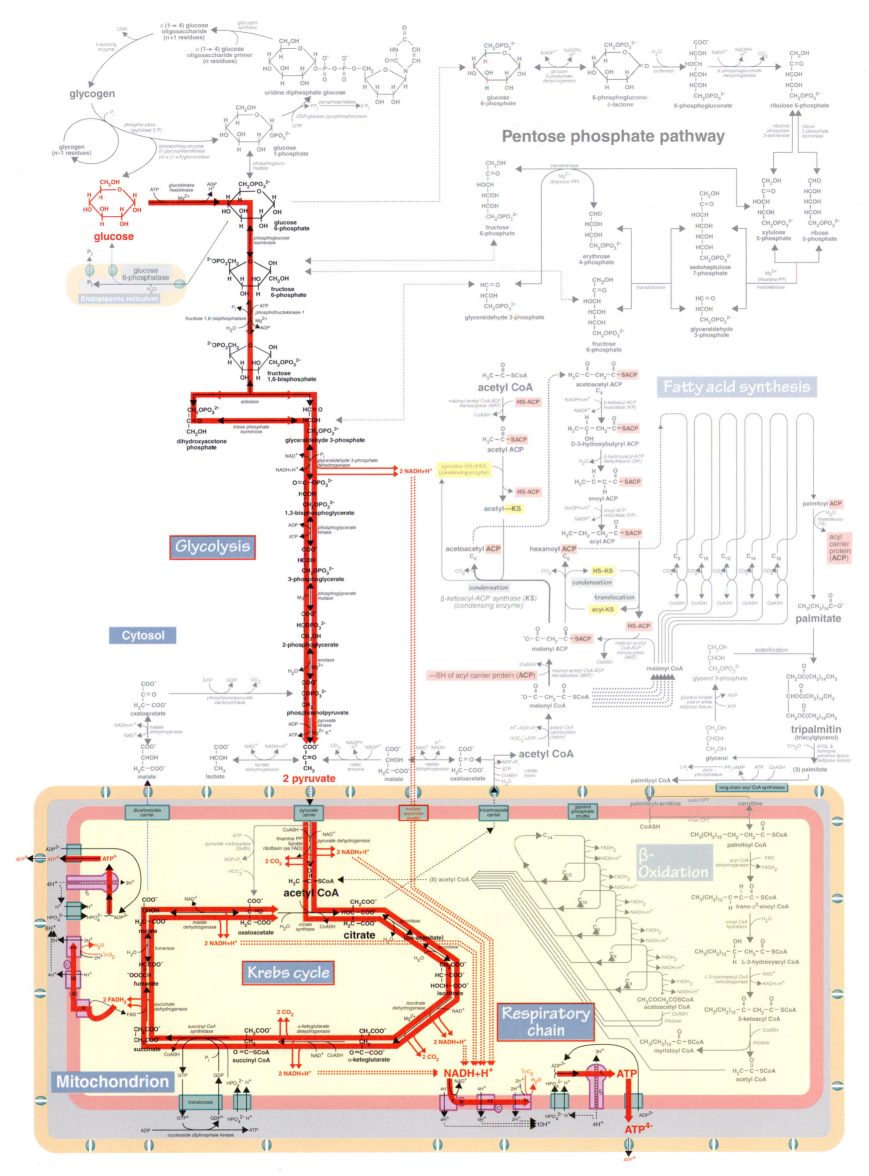

Chart 5.1 Metabolism of glucose to provide energy.

Metabolism of one molecule of glucose yields 31 (or should it be 38?) molecules of ATP

Warning! In what appears to be a conspiracy to confuse students, the yield of ATP molecules from the oxidation of glucose, traditionally quoted as **38**, is now cited as **31** in almost all the new biochemistry textbooks. This is because experimental evidence for the P/O ratios for NADH and $FADH_2$ has historically been interpreted as **whole number (i.e. integral)** values of **3** and **2** respectively. Current experimental evidence favours **non-integral** values of **2.5** for NADH and **1.5** for $FADH_2$ (see Chapter 3). Using the historic values for P/O ratios, **glucose oxidation produces 38 ATP**. Using the modern concept that P/O values for NADH and $FADH_2$ are 2.5 and 1.5; the **yield from glucose is only 31 molecules of ATP**.

Chart 6.1: oxidation of glucose yields 38 ATP molecules assuming the 'historic' P/O ratios of 3 for NADH and 2 for FADH₂

Glucose is phosphorylated to **glucose 6-phosphate**, a reaction that consumes one molecule of ATP. Glucose 6-phosphate is then converted to **fructose 1,6-bisphosphate**, consuming yet another ATP molecule. Thus, so far, instead of creating ATP, glycolysis has consumed two molecules of biochemical energy. This initial investment of energy, however, is necessary to activate the substrates, and as we will see, is amply rewarded by a 19-fold (or 15.5-fold?) net gain.

Fructose 1,6-bisphosphate is then split into two 3-carbon sugars, namely dihydroxyacetone phosphate and glyceraldehyde 3-phosphate. These two substances (**triose phosphates**) are biochemically interconvertible. Because two molecules of triose phosphate are formed, all subsequent reactions are doubled up and are represented in the chart by double lines.

Oxidation of glyceraldehyde 3-phosphate, and phosphorylation using inorganic phosphate, occur to form 1,3-bisphosphoglycerate. This complex oxidation reaction is catalysed by **glyceraldehyde 3-phosphate dehydrogenase**, and the NADH formed diffuses through the cytoplasm, exchanging its hydrogen through the impermeable inner membrane of the mitochondrion via one of the **shuttle systems** (see Chapter 4). In Chart 6.1 for example, the **malate/aspartate** shuttle has been used. Each NADH formed then enters the respiratory chain, and produces three molecules of ATP.

Meanwhile, back in the glycolytic pathway, **phosphoglycerate kinase** causes 1,3-bisphosphoglycerate to react with ADP to form ATP and 3-phosphoglycerate. Similarly, two stages further down the pathway, **pyruvate kinase** causes phosphoenolpyruvate to react with ADP to form ATP and pyruvate. Pyruvate then passes into the mitochondrion and enters Krebs cycle, where $FADH_2$ and NADH are formed. $FADH_2$ is the prosthetic group attached to succinate dehydrogenase and donates its electrons via ubiquinone to complex III, and thence to complex IV. Accordingly, oxidative phosphorylation of $FADH_2$ produces only two ATP molecules compared with three from NADH (see Chapter 3). Also, it should be noted that in Krebs cycle, GTP is formed by the **succinyl CoA synthetase** reaction. GTP is energetically similar to ATP, to which it is readily converted by **nucleoside diphosphate kinase**.

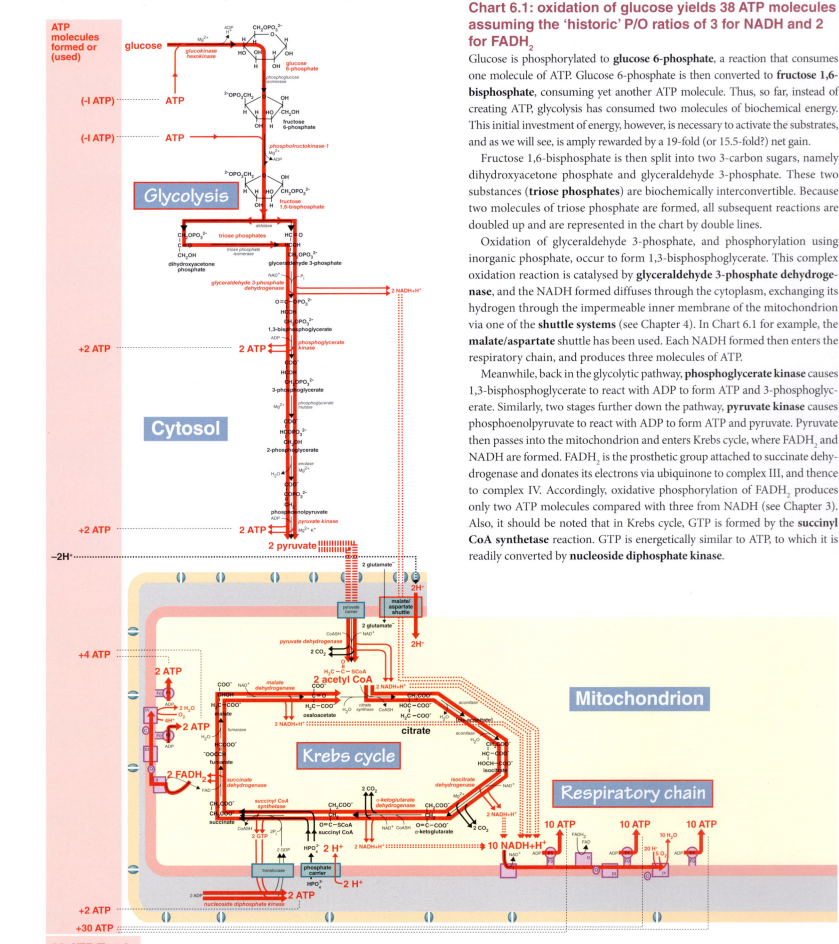

Chart 6.1 Oxidation of glucose yields 38 molecules of ATP.

Metabolism at a Glance, Fourth Edition. J. G. Salway. © 2017 John Wiley & Sons Ltd. Published 2017 by John Wiley & Sons Ltd.

Net yield is 36 ATP molecules in insects

To add to the confusion, biochemistry textbooks may appear to contradict each other even when quoting the traditional yields of ATP from glucose catabolism. Many books show the net energy yield for aerobic glucose metabolism to be **36** ATP molecules, and others give a value of **38** molecules as shown here.

The yield depends on which shuttle system (see Chapter 4) is used to transport cytosolic NADH into the mitochondrion. In the calculation shown in Chart 6.1, the malate/aspartate shuttle is used. However, if the glycerol phosphate shuttle is used, then 2 NADH molecules in the cytosol appear as 2 $FADH_2$ molecules inside the mitochondrion. The final yield of ATP is therefore 4 from the glycerol phosphate shuttle as opposed to 6 from the other shuttle. This accounts for the discrepancy referred to above. The glycerol phosphate shuttle is particularly active in insect flight muscle.

Chart 6.2: oxidation of glucose yields 31 ATP molecules assuming the 'modern' P/O ratios of 2.5 for NADH and 1.5 for $FADH_2$

As shown in Chart 6.2, oxidation of the 10 NADH formed is coupled to the pumping of a total of 100 protons from the matrix into the intermembrane space. The return of 4 protons is needed to synthesize 1 ATP molecule and to translocate it to the cytosol (see Chapter 3). The total yield of ATP from 100 returning protons is therefore 25 molecules.

Similarly, oxidation of the 2 $FADH_2$ formed in Krebs cycle is coupled to the pumping of a total of 12 protons from the matrix into the intermembrane space. As before, the return of 4 protons is needed to synthesize 1 ATP molecule and to translocate it to the cytosol so the total yield from 12 returning protons is therefore 3 molecules of ATP.

Formation of GTP by substrate-level phosphorylation. In Krebs cycle, 2 molecules of GTP are formed within the mitochondrial matrix by the succinyl CoA synthetase reaction. These can be exported to the intermembrane space by a transport mechanism (see Chapter 4). This includes a **phosphate carrier** that requires the import of one proton for each GTP exported. *In effect, this diverts 2 protons from ATP synthesis and is equivalent to the loss of 0.5 ATP molecules.* Nevertheless, the 2 GTP molecules are metabolized to 2 ATP molecules by the **nucleoside diphosphate kinase** reaction and so there is a net gain of 1.5 molecules of ATP.

Malate/aspartate shuttle. If the 2 NADH-reducing equivalents formed in the cytosol during glycolysis are translocated into the mitochondrion using the malate/aspartate shuttle, it must be remembered that the associated import of each glutamate anion needs the symport of a proton (see Chapter 4). *Thus a total of 2 protons is diverted from ATP synthesis, which is a loss equivalent to 0.5 molecules of ATP.* The total net gain from the oxidation of 2 molecules of NADH originating in the cytosol is therefore: $5 - 0.5 = 4.5$ molecules of ATP.

The net production of ATP molecules from the oxidation of one molecule of glucose when the malate/aspartate shuttle is used is 31.

Glycerol phosphate shuttle. The reducing power of NADH when translocated into the mitochondrion via the glycerol phosphate shuttle is transformed into $FADH_2$ (see Chapter 4). Two molecules of $FADH_2$ yield a total of only 3 ATP molecules, which is $4.5 - 3 = 1.5$ less than the total via the malate/aspartate shuttle.

The net production of ATP molecules from the oxidation of one molecule of glucose, when the glycerol phosphate shuttle is used, is $31 - 1.5 = 29.5$.

Should the 'historic yield' be 37 ATP molecules? I had an email from Felicity McIvor who was puzzled by the value of 38 ATPs quoted in previous editions of this book. Felicity pointed out this did not allow for the two protons used each by the phosphate carrier and the malate/aspartate shuttle. Mmm, a good point which has been overlooked by the textbooks. **If Felicity's correction is applied, the 'historic yield' should have been 37!** Best quickly to move on and use the modern P/O ratios!

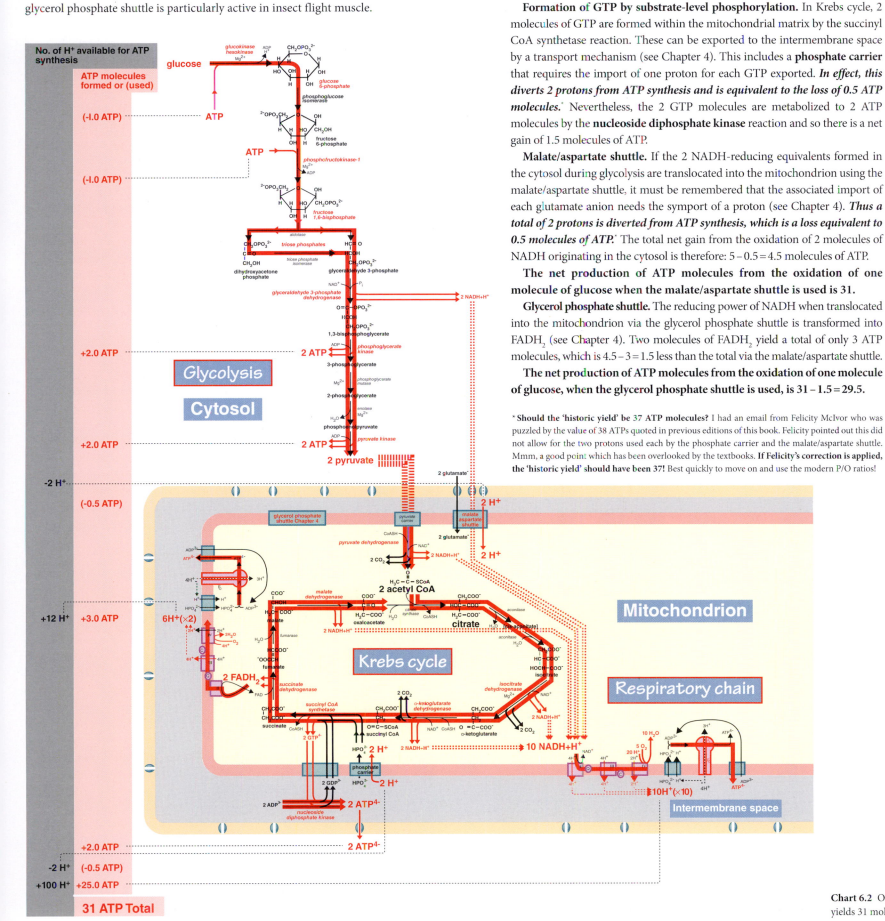

Chart 6.2 Oxidation of glucose yields 31 molecules of ATP.

Anaerobic metabolism of glucose and glycogen to yield energy as ATP

7

Anaerobic glycolysis

We have already seen how, in the presence of oxygen, glucose and glycogen are oxidized to carbon dioxide and water, with energy being conserved as ATP (see Chapter 6). However, glucose and glycogen can also be oxidized **anaerobically**: that is, without oxygen. This process is particularly important in exercising muscle. It enables muscle to generate ATP very rapidly and at a rate faster than would be permitted by the availability of oxygen from the air. In practice, this means that eventually we become 'out of breath' and then have to rest to repay the 'oxygen debt'.

Anaerobic glycolysis is also very important in the retina, kidney medulla and, paradoxically, in red blood cells in spite of the abundance of oxygen in the latter (see below).

Chart 7.1: glucose is metabolized to lactate

Anaerobic oxidation proceeds as shown in the chart. **Glucose** and **glycogen** are metabolized by glycolysis to **pyruvate** and 4 ATP molecules are produced. However, NAD⁺ is reduced to NADH by **glyceraldehyde 3-phosphate dehydrogenase**. Normally, in the presence of oxygen, this NADH equivalent (see Chapter 4) would enter the mitochondria and be oxidized to regenerate NAD⁺. Since glycolysis needs a constant supply of NAD⁺, the problem is how is NAD⁺ regenerated without oxygen?

The enzyme **lactate dehydrogenase** provides the answer. This enzyme catalyses the reduction of pyruvate to **lactate**, and simultaneously NADH is oxidized to NAD⁺. The regenerated NAD⁺ is thus free to serve glyceraldehyde 3-phosphate dehydrogenase as a coenzyme. In this way, glycolysis continues but lactate accumulates. This represents the 'oxygen debt', which must be repaid, when oxygen is available, by oxidizing the accumulated lactate to pyruvate in the liver. The pyruvate formed is converted to glucose.

ATP yield by anaerobic metabolism

Anaerobic glycolysis from glucose

Molecules of ATP formed	4
Less 2 ATP to activate glycolysis	−2
Net ATP total	2

Anaerobic glycolysis from glycogen

Molecules of ATP formed	4
Less 1 ATP to initiate glycolysis	−1
Net ATP total	3

Diagram 7.1 Cori cycle.

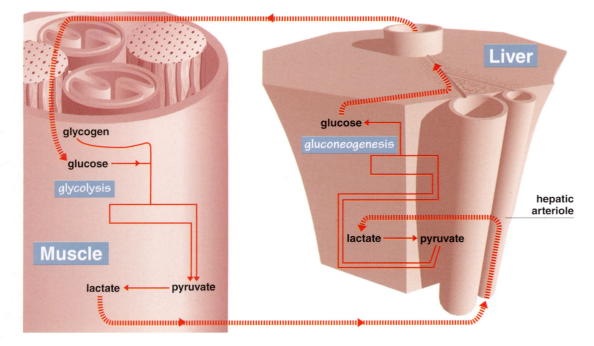

These anaerobic pathways, which produce a net yield of 2 and 3 ATP molecules respectively, are very inefficient compared with net yield from aerobic pathways, namely 31 molecules of ATP (see Chapter 6). Nevertheless, the ability to generate ATP rapidly in the absence of oxygen is vital to the survival of many species.

Physiological and clinical relevance

Anaerobic glycolysis for 'fuel-injection' performance

Adrenaline (epinephrine), as part of the 'fight or flight' response, stimulates the breakdown of glycogen and thus glycolysis. This pathway is especially important in fast-twitch (white) muscle, which is relatively deficient in oxidative metabolism due to a poor blood supply and few mitochondria. White muscle is found, for example, in the flight muscles of some game birds (e.g. grouse). It is well adapted for an explosive burst of energy, thus helping these animals to evade predators. Human skeletal muscle consists of both red and white fibres.

When oxygen becomes more plentiful again, the rate of glycolysis falls dramatically as more efficient oxidation involving Krebs cycle is activated. This adaptation is known as the **Pasteur effect** after Louis Pasteur, who first observed this phenomenon in yeast (Chart 7.2).

Hyperlactataemia and lactic acidosis

The blood concentration of lactate is normally around 1 mmol/l. Since the pK of lactic acid is 3.86, it is completely dissociated to form lactate anions and hydrogen ions at normal blood pH. If the concentration of lactate is increased up to 5 mmol/l, this is known as hyperlactataemia. If it exceeds 5 mmol/l, and the bicarbonate buffer system is overwhelmed, the condition is described as lactic acidosis and the blood pH may decrease from the normal range of 7.35–7.45 to around pH 7 or below. Lactic acidosis may result from increased lactate production due to tissue hypoxia. Alternatively, it may also result from decreased removal of lactate by the liver for gluconeogenesis due to disease or a reduced hepatic blood supply.

Lactic acidosis and disease

Lactic acidosis is often due to the generalized tissue hypoxia associated with shock or congestive cardiac failure. Here, two factors contribute to lactate accumulation: are an inadequate oxygen supply to the tissue, causing increased anaerobic glycolysis with increased lactate production, and a decreased clearance of lactate from the blood. A mild hyperlactataemia may also occur in thiamine deficiency. This is because **pyruvate dehydrogenase** needs **thiamine** for activity and, consequently, removal of pyruvate is obstructed. Since lactate dehydrogenase activity is high in cells, it maintains pyruvate and lactate at equilibrium, so that when pyruvate accumulates so also does lactate.

Diagram 7.1: the Cori cycle – muscle/liver

If our muscles need energy in an emergency or for a sprint racing event such as a 200 m race, then most of the ATP used will be derived from anaerobic breakdown of muscle glycogen by glycolysis. The diagram shows that lactate formed during this process diffuses from the muscle into the capillaries, and is transported to the liver, entering the lobules via the hepatic arterioles. Then, provided the liver cells are adequately oxygenated, the lactate is oxidized to pyruvate, which may be reconverted to glucose by the process known as gluconeogenesis (see Chapter 18). The glucose so formed may be exported from the liver via the central vein and thus made available again to the muscle for energy purposes or for storage as glycogen. This is known as the **Cori cycle**.

Diagram 7.1: the Cori cycle – red blood cells/liver

Mature red blood cells do not contain mitochondria and are therefore exclusively dependent on anaerobic oxidation of glucose for their ATP supply. The lactate produced diffuses from the red cell into the plasma and thence to the liver, where it is oxidized to pyruvate and may then be reconverted to glucose (the Cori cycle). In laboratory medicine, fluoride is used as a preservative for blood glucose samples from diabetic patients because it inhibits the glycolytic enzyme **enolase**, which converts 2-phosphoglycerate to phosphoenolpyruvate.

Metabolism at a Glance, Fourth Edition. J. G. Salway. © 2017 John Wiley & Sons Ltd. Published 2017 by John Wiley & Sons Ltd.

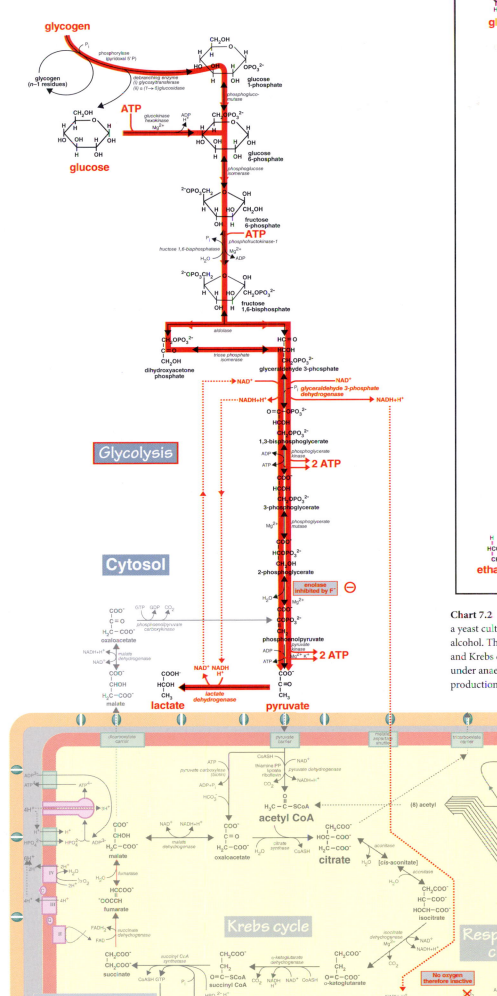

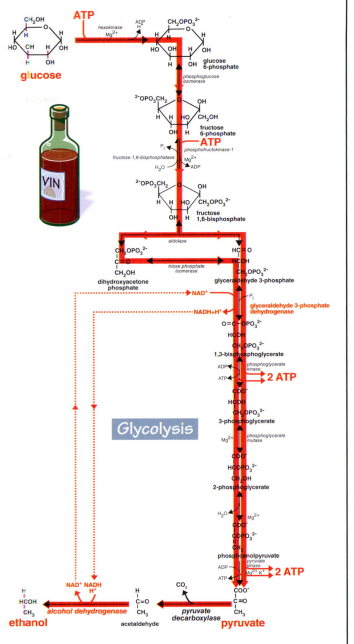

Chart 7.2 Alcoholic fermentation in yeast. Pasteur observed in 1857 that aeration of a yeast culture increased the biomass of yeast cells but prevented them from making alcohol. This is because glucose oxidation proceeds aerobically using both glycolysis and Krebs cycle, which maximizes ATP production for vigorous growth. Conversely, under anaerobic conditions, Krebs cycle cannot operate; consequently alcohol production is increased but growth of yeast cells is restricted.

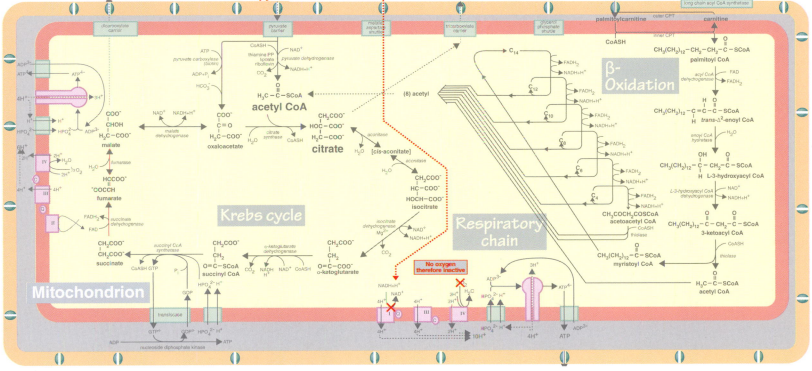

Chart 7.1 Anaerobic metabolism of glucose and glycogen to yield energy as ATP.

2,3-Bisphosphoglycerate (2,3-BPG) and the red blood cell

8

2,3-BPG helps to unload oxygen from haemoglobin

Haemoglobin, the oxygen-carrying protein found in red blood cells, has a high binding affinity for oxygen and can therefore transport oxygen to the tissues where it is needed. The problem then is that, on arrival at the tissues, haemoglobin must be persuaded to release its tightly bound cargo. It has been known since the early 1900s that the presence of H^+ ions in contracting muscle unloads oxygen from the haemoglobin. This is known as the **Bohr effect**. However, since 1967 it has been known there is another factor, **2,3-BPG** (2,3-bisphosphoglycerate) – also known as 2,3-DPG (2,3-diphosphoglycerate) in medical circles – which is an allosteric effector that binds to deoxyhaemoglobin, thereby lowering its affinity for oxygen.

Whereas the response to H^+ ions is very rapid, 2,3-BPG operates over longer periods, allowing adaptations to gradual changes in oxygen availability.

Chart 8.1: the 2,3-BPG shunt in red blood cells (Rapoport–Luebering shunt)

The chart shows only glycolysis and the pentose phosphate pathway, since the other pathways shown in previous and subsequent chapters are not present in mature red blood cells.

The shunt consists of **bisphosphoglycerate mutase** and **2,3-bisphosphoglycerate phosphatase**. Bisphosphoglycerate mutase is stimulated by 3-phosphoglycerate causing increased production of 2,3-BPG. **NB:** When this shunt operates, ATP is not produced by the phosphoglycerate kinase reaction. This means that ATP is produced exclusively by the pyruvate kinase reaction, but there is no net gain of ATP from glycolysis under these circumstances.

Physiological significance of 2,3-BPG

Fetal haemoglobin has a low affinity for 2,3-BPG

Fetal haemoglobin is a tetramer of two α-chains and two γ-chains, unlike adult haemoglobin, which comprises two α- and two β-chains. Fetal haemoglobin has a lower affinity for 2,3-BPG than adult haemoglobin, and consequently has a higher affinity for oxygen. This facilitates placental exchange of oxygen from the mother to the fetus.

2,3-BPG and adaptation to high altitude

Anyone accustomed to living at low altitude who has flown to a high-altitude location will be aware that even moderate exertion will cause breathlessness. Within a few days, adaptation occurs as the concentration of 2,3-BPG in red cells increases, enabling the tissues to obtain oxygen in spite of its relatively diminished availability in the thin mountain air. On returning to low altitude the concentration of 2,3-BPG, which has a half-life of 6 hours, returns rapidly to normal.

Importance of 2,3-BPG in medicine

Blood transfusions

Haematologists have long known that blood which has been stored prior to transfusion has an unusually high affinity for oxygen. This is because 2,3-BPG, which forms 65% of the organic phosphates of red cells, disappears on storing in acid citrate–glucose medium, the concentration falling from about 5 to 0.5 mmol/l in 10 days. Consequently, in theory, it would be expected that if a patient is given a large volume of stored blood, the red cells would be unable to unload their oxygen and so, in spite of the presence of oxygen, tissue hypoxia would result. However, in modern clinical practice this is prevented by using anticoagulants and additives (e.g. saline, adenine, glucose, mannitol), which minimize the depletion of 2,3-BPG.

Deficiency of red-cell glycolytic enzymes

Patients with inherited diseases due to deficiencies of red-cell glycolytic enzymes are unable to transport oxygen normally. However, the nature of the effect on 2,3-BPG concentrations depends on whether the deficiency is proximal or distal to the 2,3-BPG shunt. In patients with proximal deficiencies, for example **hexokinase**, **phosphoglucose isomerase**, **phosphofructokinase** and **aldolase deficiencies**, there is a reduced flow of metabolites through glycolysis, and consequently the 2,3-BPG concentration falls. There is therefore an associated tendency towards tissue hypoxia, since the haemoglobin maintains its high affinity for oxygen. In enzymopathies distal to the shunt, such as **pyruvate kinase deficiency**, the opposite situation prevails. Here, the glycolytic intermediates accumulate and, as a result, 2,3-BPG reaches about twice its normal concentration. This means that in this condition haemoglobin has a relatively low affinity for, and ability to transport, oxygen.

Finally, patients have been reported with deficiency of the shunt enzymes **BPG mutase** and **2,3-BPG phosphatase**, suggesting that both activities reside in the same protein. As would be expected, concentrations of 2,3-BPG are severely decreased in these patients, who have an increase in red-cell mass to compensate for the diminished supply of oxygen to the tissues.

Hypophosphataemia during therapy for diabetic ketoacidosis

Hypophosphataemia may result from intravenous infusion of glucose postoperatively, or may occur after insulin treatment for diabetic ketoacidosis. For example, a value of 0.3 mg/dl (normal 2.5–4.5 mg/dl) has been reported. This is because of the acute demand for phosphate by the tissues to form the phosphorylated intermediates of metabolism. Unfortunately, the fall in plasma phosphate causes low concentrations of phosphate in red cells. This results in decreased 2,3-BPG levels, which in turn causes tissue hypoxia.

It has been suggested that, during glucose infusion and during treatment for diabetic ketoacidosis, phosphate replacement might minimize tissue hypoxia and so assist recovery. Although phosphate replacement is not recommended routinely in diabetic ketoacidosis, if the patient develops distress or severe hypophosphataemia, phosphate therapy under close surveillance is indicated.

Common causes of increased red-cell 2,3-BPG concentrations

The concentration of 2,3-BPG is increased in smokers, which compensates for a diminished oxygen supply because of their chronic exposure to carbon monoxide. Also, a compensatory increase in 2,3-BPG is commonly found in patients with chronic anaemia.

Myoglobin

Myoglobin is very similar to the β-chain of haemoglobin and it also has a high affinity for oxygen. Although 2,3-BPG has no direct effect on myoglobin, this important protein and its role in oxygen transport must not be overlooked. It provides a reserve supply of oxygen and, as such, is particularly abundant in the skeletal muscle of aquatic mammals such as whales and seals, enabling them to remain submerged for several minutes.

Diagram 8.1: transport of oxygen from the red blood cell to the mitochondrion for use in oxidative phosphorylation

Diagram 8.1 shows the route by which oxygen is transported from haemoglobin to the mitochondrion. First, oxygen is dissociated from haemoglobin in red cells and diffuses through the capillary wall into the extracellular fluid, and on into the muscle cell. Here, oxygen is bound to myoglobin until required by complex IV of the respiratory chain for oxidative phosphorylation.

Reference

Liu P.Y., Jeng C.Y. (2004) Severe hypophosphataemia on a patient with diabetic ketoacidosis and acute respiratory failure. *J Chin Med Assoc*, **67**, 355–9.

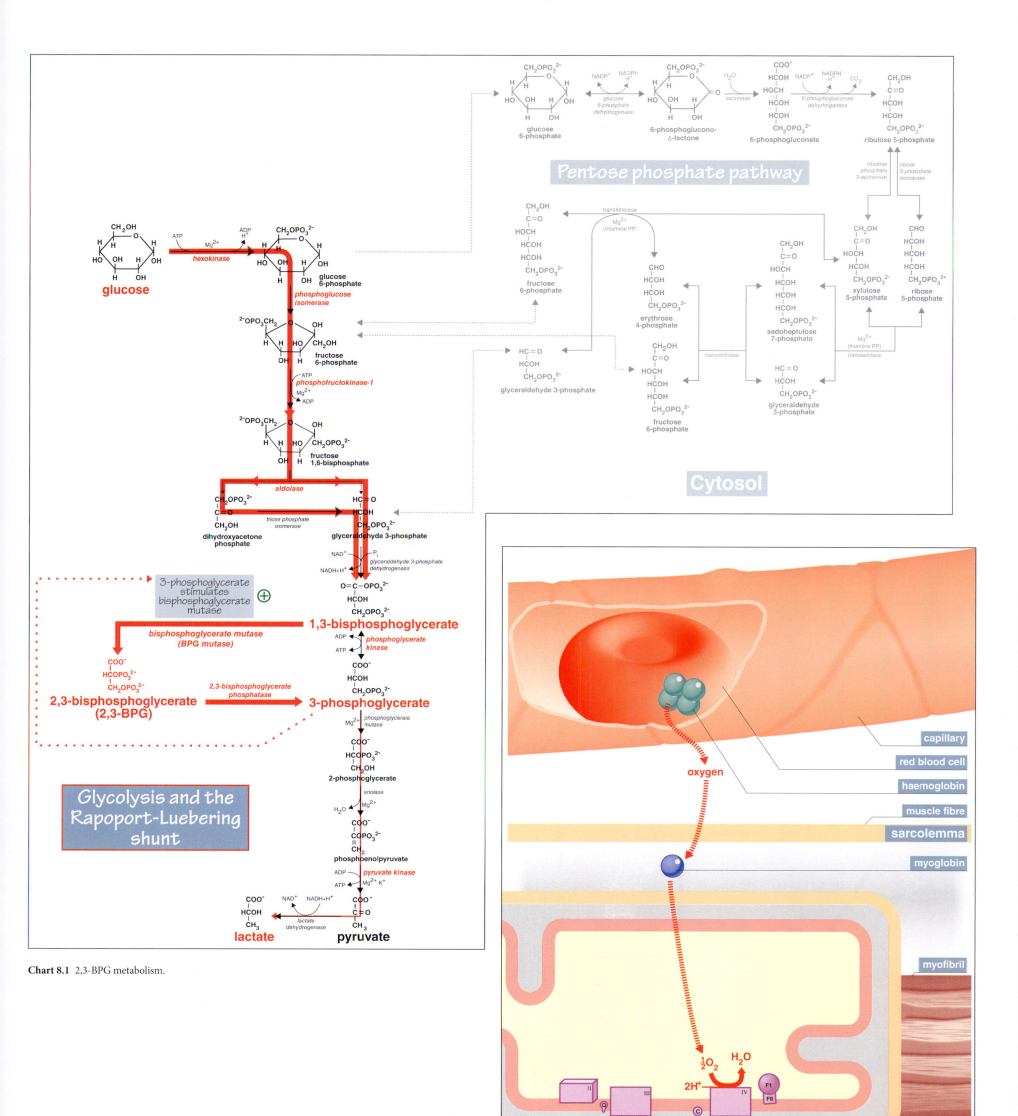

Pentose phosphate pathway

glucose 6-phosphate $\rightleftharpoons$ *glucose 6-phosphate dehydrogenase* ($NADP^+$, $NADPH$ H^+) 6-phosphoglucono-δ-lactone $\rightarrow$ *lactonase* (H_2O) 6-phosphogluconate $\rightarrow$ *6-phosphogluconate dehydrogenase* ($NADP^+$, $NADPH$ H^+, CO_2) ribulose 5-phosphate

ribulose phosphate 3-isomerase / ribose 5-phosphate isomerase

transketolase (Mg^{2+} thiamine PP)

fructose 6-phosphate

erythrose 4-phosphate

xylulose 5-phosphate

ribose 5-phosphate

transaldolase

sedoheptulose 7-phosphate

transketolase (Mg^{2+} thiamine PP)

glyceraldehyde 3-phosphate

fructose 6-phosphate

glyceraldehyde 3-phosphate

Cytosol

glucose $\rightarrow$ *hexokinase* (ATP, Mg^{2+}, ADP H^+) glucose 6-phosphate

phosphoglucose isomerase

fructose 6-phosphate

phosphofructokinase-1 (ATP, Mg^{2+}, ADP)

fructose 1,6-bisphosphate

aldolase

dihydroxyacetone phosphate

triose phosphate isomerase

glyceraldehyde 3-phosphate

glyceraldehyde 3-phosphate dehydrogenase (NAD^+, P_i, $NADH+H^+$)

1,3-bisphosphoglycerate

3-phosphoglycerate stimulates bisphosphoglycerate mutase ⊕

bisphosphoglycerate mutase (BPG mutase)

2,3-bisphosphoglycerate (2,3-BPG)

2,3-bisphosphoglycerate phosphatase

3-phosphoglycerate

phosphoglycerate kinase (ADP, ATP)

phosphoglycerate mutase

2-phosphoglycerate

enolase (H_2O, Mg^{2+})

phosphoenolpyruvate

pyruvate kinase (ADP, ATP, Mg^{2+} K^+)

lactate $\leftarrow$ *lactate dehydrogenase* (NAD^+, $NADH+H^+$) pyruvate

Glycolysis and the Rapoport–Luebering shunt

Chart 8.1 2,3-BPG metabolism.

capillary
red blood cell
oxygen
haemoglobin
muscle fibre
sarcolemma
myoglobin
myofibril

$\frac{1}{2}O_2$ H_2O
$2H^+$
II III IV F1 F0

Diagram 8.1 Transport of oxygen from the red blood cell to the mitochondrion for use in oxidative phosphorylation.

Metabolism of triacylglycerol to provide energy as ATP

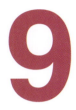

Fatty acids are oxidized and ATP is formed

Fatty acids are esterified with glycerol 3-phosphate to form triacylglycerols, which are stored in adipose tissue. They are an important respiratory fuel for many tissues, especially muscle. The complete oxidation of a typical fatty acid, palmitate, is shown in Chart 9.1.

Chart 9.1: oxidation of fatty acids with energy conserved as ATP

Three metabolic pathways are involved. These are the **β-oxidation pathway**, **Krebs cycle** and the **respiratory chain**. First of all, **adipose triacylglycerol lipase (ATGL)** and **hormone-sensitive lipase** in adipose tissue must liberate fatty acids from **triacylglycerol** (Diagram 9.1). The chart shows the hydrolysis of the triacylglycerol tripalmitin to yield three molecules of **palmitate**

and one molecule of **glycerol**. Next, **palmitoyl CoA** is formed in a reaction catalysed by **long-chain acyl CoA synthetase**; ATP is consumed in the process and AMP (adenosine monophosphate) and inorganic pyrophosphate (PP_i) are formed. Thus energy equal to 2 ATP equivalents is required for this activation reaction. The palmitoyl CoA formed is transported into the mitochondrion using the carnitine shuttle (see Chapter 35). Once in the mitochondrial matrix it is successively oxidized and cleaved to yield eight 2-carbon fragments of acetyl CoA by the β-oxidation pathway. For each turn of the β-oxidation cycle, 1 $FADH_2$ and 1 NADH are formed, thus 7 $FADH_2$ and 7 NADH are formed from palmitate. The eight molecules of acetyl CoA then enter Krebs cycle, where they are oxidized as shown. The ATP yield using the 'modern' non-integer values for the P/O ratios is as follows: the NADH and $FADH_2$ formed by both β-oxidation and Krebs cycle are oxidized by the respiratory chain and yield a total of 100 ATP by oxidative phosphorylation. A further net gain of 6 ATP is derived from the 8 GTP molecules produced by substrate-level phosphorylation in Krebs cycle.

By inspecting Chart 9.1, we can now take stock of the ATP net yield from one molecule of palmitate (Table 9.1).

For comparison, the ATP net yield from palmitate using the historic integer values for P/O ratios is shown in Table 9.2.

Table 9.2 Historic method for calculating ATP net yield from palmitate using integer values for the P/O ratio (see Chart 6.1).

From β-oxidation	ATP yield
By oxidative phosphorylation of 7 $FADH_2$	14
By oxidative phosphorylation of 7 NADH	21
	35 ATP

From Krebs cycle	ATP yield
By substrate-level phosphorylation via GTP	8
By oxidative phosphorylation of 8 $FADH_2$	16
By oxidative phosphorylation of 24 NADH	72
	96 ATP

The total yield is therefore 35 + 96 = 131 ATP. We must remember, however, to subtract the 2 ATP equivalents consumed in the initial acyl CoA synthetase reaction. **Therefore the net yield from the oxidation of one molecule of palmitate is 129 molecules of ATP**

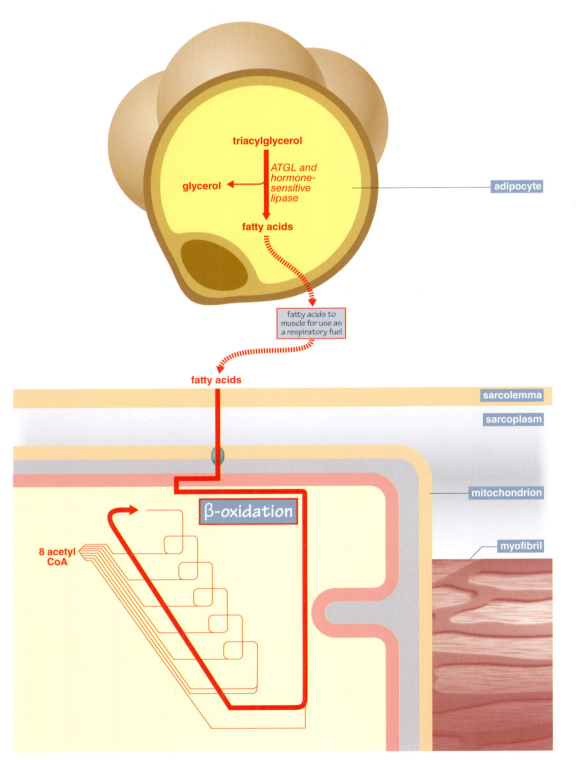

Diagram 9.1 Liberation of fatty acids from triacylglycerol. When energy is required under conditions of stress such as 'fight or flight', exercise or starvation, hormones stimulate triacylglycerol mobilization by activating adipose triacylglycerol lipase (ATGL) and hormone-sensitive lipase in adipose tissue (see Chapter 30); fatty acids and glycerol are released. The fatty acids are bound to albumin and transported in the blood to the tissues for oxidation, e.g. by muscle. The glycerol is converted by the liver to glucose (see Chapter 18), which in turn is released for oxidation, especially by the red blood cells and brain, neither of which can use fatty acids as a respiratory fuel.

Metabolism at a Glance, Fourth Edition. J. G. Salway. © 2017 John Wiley & Sons Ltd. Published 2017 by John Wiley & Sons Ltd.

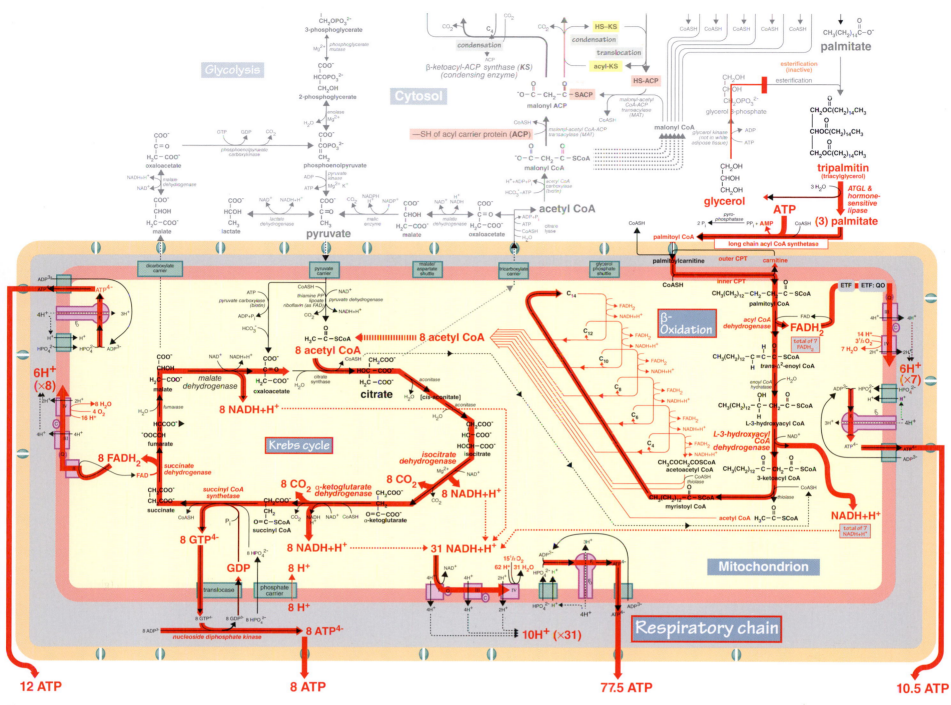

Chart 9.1 Metabolism of triacylglycerol to provide energy as ATP.

Table 9.1 ATP net yield from the oxidation of hexadecanoate (palmitate) assuming non-integer values for P/O ratios (see Chart 6.2).

Origin	Mechanism	Number of protons	ATP yield (loss)
Mitochondrion	**Oxidative phophorylation**	310	**77.5 ATP**
31 molecules of NADH	The β-oxidation spiral and Krebs cycle yield 31 molecules of NADH which, when oxidized, provide energy to pump 31×10 protons (i.e. 310). Since four protons are used to synthesize and translocate 1 ATP, therefore $310 \div 4 = 77.5$ ATP are made		
Acyl CoA dehydrogenase forms 7 FADH$_2$	Acyl CoA dehydrogenase forms 7 FADH$_2$ which, when oxidized, provide energy to pump 7×6 protons (i.e. 42). Since four protons are used to synthesize and translocate 1 ATP, therefore $42 \div 4 = 10.5$ molecules of ATP are made	42	**10.5 ATP**
Succinate dehydrogenase forms 8 FADH$_2$	Succinate dehydrogenase forms 8 FADH$_2$ which provides energy to pump 8×6 protons (i.e. 48) from the matrix, equivalent to the formation of $48 \div 4 = 12$ ATP	48	**12 ATP**
Mitochondrion	**Substrate-level phosphorylation**		**8 ATP**
Succinyl CoA synthetase forms 8 GTP	8 GTP yield 8 ATP in the nucleoside diphosphate kinase reaction		
Phosphate carrier	Phosphate/proton symport. Import of eight phosphate anions uses eight protons from the electrochemical gradient (equivalent to losing 2 ATP)	−8	**(−2 ATP)**
Cytosol	**Activation of fatty acids**		**(−2 ATP)**
Acyl CoA synthetase	Acyl CoA synthetase uses ATP and forms AMP and pyrophosphate. This is equivalent to the loss of two molecules of ATP forming ADP		
	ATP net yield from oxidation of palmitate = 104 ATP		

Metabolism of glucose to glycogen

10

Glycogen is stored in the fed state

If we consume large quantities of carbohydrate-rich food in excess of our immediate requirements, then we might expect the concentration of glucose in the blood to rise higher and higher until it eventually assumed the consistency of syrup. If this happened, there would be serious osmotic implications, with water being drawn from the body's cells into the hypertonic blood, causing the former to become dehydrated.

Fortunately, apart from in the diabetic state, this sequence of events does not happen. We have evolved an elaborate control mechanism so that, when provided with a surplus of carbohydrate fuel, it is stored for less bountiful occasions either as **glycogen** or as fat. Glycogen is made from many glucose molecules joined together to form a compact, highly branched, spherical structure.

Chart 10.1: overview of glycogen synthesis (glycogenesis)

The chart opposite shows how the metabolic fate of glucose can vary according to the energy status of the cell. As we saw Chapter 6, if the cell needs energy and glucose is available, then the glucose will be oxidized by the glycolytic pathway, Krebs cycle and the respiratory chain, with the formation of ATP. If, however, the cell is supplied with surplus glucose, causing a high-energy state in the mitochondrion, then the capacity for metabolic flux through Krebs cycle is overwhelmed and certain metabolites accumulate. Some of these metabolites, such as **citrate**, and **ATP** from the respiratory chain, symbolize an energy surplus and act as messengers (allosteric inhibitors) that inhibit glycolysis. Thus in liver and muscle some of the excess glucose is channelled along the metabolic pathway to glycogen, a process known as **glycogenesis**.

Glycogen as a fuel reserve

The liver and muscles are the major depots for this important energy reserve. The average man who has been well fed on a diet rich in carbohydrate stores 70 g of glycogen in his liver and 200 g in his muscles. The liver glycogen reserves are sufficient only for an overnight fast at the longest. Accordingly, fat reserves must also be used, especially during long periods of fasting or strenuous exercise.

As we will see later, the brain cannot use fat directly as a fuel and is mainly dependent upon a steady supply of glucose via the blood. If the brain is denied glucose it ceases to function properly. The symptoms of a low plasma glucose level include a feeling of dizziness, faintness or lethargy. In hypoglycaemia, defined as a plasma glucose of less than 2.5 mmol/l, these symptoms can progress to unconsciousness, coma and, unless glucose is provided rapidly, death.

We can now appreciate the great importance of the reserves of glucose stored as glycogen in the liver. We survive between meals because the liver is able to keep the blood glucose 'topped up' and can maintain a fasting blood concentration of 3.5–5.5 mmol/l, which satisfies the pernickety fuel requirements of the brain.

Glycogen is also an important energy source when confronted with a 'fight or flight' situation. This role will be discussed fully later (see Chapters 11–14) but, as we will see below, the structure of the glycogen molecule is beautifully adapted for the rapid mobilization of glucose in an emergency.

Diagram 10.1: glycogen, a molecule that is well designed for its function

Glycogen is a complex, hydrated polymer of glucose molecules that form a highly branched, spherical structure. The very large molecular weight, which ranges over several million daltons, enables glucose to be stored without the osmotic complications associated with free glucose molecules. The size of the glycogen molecule varies with the prevailing nutritional status, being larger (up to 40 nm in diameter) in the fed state, and progressively shrinking to around 10 nm or less between meals.

The glucose chain is attached to the protein **glycogenin**. The glucose molecules are joined by $\alpha(1 \rightarrow 4)$ glycosidic bonds, except at the branch points, which are $\alpha(1 \rightarrow 6)$ glycosidic bonds. A branch occurs, on average, every 10 glucose units along the chain. This highly branched, spherical structure creates a large number of exposed terminal glucose molecules, which are accessible to the enzymes involved in glycogen breakdown (glycogenolysis). This ensures an extremely rapid release of glucose units from glycogen in the 'fight or flight' emergency situation, which can sometimes be vital for survival.

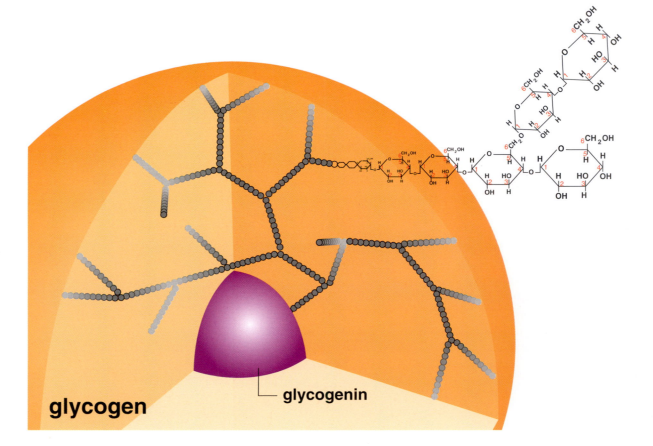

glycogen

glycogenin

Diagram 10.1 Diagrammatic representation of a glycogen molecule.

Metabolism at a Glance, Fourth Edition. J. G. Salway. © 2017 John Wiley & Sons Ltd. Published 2017 by John Wiley & Sons Ltd.

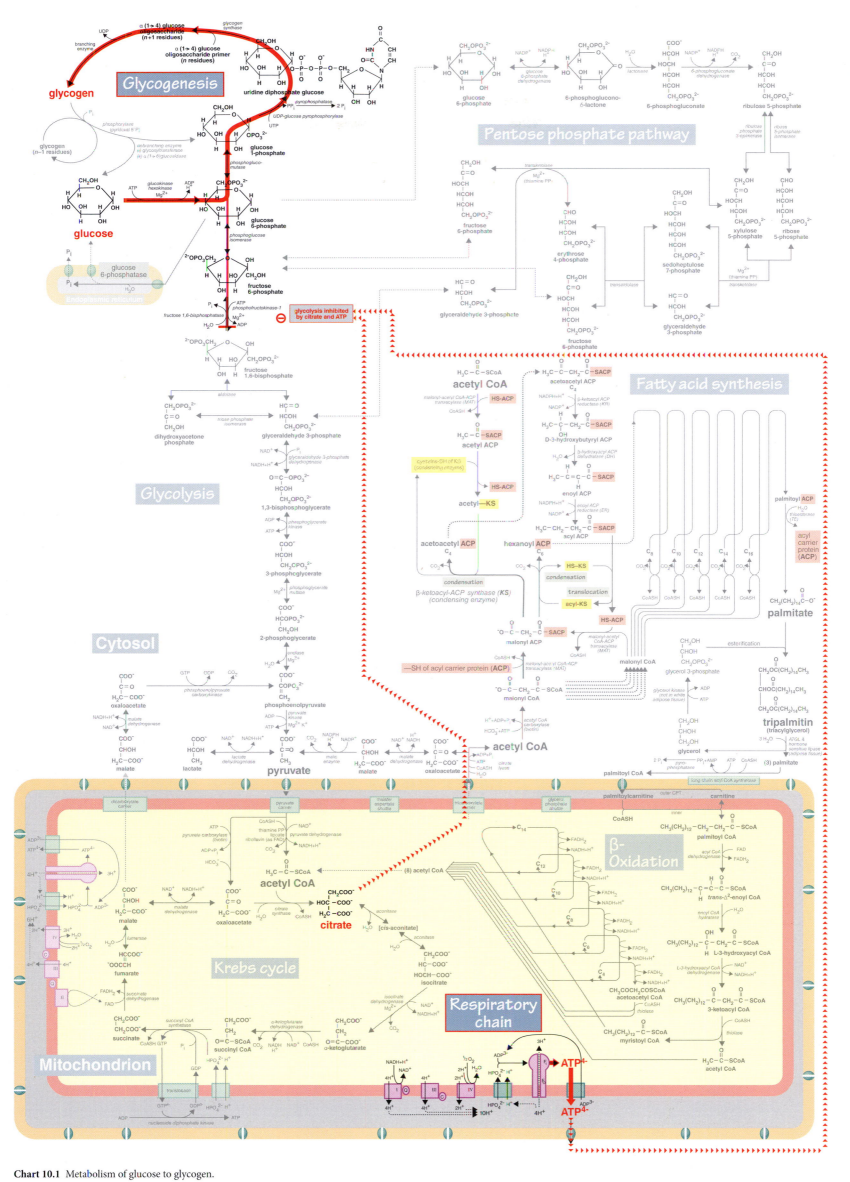

Chart 10.1 Metabolism of glucose to glycogen.

Glycogen metabolism I

11

Different roles of glycogen in liver and muscle

Glucose is stored as glycogen. Although both liver and muscle store glycogen, there are major differences between the two in the way that glycogen metabolism is deployed and controlled. The liver exports glucose derived from glycogen for use by other tissues. In skeletal muscle, the glucose is particularly important as a fuel that is immediately available during periods of extreme activity, as in the adrenaline-driven 'fight or flight' response.

Metabolic demands made on glycogen metabolism

The simplistic approach to glycogen metabolism is to consider glycogen synthesis in the fed state, followed by glycogen breakdown during fasting or 'fight or flight', followed by glycogen synthesis after feeding to complete the cycle. However, nature does not order periods of feeding, fasting and fight or flight with carefully planned transition periods in between. Indeed, in nature, animals are very vulnerable to attack by a predator when they are feeding. The prey's muscles must then respond to the crisis by instantly diverting the flux of glucose metabolites from the feeding state of glycogen **synthesis** to glycogen **breakdown** for anaerobic glycolysis. Furthermore, this instantaneous metabolic U-turn must be achieved in spite of the lingering presence of insulin secreted during feeding, which tends to promote glycogen synthesis. Next, after a strenuous chase, the prey (assuming it has survived) must quickly replenish its glycogen reserves for the next emergency, whether food is available or not. Moreover, this must be done without excessively draining blood glucose concentrations and causing hypoglycaemia. Not surprisingly, the complicated physiological demands made on glycogen metabolism are matched by a complicated regulatory mechanism. The details of this mechanism are still not fully understood, but it involves an **amplification cascade** dramatically enhancing the effects of the hormones that initiate this series of reactions (see Chapter 12).

Glycogen metabolism: an overview

Liver and muscle share some general features during the processes of glycogen synthesis from glucose 1-phosphate, and glycogenolysis back to glucose 1-phosphate; these are summarized below.

Glycogenesis

Glucose 1-phosphate reacts with **uridine triphosphate (UTP)** (Chart 11.2) to form **uridine diphosphate glucose (UDP-glucose)**. This is an activated form of glucose used for glycogen synthesis. A **primer**, in the form of an $\alpha(1 \rightarrow 4)$ glucose oligosaccharide attached to the protein glycogenin, is also needed. The glucosyl group from UDP-glucose is added to the polysaccharide chain by **glycogen synthase** provided it consists of four or more glucose residues. Once the chain contains 11 or more residues, the **branching enzyme** becomes involved. The branching enzyme forms the many branches of glycogen by severing a string of seven residues from the growing chain and rejoining it by an $\alpha(1 \rightarrow 6)$ linkage to an interior point at least four residues from an existing branch.

Glycogenolysis

The enzyme controlling glycogenolysis is **phosphorylase** (Chart 11.1). It requires pyridoxal phosphate and inorganic phosphate and exists in both active and inactive forms. Phosphorylase progressively nibbles its way along the chain of $\alpha(1 \rightarrow 4)$ glucose molecules, releasing molecules of **glucose 1-phosphate**. Its progress is obstructed when it reaches a stage on the chain four glucose residues away from a branch point. Now the bifunctional debranching enzyme is needed, one component of which, **glycosyltransferase**, rescues the situation by transferring the terminal three (of these four) glucose molecules to the end of another chain so that phosphorylase activity can continue. The remaining glucose molecule, which now forms an $\alpha(1 \rightarrow 6)$-linked stump at the branching point, is removed as free glucose by $\alpha(1 \rightarrow 6)$ **glucosidase**, the second component of the debranching enzyme.

The glucose 1-phosphate formed by phosphorylase is converted to glucose 6-phosphate by **phosphoglucomutase**.

Glycogen metabolism in liver

Liver stores glycogen as a reserve fuel for periods of fasting or 'fight or flight'. Liver does not usually use the glycogen-derived glucose itself for energy; instead it is exported for use by the brain, erythrocytes and muscle.

Glycogenolysis in liver

Glycogenolysis (Chart 11.1) is stimulated by glucagon in response to fasting, and by adrenaline for 'fight or flight'. Both of these hormones stimulate the **glycogenolysis cascade** (see Chart 12.1) to produce glucose 6-phosphate. Liver (unlike muscle) has **glucose 6-phosphatase**, which enables mobilization of glucose into the blood.

NB: In liver, in contrast to muscle, cyclic AMP-mediated phosphorylation **inhibits** glycolysis and stimulates hepatic gluconeogenesis (see Chapter 18). In the physiological context this means that during fasting, when glucagon is present, both glycogenolysis and gluconeogenesis will be active.

Glycogen synthesis in liver
Glycogenesis: the 'direct' pathway from dietary glucose
Traditionally it was thought that glucose from dietary carbohydrate is transported **directly** to the liver for metabolism to glycogen, i.e. by the '**direct**' **pathway** for glycogenesis (Chart 11.2). However, evidence suggests that following a fast, during the period immediately after refeeding, glycogen synthesis proceeds via an '**indirect**' **pathway** involving skeletal muscle (see below).

Glycogenesis: the 'indirect' pathway from dietary glucose via muscle lactate
During refeeding after fasting, glucose is metabolized anaerobically to lactate by muscle even though the conditions are aerobic. This is because, immediately after refeeding, the high ratio of acetyl CoA/CoA caused by the lingering β-oxidation of fatty acids results in pyruvate dehydrogenase remaining inhibited (see Chapter 47). Consequently, glucose in muscle is metabolized to pyruvate, which is reduced to lactate. This lactate is transported in the blood to the liver for gluconeogenesis and glycogen synthesis.

Liver glycogen storage diseases (GSDs)
Type I glycogen storage disease (von Gierke's disease)
In type I glycogen storage disease (GSD), glycogen accumulates in the liver, kidneys and intestines. It has been divided into subtypes, of which **types Ia, Ib and Ic** are shown in Chart 11.3. The basic defect is glucose 6-phosphatase deficiency either from loss of the catalytic enzyme unit itself (Ia), or of either the endoplasmic reticulum glucose 6-phosphate translocator (Ib) or the phosphate translocator (Ic) (see also Diagram 18.1).

In all cases the clinical features are identical and are a consequence of the substrate cycling of glucose 6-phosphate shown in Chart 11.3. Patients have low levels of blood glucose, and raised levels of lactate, ketone bodies, lipids and urate. Lactate supplied by the extrahepatic tissues is metabolized to glucose 6-phosphate, which in the absence of glucose 6-phosphatase cannot be metabolized to glucose. The result is hypoglycaemia, which is potentially fatal. Instead, the glucose 6-phosphate is diverted into glycogen synthesis causing hepatomegaly, and into the pentose phosphate pathway forming ribose 5-phosphate, which is a precursor of purine synthesis. Purine catabolism forms uric acid, which can cause gout.

Type VI glycogen storage disease (Hers' disease)
This condition is due to a deficiency of liver phosphorylase (or phosphorylase kinase) as shown in Chart 11.1. Similarly to type I disease, this causes hepatomegaly due to glycogen accumulation. However, because normal blood glucose levels can be maintained by gluconeogenesis from lactate, alanine, glycerol, etc., ketosis is moderate and hyperlactataemia does not occur.

Type III debranching enzyme deficiency (Cori's disease)
Patients are deficient in $\alpha(1 \rightarrow 6)$ glucosidase (AGL) activity and present with hypoglycaemia and hyperlipidaemia (Chart 11.1). Usually, both liver and muscle AGL is affected (subtype IIIa) but, in 15% of cases, the muscle enzyme is intact while the liver enzyme is deficient (subtype IIIb).

Metabolism at a Glance, Fourth Edition. J. G. Salway. © 2017 John Wiley & Sons Ltd. Published 2017 by John Wiley & Sons Ltd.

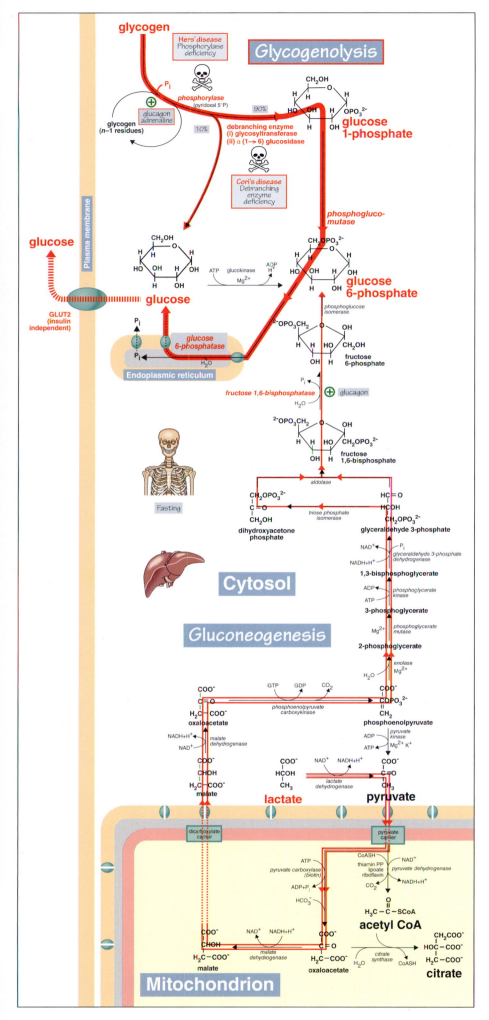

Chart 11.1 Glycogenolysis in liver.

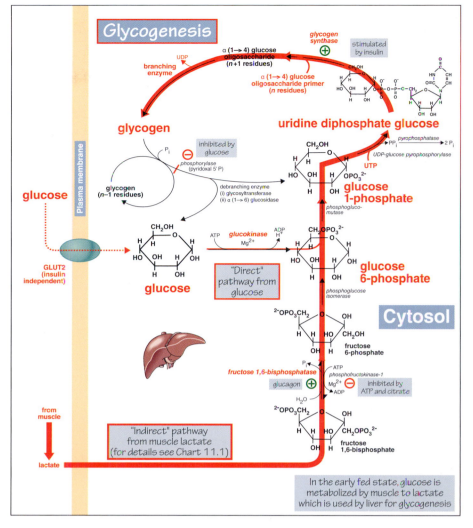

Chart 11.2 Glycogenesis in liver from glucose (direct pathway) and from lactate (indirect pathway).

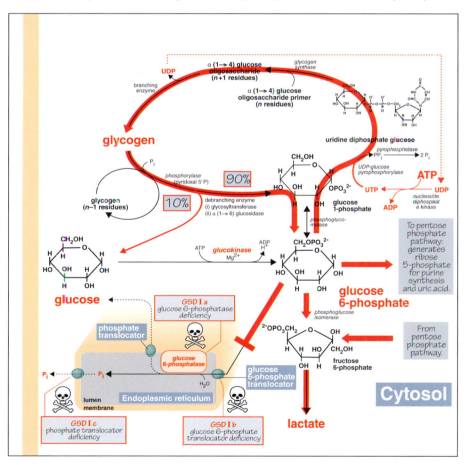

Chart 11.3 Glycogenolysis in type I glycogen storage disease (GSD I).

Glycogen metabolism II

12

Glycogen metabolism in skeletal muscle

In muscle, the main function of glycogen is to serve as a reserve of respiratory fuel by rapidly providing glucose during periods of extremely vigorous muscle contraction, such as occur in moments of danger, i.e. in the 'fight or flight' response.

Glycogenolysis in skeletal muscle

Glycogenolysis in skeletal muscle is stimulated by adrenaline via the amplification cascade shown in Chart 12.1. **Phosphorylase** produces **glucose 1-phosphate**, which is converted into **glucose 6-phosphate**. Because muscle lacks glucose 6-phosphatase, glucose 6-phosphate is totally committed to glycolysis for ATP production. Also, since muscle hexokinase has a very low K_m for glucose (0.1 mmol/l), it has a very high affinity for glucose and will readily phosphorylate the 10% of glucose units liberated from glycogen by the debranching enzyme, $\alpha(1 \rightarrow 6)$ glucosidase, as free glucose, thus ensuring its use by glycolysis. It should be remembered that adrenaline increases the cyclic AMP concentration, which not only stimulates glycogenolysis but **in muscle** also stimulates glycolysis (see Chapter 16).

Glycogen synthesis in skeletal muscle

In the fed state in resting muscle, insulin is available to facilitate glucose transport into the muscle cell using the GLUT4 transporter (Charts 12.2 and 12.3). Remember that, in the fed state, phosphofructokinase-1 is inhibited (see Chapter 16) and so glucose 6-phosphate will be used for glycogen synthesis. It should be noted that glycogen synthesis and glycogenolysis are regulated in a reciprocal way (Chart 12.1).

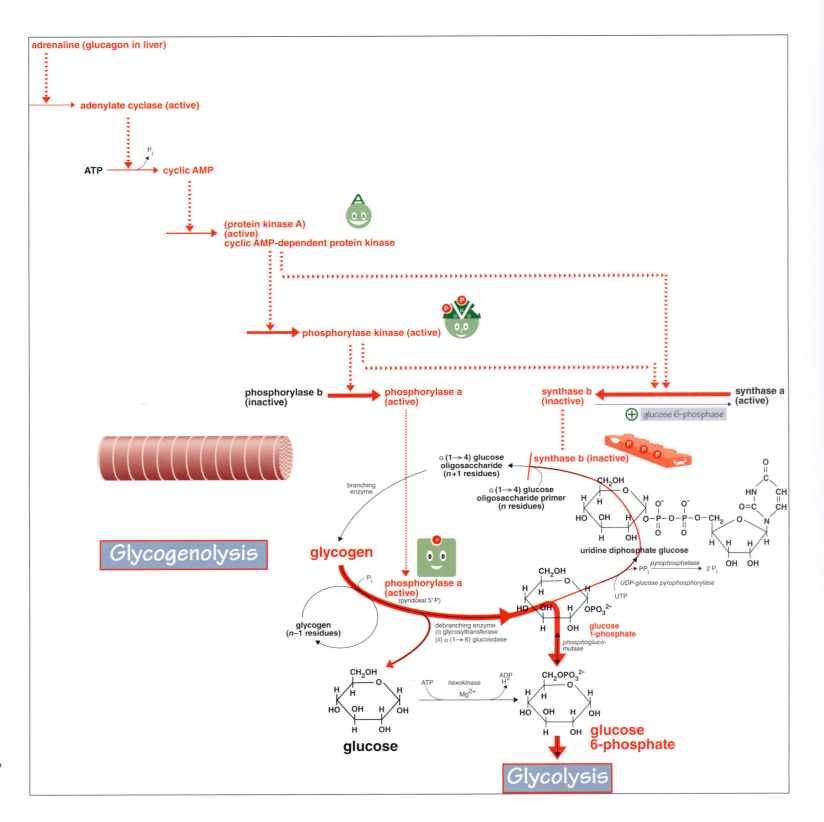

Chart 12.1 Activation of the glycogenolysis cascade is linked to the inactivation of glycogen synthesis.

Metabolism at a Glance, Fourth Edition. J. G. Salway. © 2017 John Wiley & Sons Ltd. Published 2017 by John Wiley & Sons Ltd.

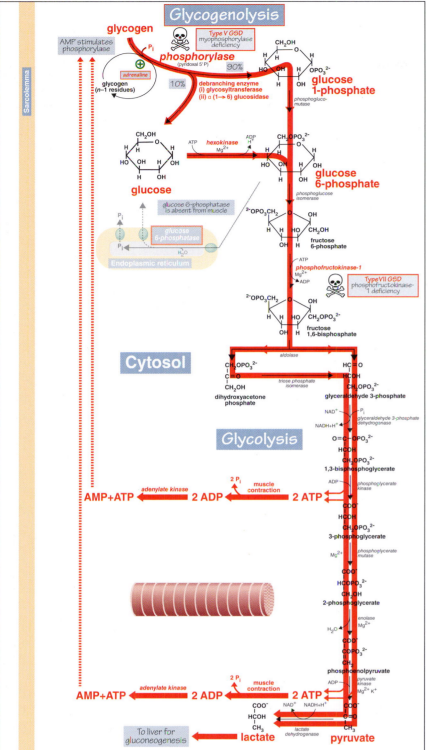

Chart 12.2 Glycogenolysis in skeletal muscle.

At this point, *reciprocal regulation of glycogen synthesis and breakdown occurs. First, let us continue with glycogenolysis before concluding with the inactivation of glycogen synthesis.*

4 One molecule of phosphorylase kinase phosphorylates several inactive molecules of **phosphorylase b** to give the active form, **phosphorylase a**, and so glycogen breakdown can now proceed.

Inactivation of glycogen synthesis

To maximize glycogen breakdown, synthesis is reciprocally inactivated by phosphorylase kinase, which is one of several protein kinases, including protein kinase A, that can cause **glycogen synthase a** to produce its low-activity **synthase b** form (Chart 12.1).

Muscle glycogen storage diseases (glycogenoses)
Type V glycogen storage disease (McArdle's disease)

In this disease, patients suffer severe muscle cramps after exercise. It is due to deficiency of muscle phosphorylase (myophosphorylase) (Chart 12.2) so that glycogen accumulates within the muscles of patients. Whereas after exercise blood lactate levels normally increase, in patients with type V glycogenosis, blood lactate concentration decreases after exertion.

Type VII glycogen storage disease (Tarui's disease)

This condition is due to deficiency of phosphofructokinase-1 in muscle (Chart 12.3), and the symptoms are induced by exercise in a similar manner to those in type V glycogenosis. Accordingly, the muscles are almost completely dependent on fatty acids as their respiratory fuel. In this disease there is an increased concentration of glucose 6-phosphate, which stimulates glycogen synthase causing accumulation of glycogen.

Glycogenolysis cascade

Chart 12.1 shows how the original signal provided by a single molecule of adrenaline is amplified during the course of a cascade of reactions that activate a large number of **phosphorylase** molecules, ensuring the rapid mobilization of glycogen as follows:

1 A molecule of adrenaline stimulates adenylate cyclase to form several molecules of **cyclic AMP**.

2 Each molecule of cyclic AMP dissociates an inactive tetramer to free two catalytically active monomers of **protein kinase A** (also known as **cyclic AMP-dependent protein kinase**) from their regulatory monomers (see Chapter 13). **NB:** This gives a relatively modest amplification factor of 2.

3 Each active molecule of protein kinase A phosphorylates and activates several molecules of **phosphorylase kinase**.

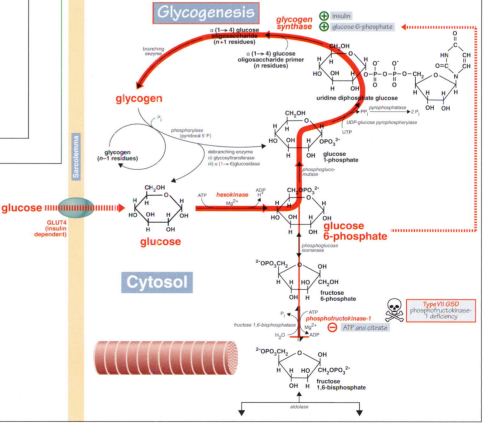

Chart 12.3 Glycogenesis in skeletal muscle.

Glycogen metabolism III: regulation of glycogen breakdown (glycogenolysis)

13

Hormonal control: the role of adrenaline and glucagon in the regulation of glycogenolysis

In liver, glycogenolysis is stimulated by both glucagon and adrenaline, whereas **in muscle** only adrenaline is effective. In a crisis, when mobilization of glycogen is stimulated by adrenaline, the response must happen **immediately!** This occurs through the remarkable amplification cascade described earlier (see Chapter 12), in which cyclic AMP plays an important role. In this way, small, nanomolar concentrations of adrenaline can rapidly mobilize a vast number of glucose residues for use as respiratory fuel.

NB: The regulation of glycogen metabolism, which is complex, is still the subject of extensive research and full details are beyond the scope of this book. **The descriptions provided here and in the next chapter are based on current knowledge, largely relating to the regulation of glycogen metabolism in skeletal muscle.** *Whereas many details of the mechanisms may be common to both liver and muscle, there are several differences stemming from the different functions of the two tissues; for example, as mentioned earlier, whereas both liver and muscle are responsive to adrenaline (albeit through different mechanisms), only liver has receptors for glucagon.*

Diagram 13.1: regulation of glycogenolysis

Formation of cyclic AMP

When adrenaline docks with its receptor, the signal is transduced through the G protein, **adenylate cylase** is activated, and ATP is converted to **cyclic AMP**, which activates **protein kinase A** (Diagram 13.2). Protein kinase A is compartmentalized at its metabolically active locations, for example on the plasma membrane, within the nucleus, mitochondria, etc., by an **A-kinase anchoring protein (AKAP)** (Diagram 13.3).

Protein kinase A

When inactive, protein kinase A exists as a complex of two catalytic subunits plus two regulatory (R) subunits and AKAP (Diagram 13.4). Cyclic AMP binds to the two regulatory units and liberates the two active catalytic subunits.

NB: The active monomers of protein kinase A (and their metabolic opponents, the protein phosphatases) (see Chapter 14) **play a key role in regulating not only glycogen metabolism, but also many other metabolic pathways** (see Chapters 16, 18 and 30).

Returning to glycogen metabolism, note that protein kinase A both **activates** glycogenolysis and concurrently **inhibits** glycogen synthesis.

Roles of protein kinase A in regulating glycogenolysis

Protein kinase A phosphorylates several enzymes involved in glycogen metabolism, and these covalent modifications persist until the enzymes are dephosphorylated by protein phosphatases (see Chapter 14). The effects of protein kinase A, shown in the diagram opposite, are:

1 **Activation of phosphorylase kinase.** Protein kinase A phosphorylates phosphorylase kinase to the active form. However, full activity requires Ca^{2+} ions, which are released into the sarcoplasm when muscle is contracting (or following α-adrenergic stimulation of liver). The fully activated phosphorylase kinase now has a double action: not only does it activate phosphorylase by forming **phosphorylase a**, but it also participates in phosphorylating (and thus inactivating) glycogen synthase.

2 **Inactivation of protein phosphatase-1.** Protein phosphatase-1 (see Chapter 14) plays a major role in switching off glycogenolysis by dephosphorylating phosphorylase a. Clearly this must be stopped. Accordingly, protein phosphatase-1 is inactivated by two assassins in the forms of **protein kinase A** and **protein phosphatase inhibitor-1** (see below). The first attack is by protein kinase A, which phosphorylates site 2 of the regulatory subunit of the protein phosphatase-1G complex. Consequently, protein phosphatase-1 dissociates from its sanctuary in the complex and the free protein phosphatase-1 is relatively inactive. Moreover, it is now unprotected and vulnerable to a second attack by the protein phosphatase inhibitor-1, which diffuses into action and delivers the *coup de grâce*. So, finally, with interference by protein phosphatase-1 activity well and truly

suppressed, phosphorylase a activity prevails unchallenged and glycogen breakdown can now take place.

3 **Activation of protein phosphatase inhibitor-1.** The conspiracy between protein kinase A and protein phosphatase inhibitor-1 is initiated when the latter is phosphorylated to its active form by the former. The active inhibitor can now join protein kinase A in the vendetta against protein phosphatase-1, as described in point 2 above.

4 **Resumption of glycogen synthesis after 'fight or flight'.** Rapid replacement of glycogen stores is needed after a 'fight or flight' incident to survive the next crisis. Furthermore, this must be accomplished in the absence of insulin. Protein kinase A fulfils this requirement by phosphorylating **both** sites 1 and 2 of the regulatory subunit G thereby inactivating protein phosphatase-1 during the emergency. However, during recovery when adrenaline stimulation has finished, site 2 is preferentially dephosphorylated. This leaves site 1 phosphorylated and protein phosphatase-1 active and immediately able to activate glycogen synthase (Diagram 14.1).

Phosphorylase kinase

This protein is a hexadecamer of four subunits (Diagram 13.5), each subunit being a tetramer of α-, β-, γ- and δ-monomers; the native protein thus comprises $α_4β_4γ_4δ_4$. The catalytic site is on the γ-monomer.

The α- and β-monomers are phosphorylated during modification from the inactive b form to the active phosphorylase kinase a. Although phosphorylation of the α-monomer causes some stimulation of activity, it is the subsequent rapid phosphorylation of the β-monomer that is the major activator of phosphorylase kinase activity. The δ-monomer is composed of calmodulin, which has four regulatory binding sites with different affinities for calcium ions. They can bind calcium ions at concentrations as low as 0.1 µmol/l, such as occur in resting muscle. However, they are fully occupied and maximally stimulated following the 100-fold increase in calcium ion concentration – up to 10 µmol/l – that occurs during exercise.

Phosphorylase kinase a is inhibited when **protein phosphatase**-1 removes phosphate from the β-monomer and by **protein phosphatase-2A**, which dephosphorylates the α-monomer (see Diagram 14.1).

Properties of glycogen phosphorylase

Phosphorylase a is phosphorylated (**NB:** the 'a' is a letter chosen at random to name this phosphorylase: **it does not mean active!**). **Phosphorylase b is non-phosphorylated** but can be phosphorylated at serine 14 to form phosphorylase a. Phosphorylase is a dimer of two identical 97 kDa proteins. For simplicity a monomer is shown in Diagram 13.1.

In resting muscle, phosphorylase b is in the inactive T form; in contracting muscle it is in the active R form. Adrenaline activates a signalling sequence concluding when **phosphorylase kinase** phosphorylates the **T form of phosphorylase b**. This causes a conformational change to the **very active R state of phosphorylase a**. Also, during exercise, ATP is converted to AMP, which allosterically stimulates phosphorylase b by forming the very active R state, which decreases its K_m for phosphate. Conversely, ATP and glucose 6-phosphate counter the effect of AMP so that in the resting state, as the concentrations of the former recover, phosphorylase b is converted back to the inactive T form.

Phosphorylase a is not dependent on AMP for activity, provided the concentration of P_i is sufficiently increased, as happens during muscle contraction.

Inactivation of phosphorylase a occurs when it is dephosphorylated by protein phosphatase-1 (see Diagram 14.1).

Protein phosphatase inhibitor-1

The inhibitor-1 is an 18.7 kDa protein that is modified to its active form by phosphorylation of a threonine residue in a reaction catalysed by protein kinase A (Diagram 13.6). The inhibitor inactivates protein phosphatase-1 but has no effect on protein phosphatase-2A. In resting muscle, i.e. when glycogenolysis is not active, protein phosphatase inhibitor-1 is inactivated when it is dephosphorylated by protein phosphatase-2A (see Diagram 14.1).

Diagram 13.1 (opposite) Regulation of glycogenolysis.

Diagram 13.2 Active protein kinase A.

Diagram 13.3 A-kinase anchoring protein (AKAP).

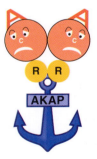

Diagram 13.4 Inactive protein kinase A bound to its regulatory proteins and AKAP.

Diagram 13.5 Very active phosphorylase kinase.

Diagram 13.6 Active protein phosphatase inhibitor-1.

Metabolism at a Glance, Fourth Edition. J. G. Salway. © 2017 John Wiley & Sons Ltd. Published 2017 by John Wiley & Sons Ltd.

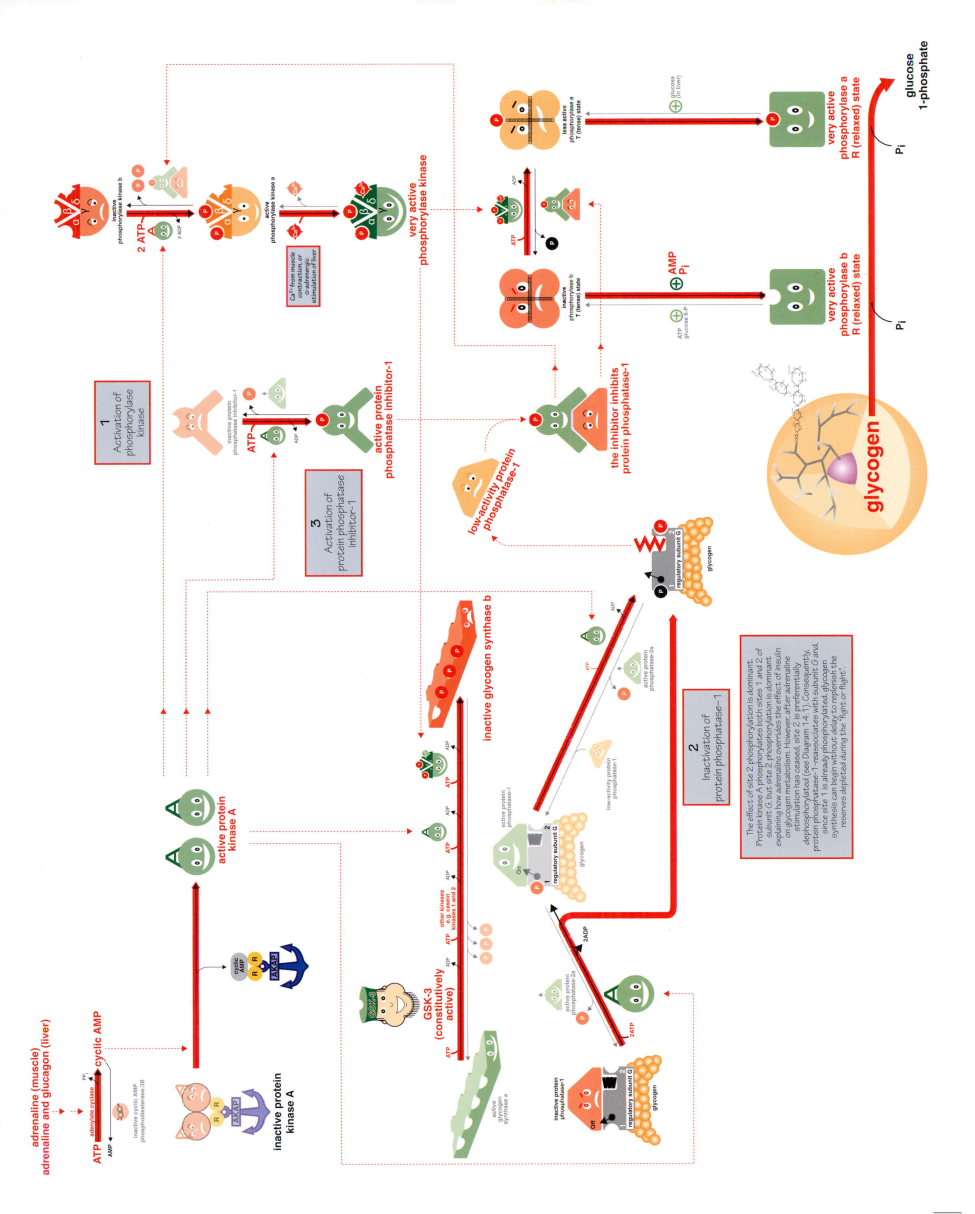

Glycogen metabolism IV: regulation of glycogen synthesis (glycogenesis)

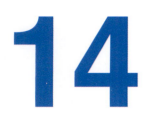

Hormonal control: role of insulin in the regulation of glycogen synthesis

Insulin is secreted by the β-cells of the pancreas following a carbohydrate meal. Insulin is needed to transport glucose into muscle cells, which means that glycogenesis is most active in the post-prandial state. The details of how insulin signals its numerous effects on cells is summarized in Chapter 59). However, fundamental to glycogen synthesis is the regulation of **glycogen synthase**, which is regulated as shown in Diagrams 13.1 and 14.1.

*Glycogen synthesis has been studied most extensively in muscle, and it is to this tissue that the following description of regulation relates. It should be noted that as we saw in Chapter 13, in the **catabolic state** of glycogenolysis, **phosphorylation by protein kinases** dominates the scene. On the other hand, in the **anabolic state** of glycogenesis, **protein phosphatase-1** and **-2A** dominate and **protein dephosphorylation** occurs.*

Diagram 14.1 (opposite) Regulation of glycogenesis.

Protein phosphatases

Protein phosphatase-1 and -2A are the protein phosphatases in skeletal muscle involved in the regulation of glycogen metabolism.

Protein phosphatase-1 (PP-1)

Experiments suggest it is a 37 kDa protein that is inhibited by protein phosphatase inhibitor-1 and okadaic acid. There are several forms of PP-1, but the major active form associated with glycogen is known as PP-1G. This is a complex of PP-1 and a large, 160 kDa **regulatory subunit G**, which is bound to glycogen.

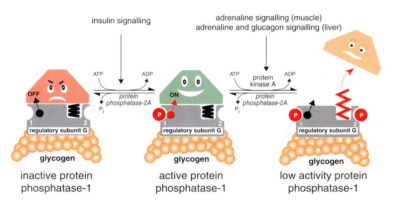

inactive protein phosphatase-1 · active protein phosphatase-1 · low activity protein phosphatase-1

Regulation of PP-1G activity

PP-1G is active when phosphorylated at site 1 by insulin-generated signals via phosphatidylinositol-3 kinase (**PI-3 kinase**) (see Chapter 59). Conversely, it is slowly inactivated by dephosphorylation of site 1 by **protein phosphatase-2A**. However, PP-1 is also inactivated by phosphorylation at site 2 by **protein kinase A**, which causes the catalytic subunit to dissociate from the regulatory subunit G. The latter process is reversed by protein phosphatase-2A, which dephosphorylates site 2 permitting re-association of the subunits to form active PP-1G.

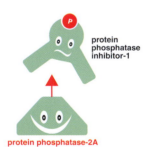

protein phosphatase inhibitor-1

protein phosphatase-2A

Diagram 14.2 Protein phosphatase-2A is not inhibited by protein phosphatase inhibitor-1.

Protein phosphatase-2A (PP-2A)

Several forms of PP-2A have been identified in eukaryotic cells, some containing two subunits and some three subunits. It is inhibited by okadaic acid but is not inhibited by inhibitor-1 (Diagram 14.2).

Diagram 14.1: regulation of glycogen synthesis
Removal of cyclic AMP

We have seen in Chapter 13 how hormone-stimulated mobilization of glycogen is mediated by cyclic AMP. Obviously, if glycogen synthesis is to occur, glycogen breakdown must stop, and so cyclic AMP must be destroyed. There is evidence based on studies of adipose tissue suggesting the presence of an insulin-stimulated series of reactions resulting in the activation of

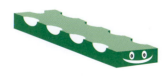

Diagram 14.3 Active glycogen synthase a.

cyclic AMP phosphodiesterase-3B (PDE-3B) and the conversion of cyclic AMP to AMP.

Role of protein phosphatase-1 and -2A in regulating glycogenesis

With PP-1 active, glycogen synthesis can begin in earnest. Basically, PP-1 and PP-2A oppose the action of the protein kinases and have the following effects:

1 **Inactivation of PP-1 inhibitor.** In resting muscle, PP-2A inactivates the PP-1 inhibitor in an act of biochemical camaraderie that is much appreciated by its team mate, PP-1.
2 **Inactivation of phosphorylase kinase.** PP-1 dephosphorylates the β-monomer, and PP-2A dephosphorylates the α-monomer, thereby inactivating **phosphorylase kinase**. This prevents the formation of **phosphorylase a** thus inhibiting glycogen breakdown.
3 **Activation of glycogen synthase.** Finally, PP-1 dephosphorylates synthase b to form the high-activity **synthase a**, which catalyses the formation of glycogen from uridine diphosphate glucose.

Properties of glycogen synthase

Glycogen synthase is a simple tetramer of four identical 85 kDa monomers (for simplicity, a single monomer is shown in Diagram 14.3). Its activity is regulated by synergistic phosphorylation, which can occur at nine sites (serine residues) in a precise, hierarchical manner producing the inactive **glycogen synthase b**. Glycogen synthase is most active in its dephosphorylated form, known as **synthase a**.

Inactivation (phosphorylation) of glycogen synthase

Glycogen synthase has 737 amino acid residues and, of these, nine are serine residues that can be phosphorylated. Two of these are situated in the N-terminal region of the molecule (N-7 and N-10) and seven are located in the C-terminal region (C-30, C-34, C-38, C-42, C-46, C-87 and C-100). It has been demonstrated *in vitro* that at least seven protein kinases can phosphorylate glycogen synthase; five important examples are:

1 **Protein kinase A**, which phosphorylates sites C-87, C-100 and N-7.
2 **Glycogen synthase kinase-3 (GSK-3)**, which phosphorylates the cluster of serine residues at C-30, C-34, C-38 and C-42 (but not C-46). It is thought that GSK-3 plays a major role in insulin-stimulated glycogen synthesis as follows: during fasting, in the absence of insulin, GSK-3 is **constitutively active** and it phosphorylates glycogen synthase rendering it inactive. However, after feeding, insulin is present and causes the inactivation of GSK-3. This permits dephosphorylation and activation of glycogen synthase (see Chapter 50).
3 **Phosphorylase kinase**, which phosphorylates the serine residue at N-7.
4 **Casein kinase-1**, which phosphorylates at N-10.
5 **Casein kinase-2**, which phosphorylates at C-46.

Activation (dephosphorylation) of glycogen synthase by protein phosphatase-1

Protein phosphatase-1 dephosphorylates synthase b to produce **active glycogen synthase a**. PP-1 in turn is activated by insulin-generated signals mediated via PI-3 kinase (see Chapter 59). This results in **phosphorylation** of site 1 of the glycogen-bound regulatory subunit G, thereby activating PP-1. Alternatively, **dephosphorylation** of site 2 of the regulatory subunit by PP-2A allows reassociation of the catalytic and regulatory subunits to form active PP-1.

Role of glucose in the inhibition of phosphorylase in liver

Glucose, when abundant after a carbohydrate meal, is the major inhibitor of phosphorylase activity in liver. When glucose is bound to phosphorylase a, the latter acts as a better substrate for PP-1.

Metabolism at a Glance, Fourth Edition. J. G. Salway. © 2017 John Wiley & Sons Ltd. Published 2017 by John Wiley & Sons Ltd.

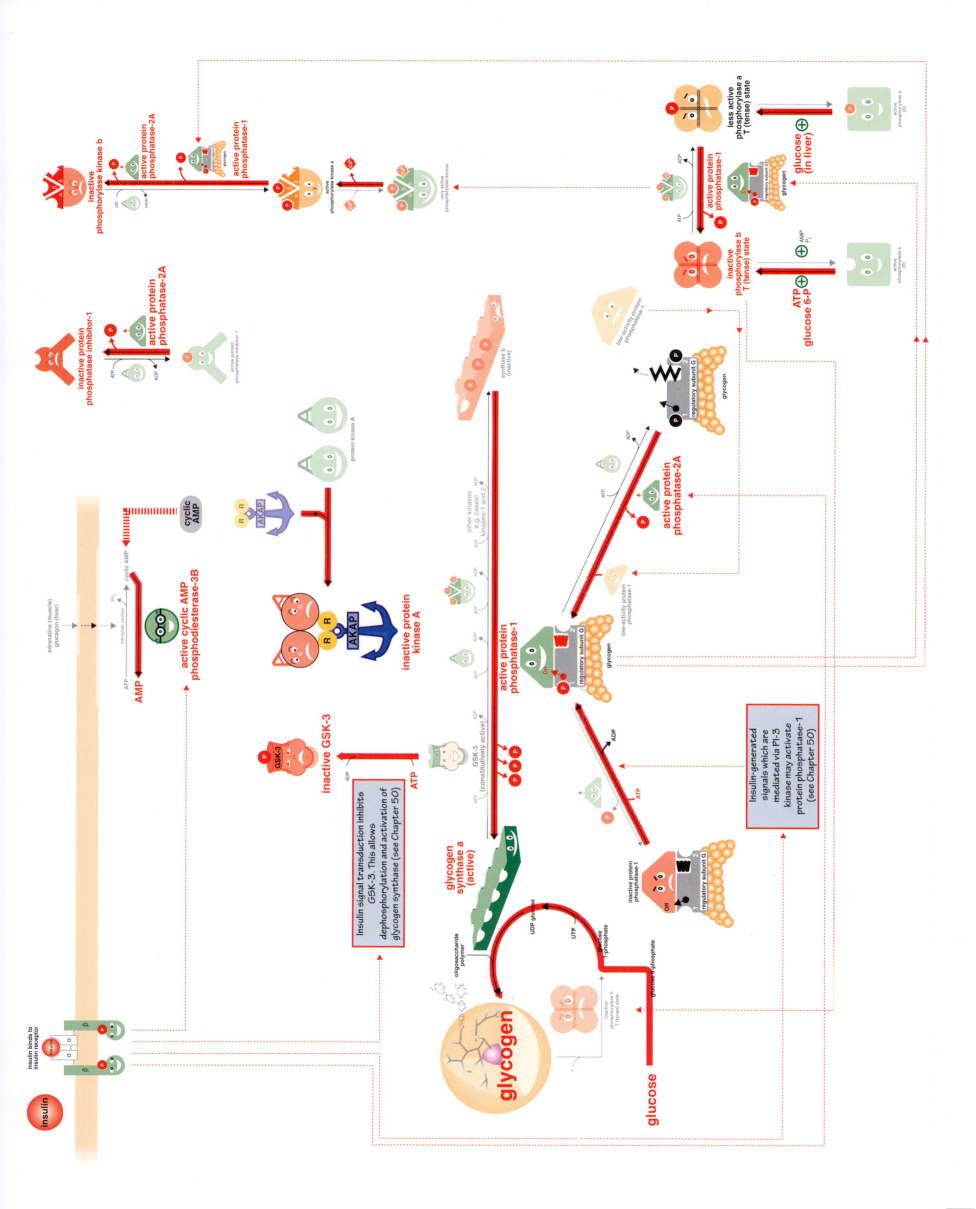

Pentose phosphate pathway: the production of NADPH and reduced glutathione

15

Pentose phosphate pathway

In mammals, the pentose phosphate pathway (also known as the hexose monophosphate shunt) is very active in liver, adipose tissue, lactating mammary gland, adrenal cortex and red blood cells. In these tissues it provides 'reducing power' in the form of NADPH. This NADPH is used for the biosynthesis of fatty acids and cholesterol and the production of reduced glutathione. The pathway is used by plants in the photosynthetic dark reaction.

Another important function is to produce ribose 5-phosphate for the biosynthesis of purines and pyrimidines, nucleotides and nucleic acids. However, as described later, only the 'reversible, non-oxidative phase' of the pathway, which is ubiquitous, is needed for this process.

Chart 15.1: pentose phosphate pathway

The pathway can be considered in two phases: (i) the **irreversible, oxidative phase** comprising the reactions catalysed by glucose 6-phosphate dehydrogenase, lactonase and 6-phosphogluconate dehydrogenase; and (ii) the **reversible, non-oxidative phase** involving the rest of the pathway.

Irreversible, oxidative phase of the pentose phosphate pathway

The stoichiometry of the pentose phosphate pathway can be studied by following the metabolic fate of three molecules of glucose. In the fed state, glucose is phosphorylated to **glucose 6-phosphate**. Remember that phosphofructokinase-1 (PFK-1) is inhibited by the abundance of ATP and citrate in the well-fed, high-energy state. Accordingly, glucose 6-phosphate enters the pentose phosphate pathway, where it is oxidized by **glucose 6-phosphate dehydrogenase** (G6-PDH) and NADPH is formed. Also produced is 6-phosphoglucono-δ-lactone, which is rapidly and irreversibly hydrolysed by **lactonase**. Next, **6-phosphogluconate dehydrogenase** irreversibly produces **ribulose 5-phosphate**, another molecule of NADPH is formed and CO_2 is evolved. Henceforth, the flux of metabolites is committed to the next 'reversible' phase of the pathway.

Reversible, non-oxidative phase of the pentose phosphate pathway

These reactions convert three molecules of **ribulose 5-phosphate** to two molecules of fructose 6-phosphate and one molecule of glyceraldehyde 3-phosphate and all the reactions are reversible. **NB: Ribose 5-phosphate** is a precursor of nucleotide synthesis (see Chapters 54 and 55). Consequently, orally administered fructose increases the production of purines and uric acid, so gout sufferers should have a low-fructose diet.

Fate of fructose 6-phosphate

In red blood cells, for example (Chart 15.1), fructose 6-phosphate is converted to glucose 6-phosphate by the equilibrium reaction catalysed by **phosphoglucose isomerase** for re-entry into the pentose phosphate pathway. This cycle is especially important in cells prone to oxidative damage, e.g. red blood cells, where NADPH is used to synthesize **reduced glutathione**.

Alternatively, **in the fed state in liver** (Chart 15.2) and **adipose tissue** where lipogenesis prevails, fructose 6-phosphate is directed via glycolysis to pyruvate and then onwards for fatty acid synthesis (see Chapter 28). However, the inhibition of PFK-1 by citrate and ATP must be overcome.

Regulation of the pentose phosphate pathway

The flow of metabolites through the pathway is regulated at the glucose 6-phosphate dehydrogenase reaction and the 6-phosphogluconate dehydrogenase reaction by the availability of NADP$^+$. Therefore, in red blood cells, for example, the flow is linked to the availability of NADP$^+$ provided by **glutathione reductase**; the latter is needed to produce **reduced glutathione**, which protects the cells from oxidative damage. In liver it is regulated by the availability of NADP$^+$ supplied by fatty acid synthesis (see Chapter 28).

Roles of glutathione: as an antioxidant, in xenobiotic metabolism and in amino acid transport

Glutathione is a tripeptide formed from **glutamate, cysteine** and **glycine** (Diagram 15.1). Glutathione protects cells against oxidative damage by removing hydrogen peroxide (Chart 15.1). Glutathione is very abundant in liver (up to 10 mmol/l), where it has many functions. In particular it conjugates with fat-soluble toxins and drug metabolites to form water-soluble products for excretion. Another role is transporting amino acids across the plasma membrane into the cytosol by the **γ-glutamyl cycle** (Diagram 15.1). Glutathione reacts with the amino acid to form the dipeptides **γ-glutamyl amino acid** and **cysteinylglycine** in a reaction catalysed by **γ-glutamyltranspeptidase (γ-GT)**. **γ-Glutamylcyclotransferase** then liberates the amino acid into the cytosol. **NB:** γ-GT is located on the outer surface of the plasma membrane. After consuming alcohol it is dislodged and appears in the plasma. Accordingly it is a sensitive test for alcohol abuse.

Glucose 6-phosphate dehydrogenase deficiency

The most common inborn error of metabolism is glucose 6-phosphate dehydrogenase (G 6-PDH) deficiency, which results in reduced production of NADPH by the pentose phosphate pathway. In affected individuals under normal circumstances, NADPH is produced in sufficient amounts to form reduced glutathione that prevents oxidative damage to red blood cells. Consequently, those people deficient in G 6-PDH are often unaware of their condition until severe oxidative stress is provoked by taking a drug such as primaquine, which precipitates acute haemolysis and can damage up to 50% of the red blood cells. Several other drugs causing acute anaemia in G 6-PDH deficiency include: sulphonamides, methylene blue and nalidixic acid. This is because the increased demand for NADPH by cytochrome P450 enzymes to metabolize such drugs renders the patient unable to maintain glutathione in its reduced state, hence the catastrophic oxidative damage to the red blood cells.

Favism

Some individuals with G 6-PDH deficiency suffer a haemolytic crisis after eating fava beans (*Vicia faba*) – also known as broad beans – which are a staple food in the Mediterranean region. This condition is known as favism. Surprisingly, sufferers from favism do not necessarily experience drug-induced haemolysis. There is no simple explanation for this apparent discrepancy.

Diagram 15.1 γ-Glutamyl cycle. This cycle forms glutathione from glutamate, cysteine and glycine. Extracellular amino acids combine with glutathione and enter the cell in the presence of the transmembrane enzyme, γ-glutamyl transpeptidase. **5-Oxoprolinuria (pyroglutamic aciduria):** although usually associated with γ-glutamyl cycle defects, 5-oxoprolinuria also occurs in patients with other inborn errors, e.g. urea cycle defects and organic acidurias. This is probably because of reduced ATP availability in these conditions since ATP is needed by 5-oxoprolinase for 5-oxoproline degradation. 5-Oxoprolinuria also occurs in hawkinsinuria secondary to glutathione depletion (see Chapter 49).

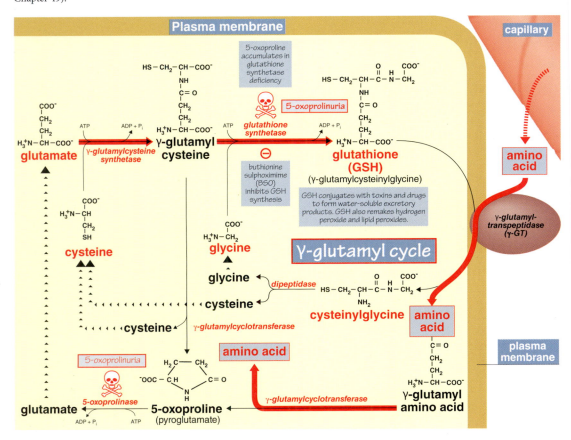

Metabolism at a Glance, Fourth Edition. J. G. Salway. © 2017 John Wiley & Sons Ltd. Published 2017 by John Wiley & Sons Ltd.

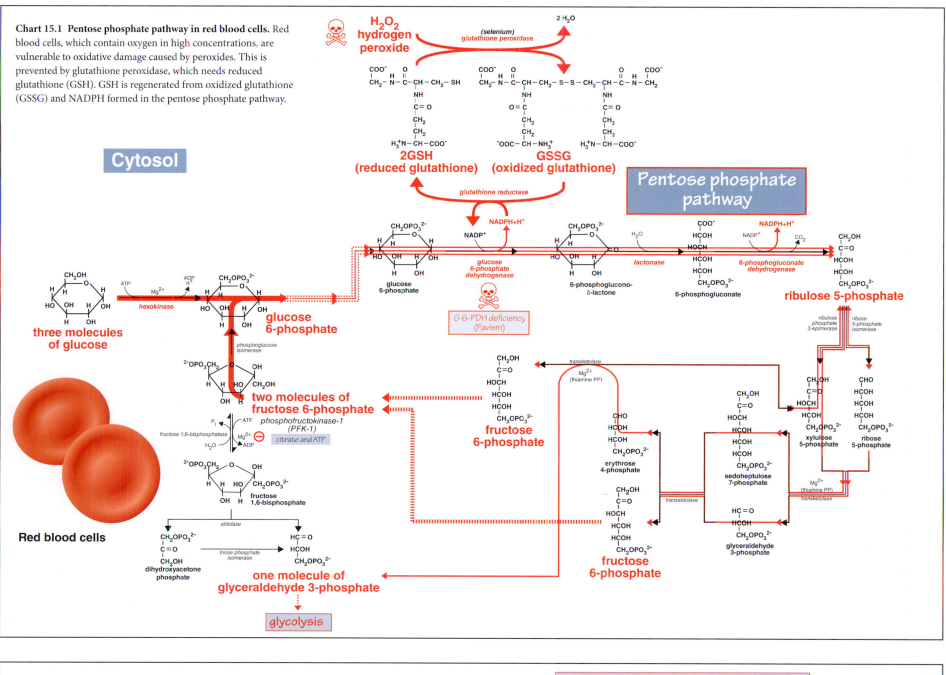

Chart 15.1 Pentose phosphate pathway in red blood cells. Red blood cells, which contain oxygen in high concentrations, are vulnerable to oxidative damage caused by peroxides. This is prevented by glutathione peroxidase, which needs reduced glutathione (GSH). GSH is regenerated from oxidized glutathione (GSSG) and NADPH formed in the pentose phosphate pathway.

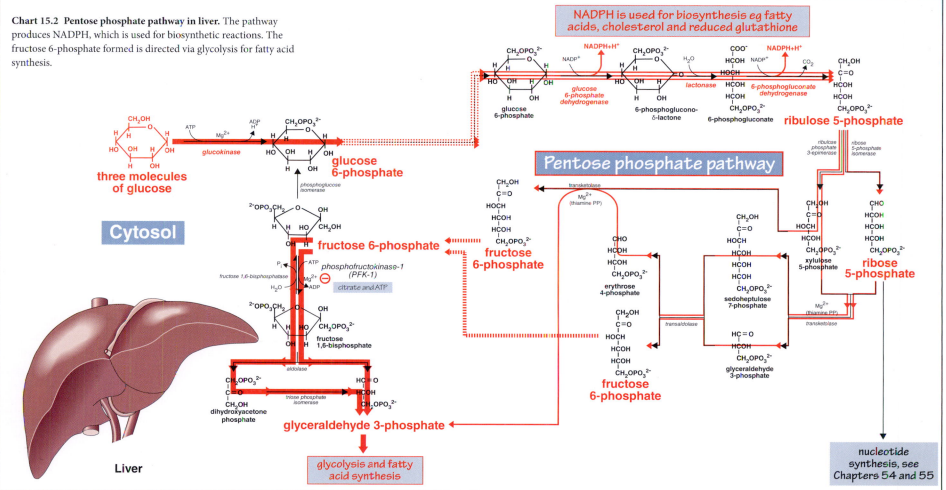

Chart 15.2 Pentose phosphate pathway in liver. The pathway produces NADPH, which is used for biosynthetic reactions. The fructose 6-phosphate formed is directed via glycolysis for fatty acid synthesis.

Regulation of glycolysis: overview exemplified by glycolysis in cardiac muscle

16

The regulatory mechanisms for glycolysis in cardiac muscle, skeletal muscle and liver are different. The glycolytic pathway is ubiquitous but its physiological functions vary between different cell types. For example, whereas glycolysis can be very important for energy metabolism in cardiac and skeletal muscle, glucose is not a major source of energy for the liver. On the contrary, liver in the fed state tends to convert glucose to the fuel reserves glycogen and triacylglycerols. Indeed, apart from during the phase of food absorption in the fed state, liver is usually not in glycolytic (i.e. glucose **consuming**) mode, but instead **produces** glucose by either glycogenolysis or gluconeogenesis. Accordingly, regulation of glycolysis in **liver** is described in Chapters 28 and 18, and glycolysis in **skeletal muscle** is outlined in Chapter 17. Meanwhile, a general description of glycolysis is given below, while the chart opposite emphasizes the regulation in **cardiac muscle**.

Chart 16.1: regulatory stages in glycolysis
Transport of glucose into the cell
Glucose in the surrounding fluid must cross the plasma membrane into the cell. This occurs by facilitated diffusion mediated by a family of proteins known as **glucose transporters (GLUTs)**, which are distributed in different types of cells. **Skeletal muscle cells**, **cardiomyocytes** and **adipocytes**, which are sensitive to insulin, have a transporter known as GLUT4. In response to insulin these transporters are recruited from vesicles within the cell to the plasma membrane, where they increase glucose uptake (see Chapters 5 and 59). It should be noted that the transporters in **liver** (GLUT2) and in **red blood cells** (GLUT1) are constitutively located in the plasma membrane and so do not need insulin to be active. In cardiomyocytes, cardiac work also increases translocation of GLUT4 to the sarcolemma.

Phosphorylation of glucose by hexokinase and glucokinase
Phosphorylation of glucose to glucose 6-phosphate in the **liver** (see Chapters 18 and 28) is catalysed by the glucose-phosphorylating isoenzyme **glucokinase**, whereas in **muscle** the isoenzyme is **hexokinase**. Glucokinase (also known as hexokinase-4) is found only in **liver** and the **β-cells of the pancreas**, whereas hexokinase is widely distributed. The major difference between the isoenzymes is in their affinity for glucose. For glucokinase, the $K_{0.5}$ (glucose) is 10 mmol/l, whereas hexokinase has a K_m for glucose of 0.1 mmol/l. Thus the **liver** isoenzyme glucokinase is well adapted to cope with the high concentration surges of glucose in the blood during feeding. It should be remembered that dietary glucose from the intestines is absorbed into the hepatic portal vein, which transports the glucose directly to the liver at concentrations that can exceed 15 mmol/l. On the other hand, the high affinity of hexokinase for glucose ensures that, even if the intracellular concentration of glucose in **muscle** should fall as low as 0.1 mmol/l during a burst of strenuous exercise, the hexokinase reaction can still proceed at half its maximum velocity.

Another difference between hexokinase and glucokinase is that the former is inhibited by its product, **glucose 6-phosphate**, whereas glucokinase is not inhibited in this way. This ensures that, when **liver** is presented with a large load of glucose after feeding, it can be phosphorylated to glucose 6-phosphate prior to glycogenesis or lipogenesis. On the other hand, if glucose 6-phosphate accumulates in **muscle**, it inhibits hexokinase, decreases the glycolytic flux and thereby conserves glucose.

Glucokinase regulatory protein
It has been shown in **liver** glucokinase is inactivated by sequestration with the **glucokinase regulatory protein (GKRP)**, which is bound within the hepatocyte nucleus. Very low concentrations of fructose liberate glucokinase from its regulatory protein and the active glucokinase molecule is translocated into the cytosol. This dramatic and novel control mechanism is described in Chapter 23.

Phosphofructokinase-1
Phosphofructokinase-1 (PFK-1) must be distinguished from phosphofructokinase-2 (PFK-2). PFK-2 produces **fructose 2,6-bisphosphate (F 2,6-bisP)**, which is a potent allosteric stimulator of PFK-1 (see below).

ATP, although a substrate for PFK-1, is also an allosteric inhibitor when present in increased concentrations, for example in the fed state. Inhibition by ATP is potentiated by **citrate** (see Chapter 27). However, this inhibition can be overcome by F 2,6-bisP (see below).

Fructose 2,6-bisP is an important allosteric stimulator of glycolysis in muscle and inhibitor of gluconeogenesis in liver
Since F 2,6-bisP stimulates PFK-1, it has an important stimulatory effect on glycolysis. Furthermore, in **liver**, it **stimulates** PFK-1 (glycolysis) but **inhibits** fructose 1,6-bisphosphatase (F 1,6-bisPase) thereby decreasing gluconeogenesis (see Chapters 18 and 28). The concentration of F 2,6-bisP in **liver** is down-regulated by glucagon, is up-regulated in **cardiac muscle** by adrenaline, and in **skeletal muscle** is simply regulated by the concentration of fructose 6-phosphate (Diagrams 16.1, 16.2 and 16.3). In liver and cardiac muscle, the hormones stimulate the production of cyclic AMP, which frees the active catalytic monomers of **protein kinase A (PKA)** (see Chapter 13), which in turn phosphorylates the 'bifunctional enzyme' phosphofructokinase-2/fructose 2,6-bisphosphatase (PFK-2/F 2,6-bisPase). Following phosphorylation, in **cardiac muscle**, PFK-2 is active and F 2,6-bisPase is inactive. This causes an increase in the concentration of F 2,6-bisP, which stimulates PFK-1, thereby increasing the rate of glycolysis.

The bifunctional enzyme, phosphofructokinase-2/fructose 2,6-bisphosphatase (PFK-2/F 2,6-bisPase)
The isoenzymes of PFK-2/F 2,6-bisPase found in cardiac muscle, liver and skeletal muscle are represented in Diagrams 16.1, 16.2 and 16.3. The **cardiac isoenzyme** consists of 530 amino acids with a phosphorylation site at serine 466. Adrenaline through PKA phosphorylates this site and activates PFK-2, which favours the production of F 2,6-bisP, which stimulates PFK-1 and thus increases glycolysis (Chart 16.1).

The **liver isoenzyme** comprises 470 amino acids with a regulatory site at serine 32. Glucagon through PKA phosphorylates the bifunctional enzyme and **inactivates PFK-2** and **activates F 2,6-bisPase**. Thus in summary, in **liver** during fasting, glucagon causes concentrations of **F 2,6-bisP** to be decreased; **thus PFK-1** activity is **decreased**, the inhibition of F 1,6-bisPase by F 2,6-bisP is relieved, and so gluconeogenesis is stimulated (see Chapter 18). On the other hand, in the fed state when the insulin/glucagon ratio is high, dephosphorylation of PFK-2/F 2,6-bisPase occurs, PFK-2 is active, and F 2,6-bisP is formed, which stimulates PFK-1 and therefore glycolysis, providing pyruvate for fatty acid synthesis (see Chapter 28).

The **skeletal muscle isoenzyme** is the poor relation of the trio. It consists of only 450 amino acids and has no phosphorylation sites at either serine 32 or serine 466. Instead it is regulated simply by the availability of fructose 6-phosphate (F 6-P). When F 6-P is abundant, PFK-2 is active, **F 2,6-bisP** is formed, PFK-1 is stimulated and glycolysis is increased (see Chapter 17).

Pyruvate kinase
The inhibitory effects of alanine (allosteric) and glucagon (cyclic AMP/PKA-mediated phosphorylation) on the **liver isoenzyme** of pyruvate kinase are mainly concerned with directing the glycolytic pathway to the gluconeogenic mode (see Chapter 18). **NB:** The **muscle isoenzyme** of pyruvate kinase is not inhibited by alanine and so pyruvate, and thus alanine, can be formed when the glucose alanine cycle is operating (see Chapter 45). Also, the **muscle** isoenzyme is not subject to regulation by phosphorylation.

Fructose 1,6-bisphosphate activates pyruvate kinase allosterically by feed-forward stimulation. This has obvious advantages for energy metabolism in exercising **muscle** by enhancing the glycolytic flux at the end of the pathway. In **liver**, this feed-forward stimulatory effect of fructose 1,6-bisphosphate can overcome the inhibitory effect of alanine on pyruvate kinase.

Reference
For a review of the PFK-2/F 2,6-bisPase bifunctional enzyme see:
El-Maghrabi R.M., Noto F., Wu N., Manes N. (2001) 6-Phosphofructo-2-kinase/fructose-2,6-bisphosphatase: suiting structure to need, in a family of tissue-specific enzymes. *Curr Opin Clin Nutr Metab Care*, **4**, 411–18.

Metabolism at a Glance, Fourth Edition. J. G. Salway. © 2017 John Wiley & Sons Ltd. Published 2017 by John Wiley & Sons Ltd.

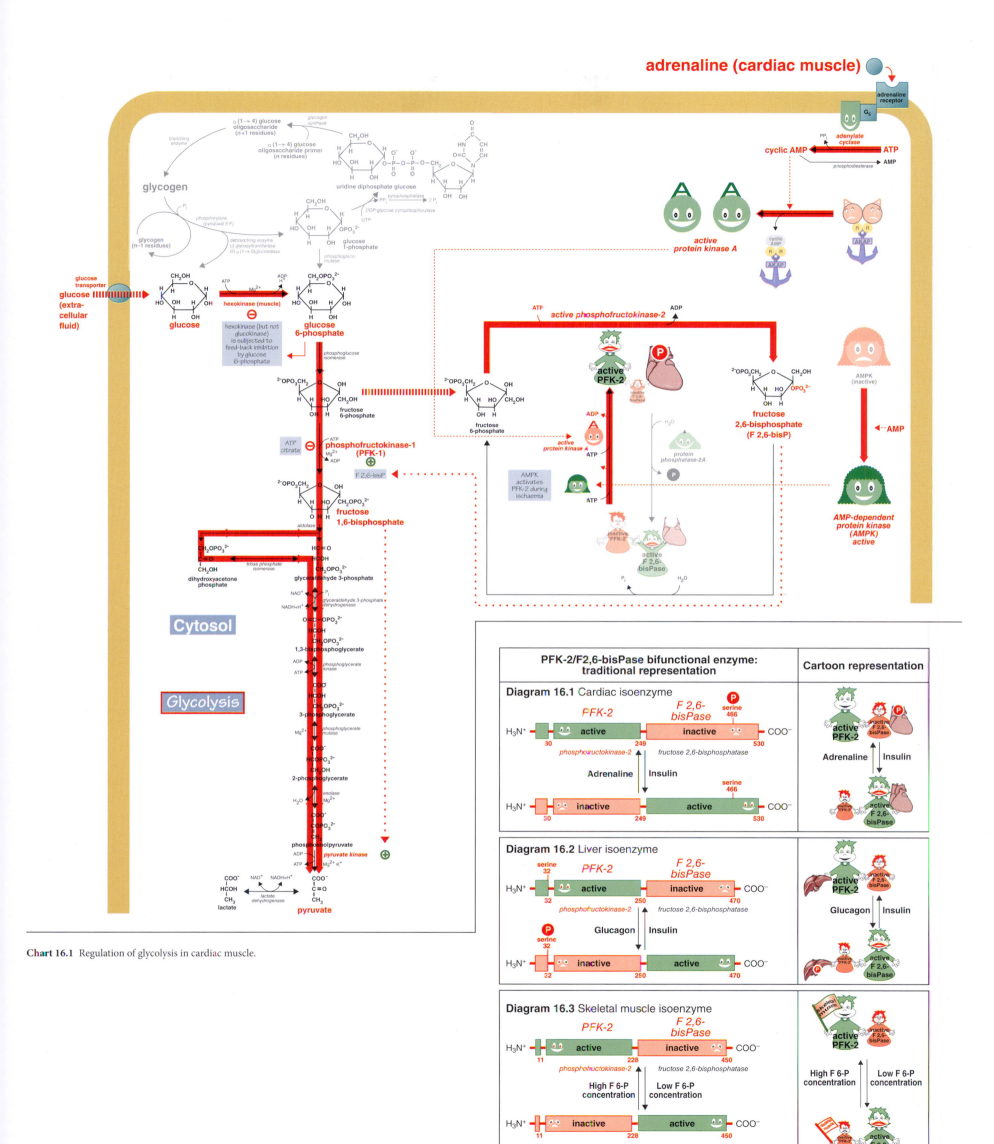

Chart 16.1 Regulation of glycolysis in cardiac muscle.

Glycolysis in skeletal muscle: biochemistry of sport and exercise

17

Anaerobic ATP production

The ATP used for contraction by the white, type II (fast-twitch) muscle fibres is provided anaerobically during explosive bursts of muscle activity, such as sprint races or other athletic events. In track events such as the 100 metres, ATP is provided both by the phosphagen **phosphocreatine** and a 1000-fold increase in glycolysis (Chart 17.1). Phosphocreatine hydrolysis provides **inorganic phosphate (P_i)** for phosphorylase, which is activated by Ca^{2+} released from the sarcoplasmic reticulum, and also by adrenaline through the cyclic AMP signalling system (see Chapter 13). Lactate and hydrogen ions are produced, with the latter being buffered by bicarbonate in the plasma to form carbonic acid and then carbon dioxide, which is expired from the lungs.

The AMP formed by **adenylate kinase** is deaminated to form inosine monophosphate (IMP), which is a potent stimulator of phosphorylase. It is also dephosphorylated by **5′-nucleotidase** producing **adenosine**, which binds to adenosine A_2 receptors on blood vessels causing vasodilation. Accordingly, adenosine has been described as a 'retaliatory metabolite' that retaliates against hypoxia in exercising muscle by increasing the supply of oxygen via the blood.

Aerobic ATP production
Glycogen and fatty acids are used as fuel

The ATP used for contraction by the red, type I (slow-twitch) muscle fibres is generated aerobically for endurance events such as the marathon (Chart 17.2). Glycogen and fatty acids are the principal fuels used. The latter originate from three possible sources. Most important are: (i) fatty acids mobilized from adipose tissue by hormone-sensitive lipase; and (ii) fatty acids from plasma very low-density lipoprotein (VLDL) mobilized by

Chart 17.1 Anaerobic production of ATP for muscle contraction.

lipoprotein lipase; (iii) of lesser importance are fatty acids formed by hydrolysis of the intramuscular triacylglycerol.

Glycogen exhaustion causes the athlete to 'hit the wall'

Both fatty acids and glycogen form acetyl CoA, which is oxidized by Krebs cycle. ATP is generated by oxidative phosphorylation in the respiratory chain. The abundant supply of acetyl CoA condenses with a matching supply of oxaloacetate. Although this is regenerated by Krebs cycle (see Chapter 19), supplementary oxaloacetate is needed. The supply of this is maintained by **anaplerotic reactions**, notably the Krebs cycle intermediate **succinyl CoA** produced by catabolism of **isoleucine** and **valine**.

If muscle glycogen is exhausted, then fatty acids alone are used as fuel. However, their metabolism generates ATP at only half the rate of glycogen and so the long-distance runner is forced to slow down dramatically.

The sprint to the tape is fuelled by glycogen

The abundant acetyl CoA restricts the activity of pyruvate dehydrogenase. This limits glycolysis and helps to conserve glycogen throughout the race and, if reserves permit, enables a powerful **anaerobic** sprint to the finish.

Glucose transporters

The principal glucose transporter in skeletal muscle is GLUT4, which is recruited to the sarcolemma by insulin and exercise. The glucose transporter GLUT1 is probably more important for basal uptake of glucose into muscle cells, and for replenishing the glycogen reserves with glucose formed from lactate by the liver following recovery from exercise.

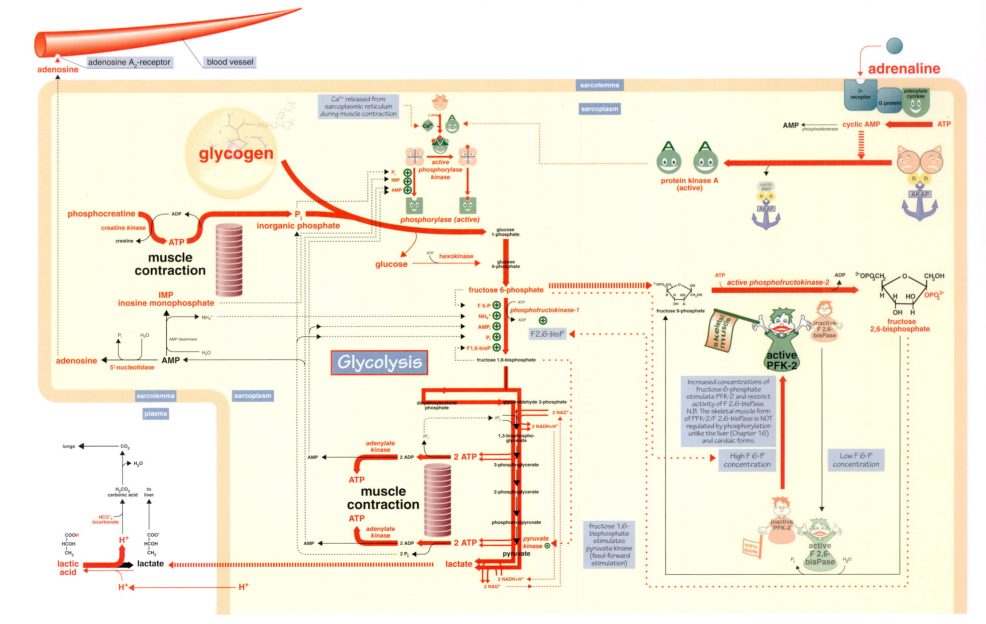

Metabolism at a Glance, Fourth Edition. J. G. Salway. © 2017 John Wiley & Sons Ltd. Published 2017 by John Wiley & Sons Ltd.

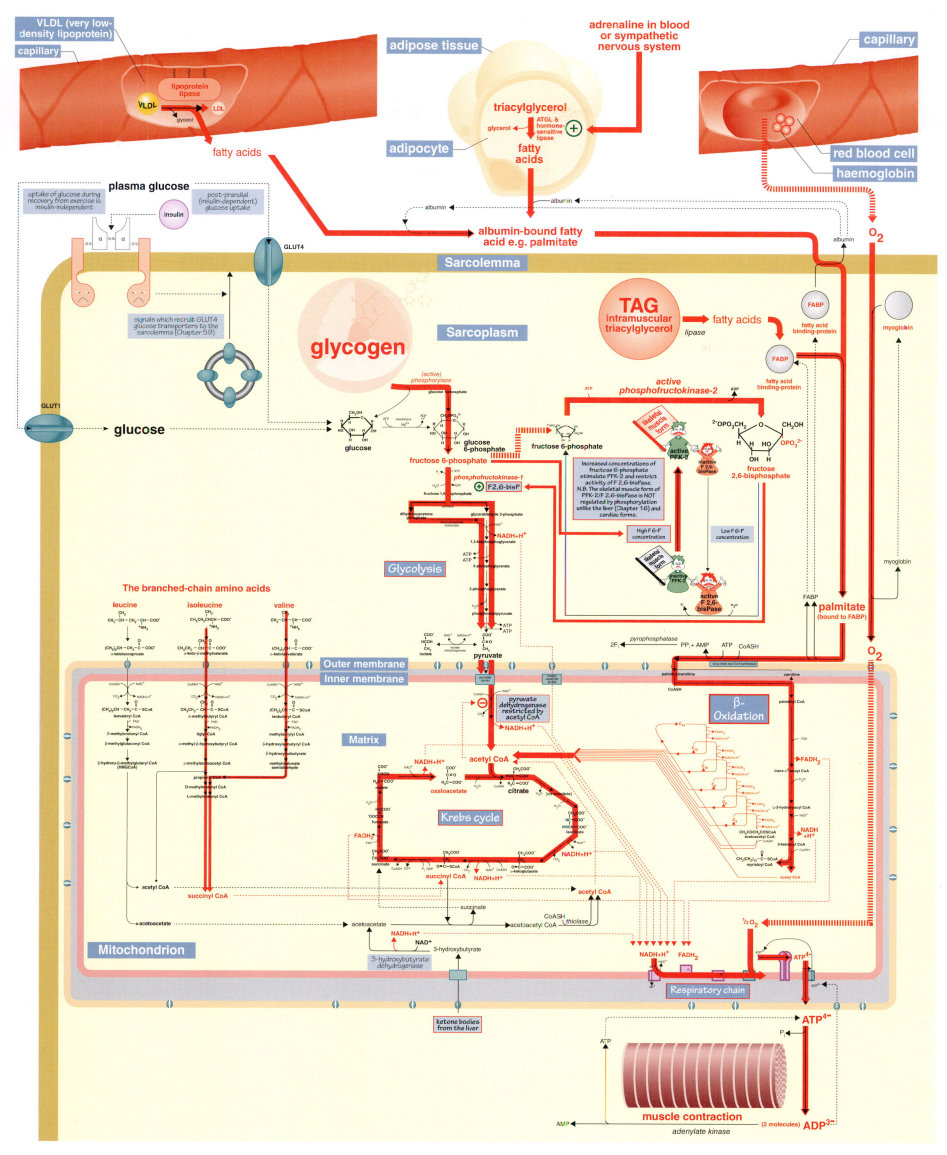

Chart 17.2 Aerobic production of ATP for muscle contraction.

Regulation of gluconeogenesis

18

Gluconeogenesis maintains the blood glucose concentration during fasting and starvation

The body's first and foremost reserve for maintaining the blood glucose concentration during fasting is liver glycogen. However, once this reserve is exhausted, glucose must be made from non-carbohydrate precursors. We have seen that the most abundant fuel reserve, the fatty acids in triacylglycerol, cannot be converted to glucose by mammals (see Chapter 20). However, glucose can be made from glycerol and lactate, and from amino acids formed by proteolysis of muscle proteins (see Chapters 7 and 45). This process is known as gluconeogenesis. It occurs mainly in liver but, during prolonged starvation, it is also active in kidney cortex.

Chart 18.1: regulation of gluconeogenesis
Dependency of gluconeogenesis on the oxidation of fatty acids

Gluconeogenesis, which operates during starvation, is linked to the mobilization of fat and the oxidation of fatty acids, e.g. **palmitate** in the mitochondrion. The latter results in the formation of large amounts of acetyl CoA, NADH and ATP, with the following effects on mitochondrial reactions:

1 **Isocitrate dehydrogenase** is inhibited by NADH.
2 **Pyruvate dehydrogenase** is inhibited by acetyl CoA, ATP and NADH.
3 **Pyruvate carboxylase** is stimulated by acetyl CoA.
4 The equilibrium of the mitochondrial **malate dehydrogenase** reaction is displaced to favour the reduction of oxaloacetate to malate.
5 **ATP** (and GTP via the nucleoside diphosphate kinase reaction) from the β-oxidation and respiratory chain pathways is used as a co-substrate for the pyruvate carboxylase, phosphoenolpyruvate carboxykinase (PEPCK) and phosphoglycerate kinase reactions.

Gluconeogenic precursors

Amino acids, particularly **alanine**, are important gluconeogenic precursors, but they must first be metabolized to cytosolic oxaloacetate (see Chapter 47). **Glycerol**, derived from triacylglycerols in white adipose tissue, is also an important gluconeogenic precursor. It is phosphorylated in liver by **glycerol kinase** to form glycerol 3-phosphate, which in turn is oxidized by glycerol 3-phosphate

dehydrogenase to form the gluconeogenic intermediate **dihydroxyacetone phosphate**. Finally, **lactate**, produced for example by anaerobic glycolysis in red blood cells or muscle, is also used for gluconeogenesis.

Hormonal regulation of gluconeogenesis

Glucagon is an important hormone in the early fasting state. It inhibits pyruvate kinase through the action of protein kinase A. Glucagon also has effects on the synthesis of certain enzymes. It increases synthesis of the aminotransferases, PEPCK and glucose 6-phosphatase, which favour gluconeogenesis.

Glucagon stimulates **ATGL** and **hormone-sensitive lipase** through protein kinase A. This mobilizes fatty acids, which are preferentially used as fuel by muscle thereby sparing glucose. Also, the fatty acids are oxidized in liver by β-oxidation to supply ATP for gluconeogenesis, and to form ketone bodies which are an alternative fuel for the brain.

Regulatory enzymes
Pyruvate carboxylase

Pyruvate carboxylase, which converts pyruvate to oxaloacetate, is stimulated by acetyl CoA. **NB:** Pyruvate dehydrogenase, which competes for pyruvate as a substrate, is inactivated by acetyl CoA.

Phosphoenolpyruvate carboxykinase (PEPCK)

PEPCK decarboxylates oxaloacetate to phosphoenolpyruvate (PEP). It requires GTP, which can be obtained from ATP by the nucleoside diphosphate kinase reaction. Hepatic PEPCK makes an important contribution to glucose homeostasis. During fasting, PEPCK activity is induced in a few minutes by glucagon. Glucocorticoids (e.g. cortisol) also induce PEPCK, which stimulates glucose production by gluconeogenesis. Conversely, after feeding, insulin rapidly inhibits expression of the PEPCK gene.

In theory, PEP could be converted to pyruvate, enter Krebs cycle as oxaloacetate and be reconverted to PEP in a futile cycle. This does not happen because liver pyruvate kinase is inactivated by protein kinase A (due to the presence of glucagon), and is inhibited by alanine, which is present in increased concentrations during gluconeogenic conditions (see Chapter 45).

Fructose 1,6-bisphosphatase (F 1,6-bisPase)

Regulation of this enzyme has been mentioned in Chapter 16. **F 1,6-bisPase is inhibited by fructose 2,6-bisphosphate (F 2,6-bisP).** Glucagon, which is secreted by the α-cells of the pancreas in response to a low blood glucose concentration, stimulates the breakdown of F 2,6-bisP in liver through the action of protein kinase A on fructose 2,6-bisphosphatase (F 2,6-bisPase) activity (see Chapter 16). Removal of the allosteric inhibitor F 2,6-bisP results in an increase in F 1,6-bisPase activity. The decrease in F 2,6-bisP also results in reduced phosphofructokinase-1 activity and a further reduction in glycolysis. F 1,6-bisPase deficiency is described in Chapter 23.

Glucose 6-phosphatase

Glucose 6-phosphatase is located on the luminal surface of the endoplasmic reticulum in liver cells (Diagram 18.1). Its substrate, glucose 6-phosphate, is transported by a translocator from the cytosol into the lumen of the endoplasmic reticulum, where it is hydrolysed to glucose and inorganic phosphate (P_i). The reaction products are then transported into the cytosol by a glucose translocator GLUT7 and a P_i translocator. Glycogen storage disease type I is due to deficiency of glucose 6-phosphatase activity (see Chapter 11).

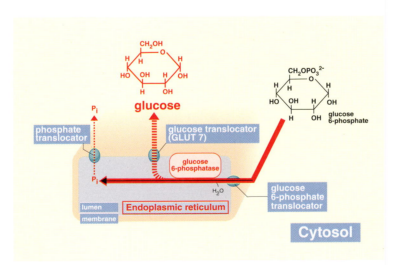

Diagram 18.1 Glucose 6-phosphatase is localized on the inside of the rough endoplasmic reticulum membrane. **NB:** The ribosomes are not shown.

Metabolism at a Glance, Fourth Edition. J. G. Salway. © 2017 John Wiley & Sons Ltd. Published 2017 by John Wiley & Sons Ltd.

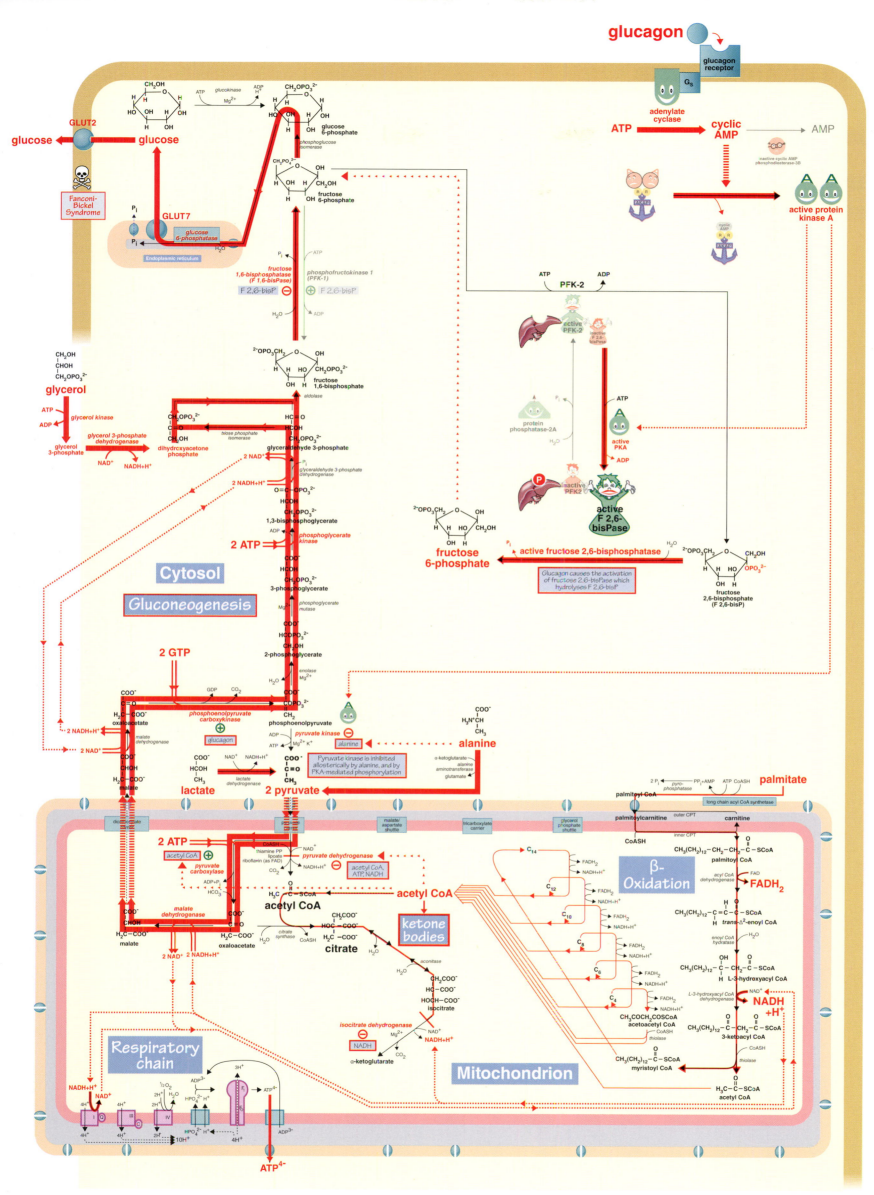

Chart 18.1
Regulation of
gluconeogenesis.

Regulation of Krebs cycle

19

Krebs cycle – the central junction of metabolism

Krebs cycle is found in nearly all mammalian cells, with the notable exception of mature red blood cells, which lack mitochondria. The cycle oxidizes acetyl CoA derived from carbohydrates, ketone bodies, fatty acids and amino acids, to produce NADH and $FADH_2$ for ATP synthesis in the respiratory chain. Furthermore, components of the cycle form essential links with the pathways for gluconeogenesis, lipogenesis and amino acid metabolism. As such, regulation of Krebs cycle must satisfy the diverse metabolic demands of these pathways in the various tissues with their different functions. For example, glucose is a premium fuel because of its vital role as a respiratory substrate for the brain and red blood cells. Because the body has a limited capacity to store carbohydrate, it must be conserved and not exhausted in a frenzied fit of exercise by the fuel-guzzling muscles, which can very happily use fatty acids as an alternative energy source. Pyruvate dehydrogenase (PDH) can therefore be thought of as the 'Minister for Glucose Conservation' since it determines whether or not pyruvate (which is mainly derived from carbohydrate or amino acids) enters Krebs cycle for oxidation.

The activity of Krebs cycle is controlled by the regulation of PDH and isocitrate dehydrogenase.

Regulation of the pyruvate dehydrogenase (PDH) complex

PDH, although not a component of Krebs cycle, has a commanding role in regulating the flux of glycolytic metabolites into the cycle. It is a multienzyme complex consisting of three component enzymes. These enzymes (E_1, pyruvate dehydrogenase; E_2, acetyl transferase; and E_3, dihydrolipoyl dehydrogenase) are responsible for decarboxylating the pyruvate, transferring the acetyl residue to CoA to form acetyl CoA, and oxidatively regenerating the intermediary lipoate involved. Associated with the complex are two enzymes that have regulatory roles (Diagram 19.1). One, PDH kinase, is a protein kinase that is specific for PDH. Its role is to phosphorylate and thus inactivate the PDH component of the complex. The other, PDH phosphatase, is a specific phosphatase that overcomes this inhibition by removing the phosphate groups, thereby activating PDH. PDH is also regulated by the availability of its coenzymes NAD^+ and CoA; i.e. its activity is decreased when high ratios of $NADH/NAD^+$ and acetyl CoA/CoA prevail.

Diagram 19.1: regulation of PDH by phosphorylation and dephosphorylation

When the energy charge of the cell is high, i.e. the ratio of ATP to ADP is increased, PDH kinase is active. E_1 is therefore phosphorylated at three sites and its activity is inhibited. Conversely, PDH kinase is inhibited by pyruvate, and this leads to activation of PDH in the presence of its substrate.

In muscle, PDH phosphatase is activated during muscle contraction, when cytosolic and mitochondrial concentrations of calcium ions are increased. In adipose tissue, PDH phosphatase is activated by insulin. In both of these cases, dephosphorylation of PDH occurs and PDH activity is stimulated.

Isocitrate dehydrogenase (ICDH)

ICDH is inhibited by the high ratio of $NADH/NAD^+$ that prevails in the high-energy state. When ICDH is inhibited, flux through this section of Krebs cycle is restricted.

Purine nucleotide cycle

When large quantities of acetyl CoA are available for oxidation by Krebs cycle, the availability of oxaloacetate for the citrate synthase reaction may become a rate-limiting factor. It is known that the purine nucleotide cycle, first described

by Lowenstein, is very active in muscle during exercise (Chart 19.1). This cycle generates **fumarate** from **aspartate** in the presence of **GTP** in circumstances when the AMP concentration is increased (e.g. when the ATP concentration is decreased, as during muscle contraction). The purine nucleotide cycle,via fumarate, thus provides an **anaplerotic** (i.e. 'topping up') supply of mitochondrial **malate** to produce **oxaloacetate** in an effort to match the abundant supply of acetyl CoA presented for oxidation by Krebs cycle.

As would be expected, patients with **muscle AMP deaminase deficiency** (myoadenylate deaminase deficiency) suffer cramps and myalgias, and fatigue easily after exercise. AMP deaminase activity in the other tissues of these patients is normal.

Glucose/fatty acid cycle

This was described in 1963 by Randle, Garland, Hales and Newsholme. However, it is not a cycle of intermediary metabolites as in Krebs cycle, but it shows that the **relationship between glucose and fatty acids is integrated and reciprocal**. It explains that if muscle has a choice between glucose and fatty acids as fuel, **muscle prefers fatty acids** and mechanisms exist to restrict glucose metabolism. This is because β-oxidation of fatty acids increases the concentration ratios of acetyl CoA/CoA, $NADH/NAD^+$ and ATP/ADP, which inhibits PDH (Chart 19.1 and Diagram 19.1) and prevents the oxidation of pyruvate (from glycolysis), thus conserving glucose. This is especially important during starvation. However, a disadvantage is that after feeding when there is an abundance of both glucose and fatty acids, this process reduces the uptake of glucose by muscle and contributes to insulin resistance (see Chapters 62 and 63).

Reference

Randle P.J., Garland P.B., Hales C.N. & Newsholme E.A. (1963) The glucose–fatty acid cycle: its role in insulin sensitivity and the metabolic disturbances of diabetes mellitus. *Lancet* **i**, 785–89.

Debating forum: Krebs cycle – is it time to change the name of the bedrock of metabolism?

Now call me a pedant if you will, but I feel the time has come to consider the nomenclature, which can confuse understanding of metabolism. Professor Sir Hans Krebs contributed to the discovery of **four** metabolic cycles* of which only one is commonly called 'the Krebs cycle', otherwise known as the tricarboxylic acid (TCA) cycle or citric acid cycle. However, the term 'tricarboxylic acid cycle' implies that a tricarboxylic acid, in particular citric acid, is cycled which, of course, does not happen. It is **oxaloacetate** (the base of a **dicarboxylic** acid) that condenses with acetyl CoA and it is **oxaloacetate** that is recycled following the oxidation of the acetyl CoA.

The reader should be aware of this and should think of this pathway as '*the Krebs oxaloacetate cycle for the oxidation of acetyl CoA*'. In the meantime, until an international nomenclature committee adopts (or ignores) this proposal, the reader should use any of the names in common use, although this author prefers 'Krebs cycle'. Finally, under no circumstances misplace an apostrophe and make the unforgivable mistake of referring to 'Kreb's cycle'!

* The four metabolic cycles associated with Krebs are:
1 The Krebs–Henseleit **urea cycle** or **ornithine cycle** (1932) (see Chapter 51).
2 The Krebs–Johnson **citric acid cycle** or **tricarboxylic acid cycle** (1937).
3 The Kornberg–Krebs **glyoxylate cycle** (1957) (see Chapter 20).
4 The Mapes–Krebs **uric acid cycle** (1978) (see Chapter 56).

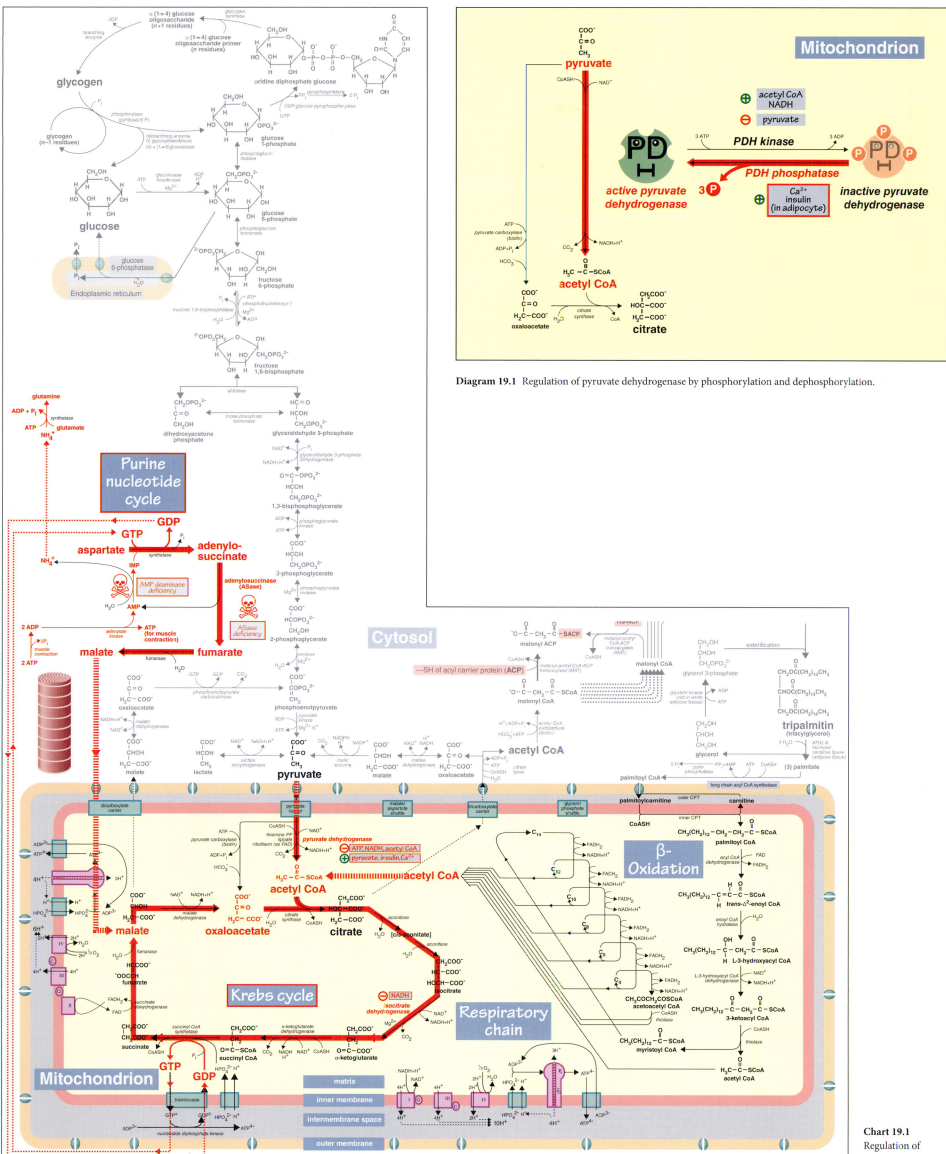

Diagram 19.1 Regulation of pyruvate dehydrogenase by phosphorylation and dephosphorylation.

Chart 19.1
Regulation of
Krebs cycle.

Mammals cannot synthesize glucose from fatty acids

20

Fatty acids cannot be used as a gluconeogenic precursor by mammals for the reasons explained below. Since glucose is a vital fuel for brain and red blood cells, this presents a serious difficulty during prolonged starvation once the glycogen reserves have been depleted (although the brain can adapt to use ketone bodies as a respiratory fuel). It is unfortunate that, because the fatty acids derived from triacylglycerol in adipose tissue cannot be used for gluconeogenesis, muscle proteins must be degraded to maintain glucose homeostasis in the starving state, thereby causing wasting of the skeletal muscles.

Chart 20.1 Two molecules of carbon dioxide are evolved when acetyl CoA is oxidized in Krebs (TCA) cycle.

Chart 20.1: in mammals, two molecules of carbon dioxide are evolved when acetyl CoA is oxidized in Krebs tricarboxylic acid (TCA) cycle

The chart illustrates why mammals cannot convert fatty acids to glucose. Fatty acids are oxidized to acetyl CoA. Because the **pyruvate dehydrogenase** and **pyruvate kinase** reactions are irreversible, acetyl CoA cannot simply be carboxylated to pyruvate and proceed to form glucose by reversal of glycolysis. Instead, the two carbon atoms contained in the acetyl group of acetyl CoA enter Krebs cycle. However, two carbon atoms are removed as carbon dioxide, as shown in the chart. Hence, in animals, there can be no **net** synthesis of glucose from acetyl CoA. Having emphasized this point, it should be noted that if fatty acids uniformly labelled with ^{14}C are fed to mammals, some of the radioactive label does become incorporated into glucose. This is because the ^{14}C-fatty acid is catabolized to ^{14}C-acetyl CoA, which enters Krebs cycle. The label is incorporated into citrate and may be retained in other intermediates of the cycle. If ^{14}C-malate is formed, it can leave the mitochondrion and the ^{14}C label may be incorporated into glucose by gluconeogenesis. **NB:** This incorporation of the ^{14}C label from acetyl CoA into carbohydrate does not represent **net** synthesis because two carbon atoms have been lost as carbon dioxide in the process.

Glycerol derived from triacylglycerol can be used for glucose synthesis

When the triacylglycerol stored in adipose tissue is hydrolysed by adipose triacylglycerol lipase and hormone-sensitive lipase, fatty acids and glycerol are released. Unlike fatty acids, glycerol **can** be used for glucose synthesis by liver (see Chapter 18). Glycerol is transported in the blood to the liver, where it is phosphorylated by **glycerol kinase** to glycerol 3-phosphate, which is reduced to dihydroxyacetone phosphate, two molecules of which are converted to glucose by gluconeogenesis, as shown in Chart 20.1.

Possible gluconeogenic pathways using fatty acid precursors in mammals

Draye and Vamecq have challenged the standard textbook dogma that mammals are unable to convert fatty acids to glucose. They point out that fatty acids with an odd number of carbon atoms, and branched-chain fatty acids, can be

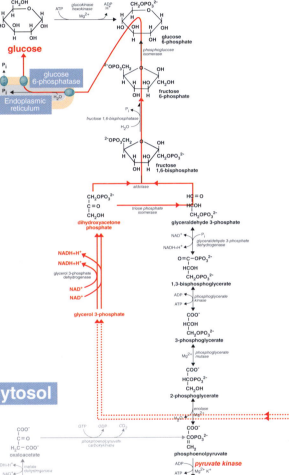

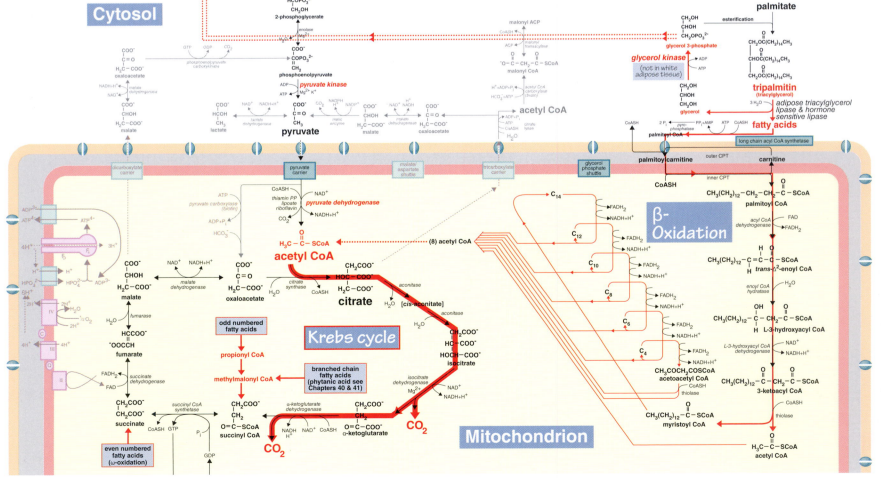

Metabolism at a Glance, Fourth Edition. J. G. Salway. © 2017 John Wiley & Sons Ltd. Published 2017 by John Wiley & Sons Ltd.

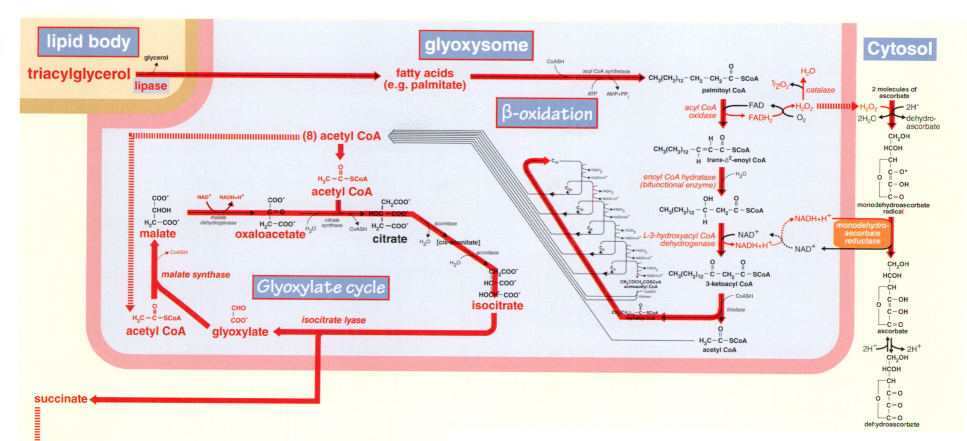

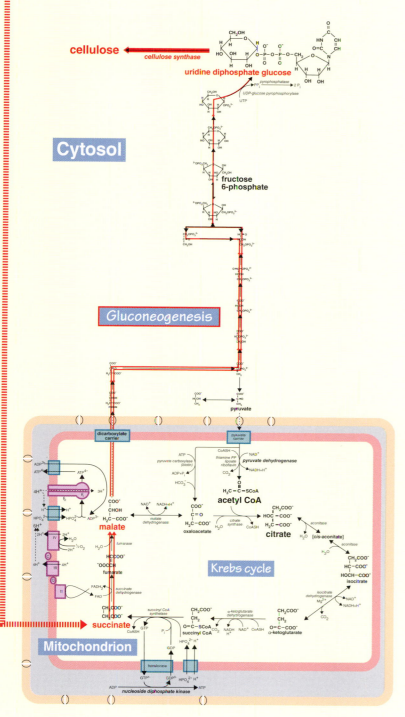

metabolized via propionyl CoA to succinyl CoA (see Chapters 40 and 41). Also, α-oxidation of phytanic acid yields succinate (see Chapter 40). Both of these products are gluconeogenic precursors. However, gluconeogenesis from these fatty acids is unlikely to be quantitatively significant in physiological terms.

Chart 20.2: the Kornberg Krebs glyoxylate cycle enables fat to be converted to sugars
Glyoxysomes in plants
During germination, oil-rich seeds can metabolize their stored fat to sugar, notably sucrose, for distribution throughout the developing seedling, and to uridine diphosphate (UDP) glucose, which is the precursor of cellulose. This process occurs in specialized peroxisomes (or microbodies) known as **glyoxysomes**. Glyoxysomes are temporary organelles present for approximately 1 week during germination. They contain all the enzymes for β-oxidation but only three of the Krebs TCA cycle enzymes, namely malate dehydrogenase, citrate synthase and aconitase. In addition they contain **isocitrate lyase** and **malate synthase**, which enable the glyoxylate cycle to proceed. The glyoxylate cycle also occurs in yeast and bacteria. More recently it has been controversially reported that the glyoxylate cycle is active in animals.

Glyoxylate cycle
The glyoxylate cycle was originally called the '**glyoxylate bypass of the citric acid cycle**'. It resembles Krebs TCA cycle, with some notable differences. In particular, the CO_2-losing stages of the latter (the isocitrate and α-ketoglutarate dehydrogenases) are absent. Instead, **isocitrate lyase** forms **glyoxylate** and **succinate**. Succinate leaves the glyoxysome, enters the mitochondrion and is oxidized to **malate**. The latter leaves the mitochondrion for gluconeogenesis in the cytosol.

Meanwhile, back in the glyoxysome, the glyoxylate combines with acetyl CoA in the presence of malate synthase to produce malate, which is oxidized to **oxaloacetate**, thereby completing the cycle (**NB**: it is **oxaloacetate** that is recycled in Krebs cycle (see Chapter 19)).

β-Oxidation in plants
Until the late 1990s, a dogma of plant biochemistry was that 'plant mitochondria lack the enzymes needed for the β-oxidation of fatty acids' and instead the pathway occurred exclusively in the peroxisomes (glyoxysomes) of higher plants. However, it is now generally accepted that plants are indeed capable of β-oxidation in both mitochondria and peroxisomes (glyoxysomes of germinating seeds). In glyoxysomes, the first oxidation reaction catalysed by **acyl CoA oxidase** uses molecular oxygen and produces hydrogen peroxide (Chart 20.2). The NADH formed by **hydroxyacyl CoA dehydrogenase** (and probably **malate dehydrogenase** of the glyoxylate cycle) is reoxidized by **monodehydroascorbate reductase**. In both cases energy is not conserved as ATP but will be dissipated as heat, which might be an advantage during the germination process.

Chart 20.2 The Kornberg Krebs glyoxylate cycle in the glyoxysome of plants.

Supermouse: overexpression of cytosolic PEPCK in skeletal muscle causes super-athletic performance

21

Rarely does experimental enzymology raise a hint of public interest but this experimental model received worldwide press and TV coverage in 2007. Hakim *et al.*, in Hanson's laboratory, overexpressed cytosolic phosphoenolpyruvate carboxykinase (PEPCK-C) in the skeletal muscle of mice to make a 'supermouse' that was seven times more physically active than the control animal. What is the explanation? (i) Supermouse is able to store massive amounts of fat in skeletal muscle for use as a fuel; and (ii) supermouse's Krebs cycle is boosted to enhance the use of this fuel for muscle contraction.

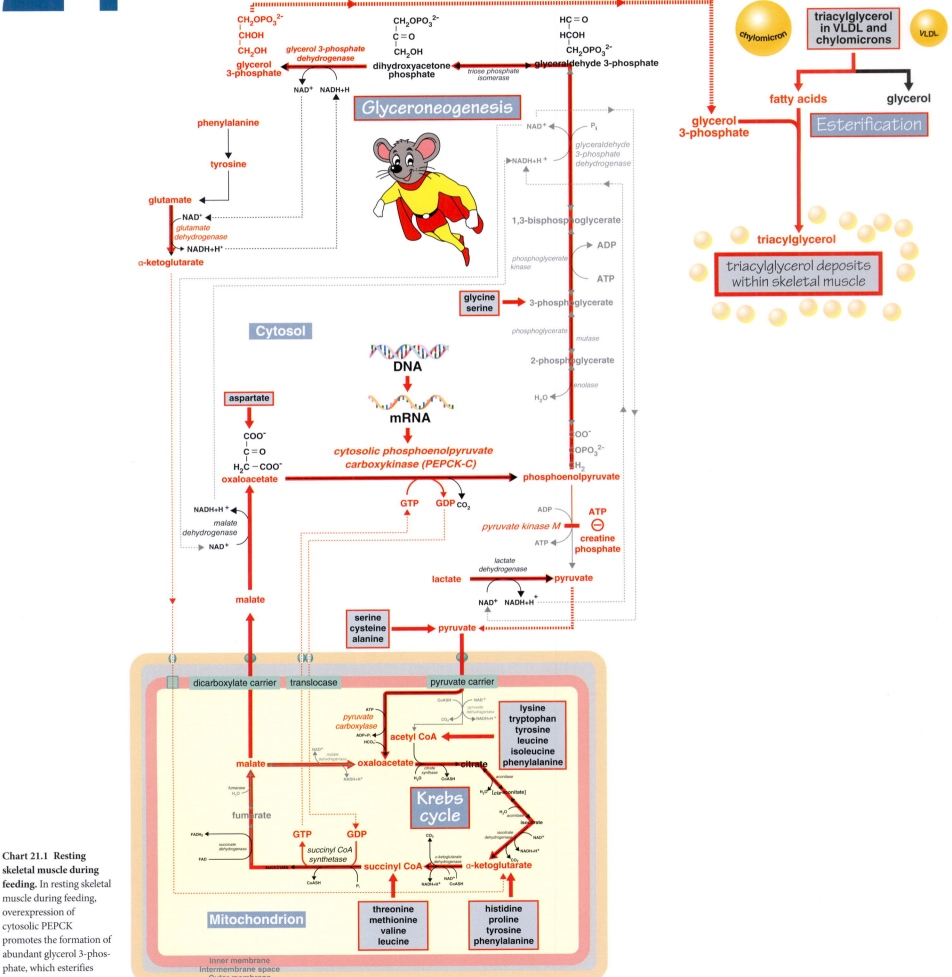

Chart 21.1 Resting skeletal muscle during feeding. In resting skeletal muscle during feeding, overexpression of cytosolic PEPCK promotes the formation of abundant glycerol 3-phosphate, which esterifies dietary fatty acids.

Metabolism at a Glance, Fourth Edition. J. G. Salway. © 2017 John Wiley & Sons Ltd. Published 2017 by John Wiley & Sons Ltd.

Metabolism of supermouse when resting and feeding: 'glyceroneogenesis increases fat reserves in muscle'

In the muscle of supermouse, it is glyceroneogenesis (see Chapter 32), **not glycolysis**, that provides an abundant supply of **glycerol 3-phosphate** for **triacylglycerol (TAG)** biosynthesis (see Chapter 29). Overexpression of PEPCK-C increases production of glycerol 3-phosphate, which esterifies ('captures') dietary fatty acids delivered to muscle by VLDL and chylomicrons producing TAG. Consequently, the concentration of TAG in skeletal muscle is 10 times that of control animals (Chart 21.1).

Regulation of pyruvate kinase. NB: (i) In **resting muscle during feeding, pyruvate kinase is inhibited** by high concentrations of ATP and creatine phosphate: this **favours glyceroneogenesis** (Chart 21.1). However, (ii) in **exercising muscle**, ATP and creatine phosphate concentrations fall, consequently the **inhibition of pyruvate kinase is relieved** promoting entry of metabolites into Krebs cycle: this **favours energy metabolism** (Chart 21.2).

Metabolism of supermouse when exercising

Remember the aphorism: '**fats burn in the flame of carbohydrates**'. In other words, a supply of glucose-derived metabolites is needed to oxidize fats; a fact familiar to long-distant runners who 'hit the wall' when they have exhausted their reserves of muscle glycogen and can no longer use fatty acids as a fuel. This is because they have depleted anaplerotic metabolites, notably **oxaloacetate**, which 'top up' the metabolites in Krebs cycle. It is thought overexpression of PEPCK-C increases the flux through Krebs cycle as follows: β-oxidation of fatty acids produces **acetyl CoA** which combines with **oxaloacetate** to form citrate for oxidation in Krebs cycle. This is coupled to the generation of ATP by oxidative phosphorylation for muscle contraction (see Chapter 9). Remember, oxaloacetate is normally present at a low concentration just sufficient to maintain an adequate flux through Krebs cycle and it is oxaloacetate that is recycled (see Chapter 19). When PEPCK-C is overexpressed, flux through Krebs cycle is stimulated because: (i) the concentration of oxaloacetate is increased; and (ii) PEPCK-C uses GTP and produces GDP needed for the succinyl CoA synthetase reaction. Also, supermouse has more mitochondria than control mice.

Reference

Hakim P., Yang J., Casadeus G., et al. (2007) Overexpression of the cytosolic form of phosphoenolpyruvate carboxykinase (GTP) in skeletal muscle repatterns energy metabolism in the mouse. *J Biol Chem* **282**, 32844–32855.
Also see 'PEPCK-C^{mus} mouse' on YouTube.

Chart 21.2 Skeletal muscle during exercise. During exercise, skeletal muscle in which cytosolic PEPCK is overexpressed produces an abundant supply of oxaloacetate for the oxidation of acetyl CoA in Krebs cycle to generate ATP for muscle contraction (see Chapter 9).

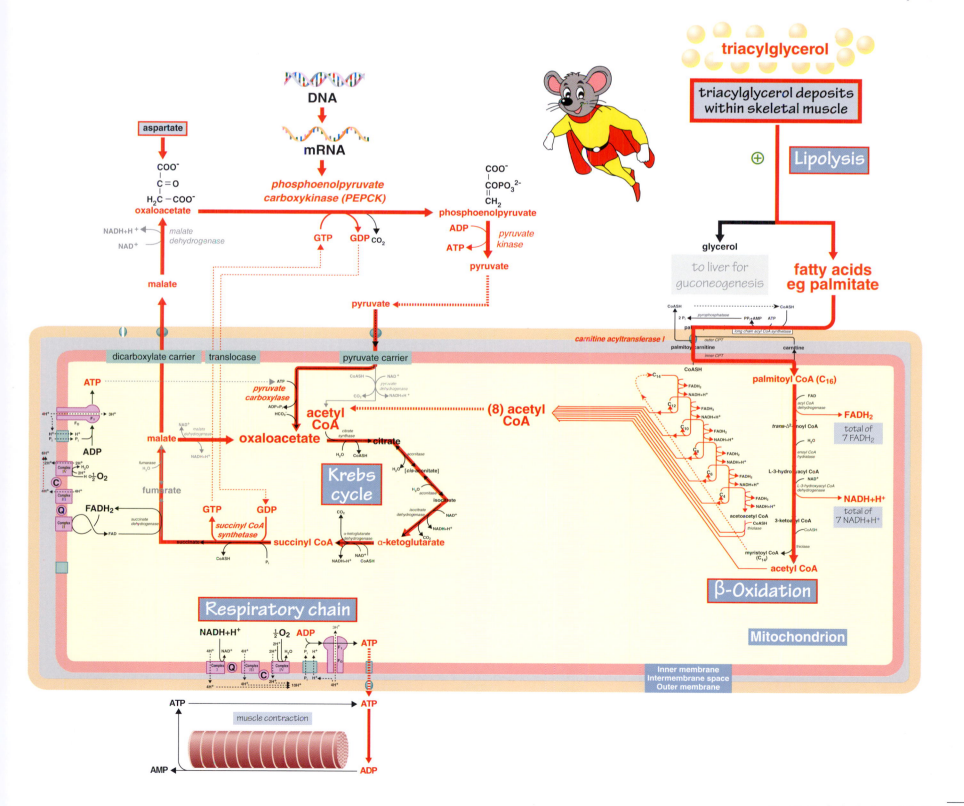

Sorbitol, galactitol, glucuronate and xylitol

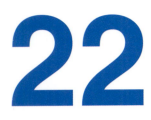

Chart 22.1: sorbitol, the dietary (exogenous) friend but endogenous foe

Dietary sorbitol as a food sweetener

Sorbitol is a sugar alcohol used as a food sweetener in diabetic diets, and has a sweetness value approximately 50% that of sucrose. Patients with diabetes can eat small quantities of sorbitol safely because it is transported relatively slowly across cell membranes, and is absorbed slowly from the intestines.

Endogenously produced sorbitol and cataracts: 'the polyol osmotic theory for the formation of diabetic cataracts'

Although the poor ability of extracellular sorbitol to cross cell membranes favours its use as a sweetener for diabetic food, paradoxically this property can also cause problems. This is because sorbitol produced **endogenously** within cells such as neurons and the optical lens, accumulates within the cell and is metabolized very slowly. Under normal circumstances this is not a problem, since **aldose reductase**, the enzyme that converts glucose to sorbitol, has a K_m for glucose of 70 mmol/l. Hence, it is relatively inactive when the blood glucose concentration is within normal limits of around 3.5–6 mmol/l. However, in uncontrolled diabetes with glucose levels of 25 mmol/l or higher, sorbitol formation occurs at a greater rate, and elevated tissue sorbitol levels have been implicated with certain complications of diabetes such as neuropathy, cataracts and vascular disease. For example, *in vitro* studies have shown that if rabbit lenses are incubated in media containing very high glucose concentrations (35 mmol/l), they accumulate sorbitol. Consequently, the intralenticular osmotic pressure increases causing the lens to swell and become opaque. This can be prevented by aldose reductase inhibitors, such as sorbinil.

Sorbitol catabolism

Sorbitol is metabolized by **sorbitol dehydrogenase** (Chart 22.1), which is particularly active in liver, to form fructose in a reaction coupled to the formation of NADH. This increases the cytosolic NADH/NAD$^+$ ratio, which both favours the reduction of dihydroxyacetone phosphate to glycerol 3-phosphate and inhibits glycolysis by favouring the reduction of 1,3-bisphosphoglycerate to glyceraldehyde 3-phosphate. Also, experiments with rat lenses incubated with glucose have demonstrated that, when the aldose reductase pathway is active, the sorbitol formed is metabolized by sorbitol dehydrogenase to form fructose. This is metabolized to **glycerol 3-phosphate**, since glycolysis is inhibited at the glyceraldehyde 3-phosphate dehydrogenase reaction. Finally, because aldose reductase generates NADP$^+$, the pentose phosphate pathway is stimulated.

Chart 22.2: galactose and galactitol metabolism

Uses of galactose

Galactose is a component of cerebrosides and glycoproteins and, during lactation, is used to synthesize lactose. The major dietary source of galactose is lactose in milk. Hydrolysis of lactose by intestinal lactase yields glucose and galactose. Surplus galactose is metabolized to glucose as shown in Chart 22.2.

Inborn errors of galactose metabolism

Classic galactosaemia is caused by a deficiency of **galactose 1-phosphate uridyltransferase (Gal-1-PUT)**. The alternative form is **galactokinase** deficiency, but both disorders have similar clinical features. In both conditions dietary galactose cannot be metabolized. Consequently, it accumulates in the blood and enters the cells of the lens, where it is reduced to **galactitol** by **aldose reductase**. It is believed that this can cause cataracts by a mechanism similar to that described for sorbitol.

Chart 22.3: glucuronate and xylitol metabolism

Glucuronate conjugates with bilirubin, steroids and drug metabolites

Uridine diphosphate (UDP) glucuronate is formed by oxidation of **UDP glucose** in the presence of UDP glucose dehydrogenase. Hydrophobic molecules such as bilirubin, steroid hormones and many drugs are conjugated with glucuronate by **UDP glucuronyltransferase** to form a water-soluble glucuronide derivative before excretion by the kidney. In Crigler–Najjar syndrome (see Chart 57.1), deficiency of UDP glucuronyltransferase causes increased levels of unconjugated bilirubin, which is bound to albumin, to accumulate in the blood. If the levels exceed the binding capacity of albumin, the unconjugated bilirubin will be taken up by the brain, causing kernicterus.

Glucuronate is the precursor of vitamin C, but not in humans

UDP glucuronate is metabolized to L-gulonate. In most animals (with the notable exception of humans, other primates, guinea-pigs and fruit bats), L-gulonate can be metabolized to ascorbate (vitamin C).

Metabolism of glucuronate and xylitol: the glucuronate/xylulose pathway

UDP glucuronate is metabolized via the ketose L-xylulose to **xylitol**. Xylitol is oxidized to D-xylulose, which is phosphorylated to **xylulose 5-phosphate**, which enters the pentose phosphate pathway before joining the glycolytic (or gluconeogenic) pathway.

Inborn error of metabolism: essential pentosuria

This is a very rare benign condition, most frequently found in Jewish people, in which large quantities (up to 4 g per day) of L-xylulose are excreted in the urine. The condition is due to deficiency of **L-xylulose reductase**.

Xylitol in chewing gum prevents dental decay

Xylitol helps to prevent dental caries and is used as a sweetener. Clinical trials indicate that 7–10 g per day of xylitol in chewing gum can provide good resistance to dental decay in children. This cariostatic effect is thought to be due to both its ability to interfere with the metabolism of *Streptococcus mutans* (the organism in plaque responsible for caries) and also its ability to stabilize solutions of calcium phosphate, which favours remineralization of enamel.

Chart 22.2 Galactose and galactitol metabolism.

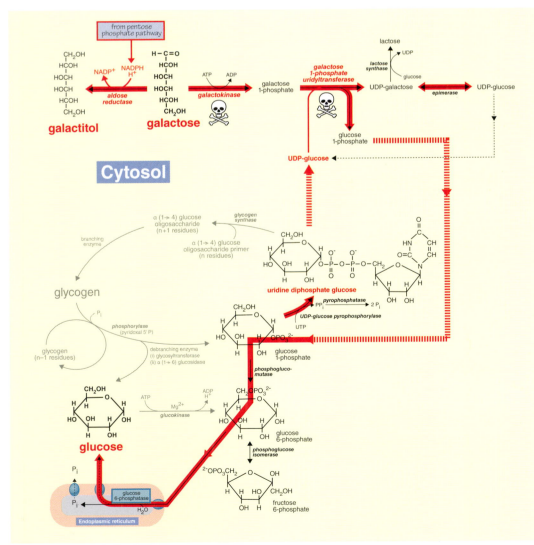

Metabolism at a Glance, Fourth Edition. J. G. Salway. © 2017 John Wiley & Sons Ltd. Published 2017 by John Wiley & Sons Ltd.

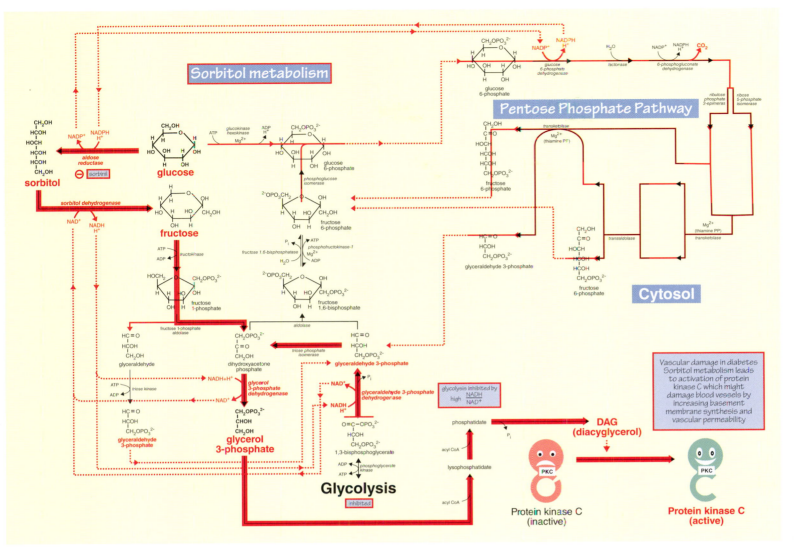

Chart 22.1 Sorbitol metabolism.

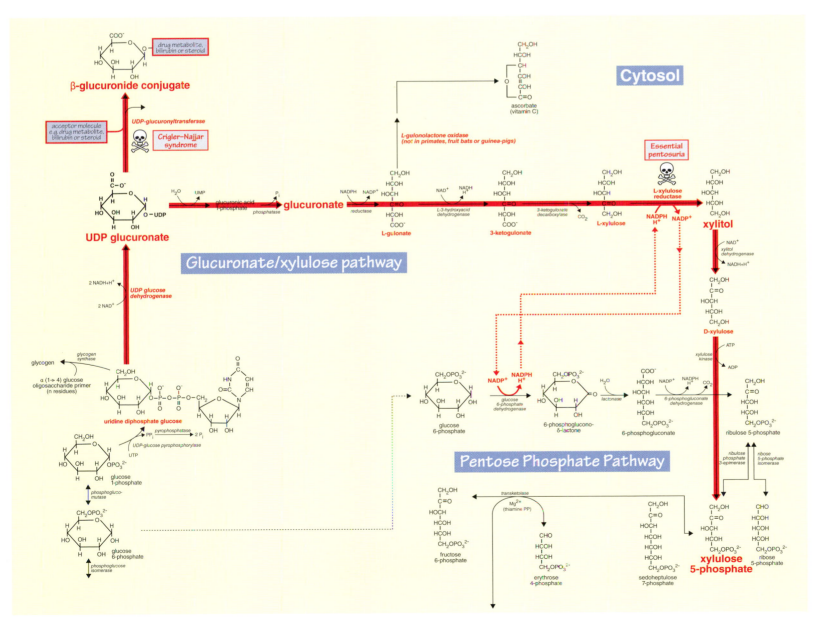

Chart 22.3 Glucuronate and xylitol metabolism.

Fructose metabolism

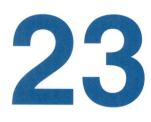

Fructose does not need insulin to enter muscle

The average daily intake of fructose in the UK is around 35–50 g, mainly as the disaccharide sucrose. This is hydrolysed by sucrase in the intestinal cells, forming glucose and fructose. Unlike glucose, however, fructose is able to enter muscle cells and adipocytes in the absence of insulin by using the (confusingly named) glucose transporter **GLUT5**. Consequently, it has been suggested that intravenous fructose should be given as an energy source in patients suffering major trauma. However, this practice is not favoured currently because of the risk of lactic acidosis, as described below.

Metabolism of fructose by liver

Fructose enters the cell via the fructose transporter GLUT5. Then, the liver enzyme **fructokinase** phosphorylates fructose to **fructose 1-phosphate** (Chart 23.1). This is cleaved by **fructose 1-phosphate aldolase** (aldolase B) to form **dihydroxyacetone phosphate** and **glyceraldehyde**. Glyceraldehyde is then phosphorylated by **triose kinase** to **glyceraldehyde 3-phosphate**. Thus the intermediary metabolites of fructose enter glycolysis as triose phosphates. Their fate now depends on the prevailing metabolic status. However, in the typical circumstances of refeeding after a period of fasting, it is most likely that gluconeogenesis will dominate in the early fed state, so

that glycogen and/or glucose will be formed. Alternatively, the substrates could be converted to acetyl CoA and used for fatty acid synthesis.

Metabolism of fructose by muscle

It is likely that the normal dietary quantities of fructose that are presented to the liver in the portal blood will be largely converted to glucose or hepatic glycogen, as described above. Consequently, relatively little fructose will remain for metabolism by muscle. However, if fructose is administered intravenously under experimental conditions, it is metabolized to fructose 6-phosphate by **hexokinase**, since fructokinase is absent from muscle (Chart 23.2). The subsequent fate of this fructose 6-phosphate will depend on the prevailing nutritional status, which will determine whether it is converted to glycogen or used as a respiratory fuel.

Dangers of intravenous fructose

Fructose is metabolized rapidly in humans, having a half-life of 18 minutes. In fact, it disappears from the circulation twice as rapidly as glucose. Although intravenous fructose was once recommended for use in parenteral nutrition, it was not without risk. This is because fructose bypasses the regulatory steps of glucose catabolism in the following ways:

1 Fructose entry into muscle uses GLUT5, which is independent of insulin.
2 Intravenous feeding with large quantities of fructose depletes cellular inorganic phosphate (P_i) and lowers the concentration of ATP. Thus phosphofructokinase is deinhibited in muscle, and uncontrolled glycolysis from fructose 6-phosphate proceeds with the production of lactic acid.
3 In liver, fructose evades the rate-limiting control mechanism by entering glycolysis as dihydroxyacetone phosphate or glyceraldehyde 3-phosphate, i.e. beyond the regulatory enzyme, phosphofructokinase-1. Consequently, in anoxic states, e.g. from the shock of severe trauma, rapid intravenous infusion of fructose may cause a massive unregulated flux of metabolites through glycolysis. In extreme circumstances this has produced excessive quantities of lactic acid and precipitated fatal lactic acidosis.

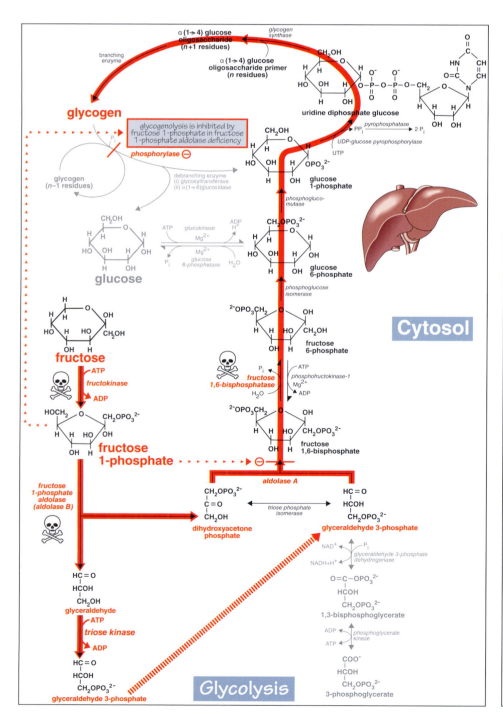

Chart 23.1 Metabolism of fructose to glycogen in liver.

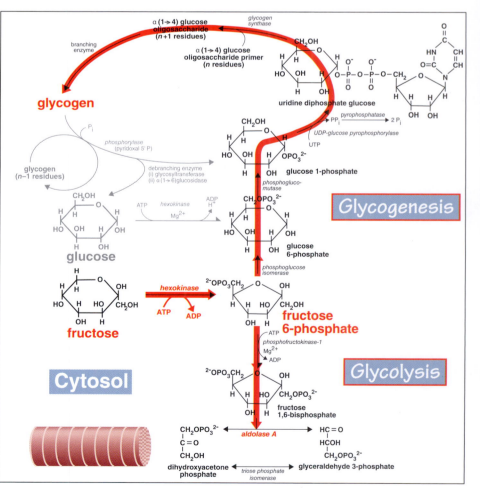

Chart 23.2 Metabolism of fructose in muscle.

Metabolism at a Glance, Fourth Edition. J. G. Salway. © 2017 John Wiley & Sons Ltd. Published 2017 by John Wiley & Sons Ltd.

Inborn errors of metabolism
Fructokinase deficiency (essential fructosuria)
This benign condition is due to a congenital absence of **fructokinase** and is most commonly found in Jewish families. The deficiency means that ingested fructose is limited to metabolism by the hexokinase route only. Consequently, fructose is metabolized much more slowly than usual, so that the blood concentration rises and fructose appears in the urine. Subjects with essential fructosuria have an entirely normal life expectancy.

Fructose 1-phosphate aldolase deficiency (hereditary fructose intolerance)
This serious condition usually presents when an infant is weaned from breast milk on to fructose-containing food. The response to fructose ingestion is a dramatic onset of vomiting and hypoglycaemia within 15–30 minutes. The disorder is due to a deficiency of **fructose 1-phosphate aldolase (aldolase B)**, which results in a massive accumulation of fructose 1-phosphate in the tissues (Chart 23.1). This process sequesters intracellular inorganic phosphate, and moreover inhibits both glycogen **phosphorylase** and fructose 1,6-bisphosphate aldolase (**aldolase A**). The resulting inhibition of glucose production by both glycogenolysis and gluconeogenesis causes the severe hypoglycaemia that is such a serious feature of this condition.

Treatment involves avoiding dietary fructose. Patients tend to develop a natural aversion to sweet foods and this usually leads to a complete absence of dental caries. If not diagnosed and treated, the disease is fatal.

Fructose 1,6-bisphosphatase deficiency
This is a disease caused by impaired hepatic gluconeogenesis due to deficiency of this enzyme (Chart 23.1). It is surprising that, given the strategic importance of fructose 1,6-bisphosphatase in maintaining gluconeogenesis, some patients are relatively unaffected by this disorder. However, in other cases, infants may be hospitalized during the first 6 months of life when the metabolic stress of an infection or fever precipitates hypoglycaemia and lactic acidosis. Although some children with this condition have hepatomegaly and are extremely ill, curiously in other cases this disorder may not be manifested until adult life.

The biochemical pathology results from the stress of trauma or infection provoking a catabolic state in which lipolysis and muscle breakdown combine to produce gluconeogenic amino acids and glycerol. Because gluconeogenesis is inhibited at the fructose 1,6-bisphosphatase reaction, the gluconeogenic metabolites accumulate and form large quantities of lactate. Similarly, ingestion of fructose leads to the formation of lactic acid, precipitating lactic acidosis.

In this condition, glycogenolysis by liver to release glucose is normal. However, once glycogen is depleted, hypoglycaemia follows due to the failure of gluconeogenesis to maintain glucose homeostasis. These patients must therefore eat frequent meals to maintain normoglycaemia.

Fructose phosphates regulate glucokinase activity
After feeding, the concentration of glucose in blood rises rapidly and must be controlled to prevent harmful consequences (see Chapter 10). In liver, **glucokinase** plays an important role in this process. However, note that glucokinase and its opposing enzyme, glucose 6-phosphatase, could operate as an ATP-wasting, futile cycle with glucose → glucose 6-phosphate → glucose. To prevent this, an elaborate mechanism occurs that inactivates glucokinase by incarcerating it within the nucleus bound to **glucokinase regulatory protein (GKRP)** (Diagram 23.1). **Fructose 6-phosphate (F 6-P)** binds GKRP to, and inactivates, glucokinase. On the otherhand, **fructose 1-phosphate** and **high concentrations of glucose** activate glucokinase by liberating it from GKRP, allowing its translocation to the cytosol. Once within the cytosol, glucokinase is bound to the non-phosphorylated form of phosphofructokinase-2/fructose 2,6-bisphosphatase (PFK-2/F 2,6-bisPase) (see Chapter 16) which maintains glucokinase in an active state.

'Fructose 6-phosphate paradox': F 6-P binds glucokinase to GKRP inactivating it within the nucleus
During fasting this makes sense when F 6-P is an intermediate in gluconeogenesis, consequently **glucokinase** must be **inactive**. However, paradoxically F 6-P is an omnipresent intermediary metabolite. *After feeding* when **glucokinase** is **active**, F 6-P is also present as an intermediate in glycolysis and the pentose phosphate pathways, which are involved in fatty acid synthesis. This tendency for F 6-P to inactivate glucokinase is overcome after feeding by **fructose 1-phosphate** and **high concentrations of glucose** that overwhelm the F 6-P effect, causing active glucokinase to dissociated from GKRP and be translocated from the nucleus to the cytosol.

Diagram 23.1 Following feeding, fructose 1-phosphate and high concentrations of glucose activate glucokinase in liver by liberating it from the nucleus where it is bound to glucokinase regulatory protein (GKRP). **During fasting,** fructose 6-phosphate binds glucokinase to GKRP within the nucleus.

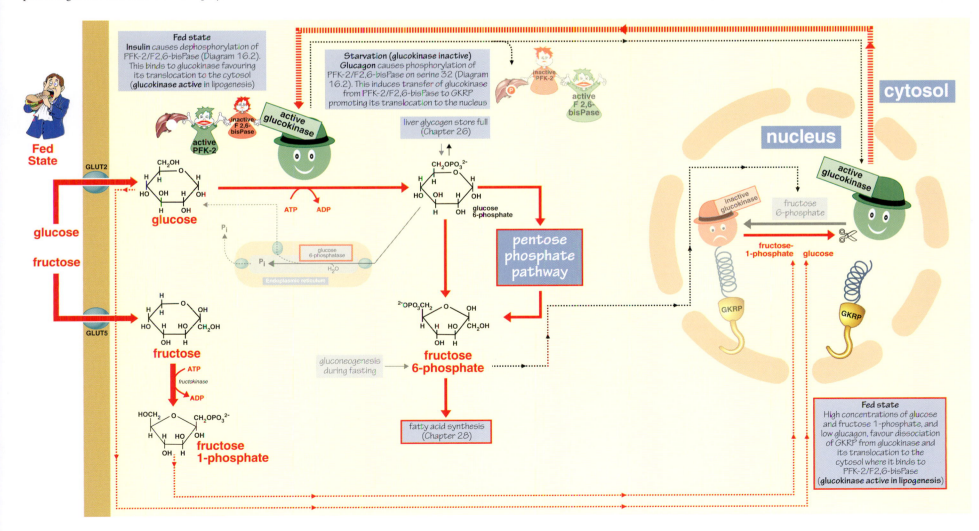

Ethanol metabolism

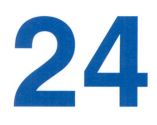

Alcohol, or more precisely ethanol, is a popular mood-altering compound that has been consumed over the centuries as wine, beer and, more recently, as spirits. Whereas there is evidence to suggest that the intake of small quantities of ethanol with food can be beneficial, excessive consumption can cause cirrhosis of the liver, or metabolic disturbances including fatty liver and hypoglycaemia.

Ethanol is metabolized by three enzyme systems

Chart 24.1 (opposite) Metabolism of ethanol.

Ethanol is rapidly oxidized in the liver by three enzyme systems, but the relative physiological importance of these is not clear (Diagram 24.1 and Chart 24.1). All three systems produce acetaldehyde, which is normally oxidized rapidly to acetate.

Alcohol dehydrogenase in the cytosol

There may be up to 20 different isoenzymes of alcohol dehydrogenase. The rate of this pathway is largely regulated by the availability of NAD⁺. This in turn depends on the ability of the malate/aspartate shuttle (see Chapter 4) to transport reducing equivalents into the mitochondrion and, moreover, on the ability of the respiratory chain to oxidize NADH to NAD⁺.

Microsomal ethanol-oxidizing system (MEOS)

This system is located in the smooth endoplasmic reticulum and involves a cytochrome P450 enzyme. These are a family of monooxygenases concerned with the detoxification of ingested drugs and xenobiotics.

Peroxisomal oxidation of ethanol

Diagram 24.1 The three enzyme systems responsible for ethanol metabolism.

Catalase uses hydrogen peroxide to oxidize alcohols such as methanol and ethanol to their corresponding aldehydes.

Metabolism of acetaldehyde

The acetaldehyde formed by any of the three systems mentioned above must now enter the mitochondrion for further oxidation by aldehyde dehydrogenase to form acetate. Finally, this acetate could, theoretically, be activated to acetyl CoA for oxidation by Krebs cycle. However, in liver, Krebs cycle is unable to oxidize this acetyl CoA, as we will see below, because of the prevailing high ratio of NADH/NAD⁺ in the mitochondrial matrix. Consequently the acetate will probably leave the liver for oxidation by the extrahepatic tissues. Evidence suggests that accumulation of acetaldehyde may be responsible for some of the unpleasant effects caused by drinking ethanol, for example the flushing and nausea that is often seen in those people who are genetically deficient in aldehyde dehydrogenase (45% of Japanese and Chinese). This phenomenon is used to discourage drinking in alcoholics, who may be given disulfiram (Antabuse), which inhibits aldehyde dehydrogenase causing the accumulation of acetaldehyde if ethanol is consumed. Finally, the sulphonylurea drug chlorpropamide inhibits aldehyde dehydrogenase and is known to cause 'chlorpropamide alcohol flushing' in diabetic patients treated with this drug.

Biochemical effects of ethanol
Increased NADH/NAD⁺ ratio

Following ingestion of ethanol, the cytosolic **alcohol dehydrogenase** reaction and the mitochondrial **aldehyde dehydrogenase** reaction both produce NADH, with relative depletion of NAD⁺ so that the ratio of NADH/NAD⁺ is significantly increased. This has the following effects:

1 **Gluconeogenesis is inhibited.** As shown in the chart opposite, the high NADH/NAD⁺ ratio in the cytosol displaces the equilibrium of the dehydrogenase reactions in favour of the reduced reactant. In particular, **pyruvate** is reduced to **lactate**, and **oxaloacetate** is reduced to **malate**, thereby preventing the flow of metabolites in the direction of gluconeogenesis. This can cause hypoglycaemia (see below).

2 **Krebs cycle is inhibited in liver.** The high NADH/NAD⁺ ratio in the mitochondrial matrix prevents the oxidation of **isocitrate** to **α-ketoglutarate**, of **α-ketoglutarate** to **succinyl CoA**, and of **malate** to **oxaloacetate**. Consequently, although acetate can be activated to acetyl CoA for metabolism in the liver, it is more likely that acetate will be exported for metabolism by the extrahepatic tissues.

Hyperlactataemia and gout

The accumulation of lactate results in hyperlactataemia. This can cause hyperuricaemia because lactate and urate share, and so compete for, the same mechanism for renal tubular secretion. Gout occurs when uric acid, which is sparingly soluble in plasma, crystallizes in the joints, particularly the toes.

Ethanol interactions with drugs

Long-term treatment with many drugs, for example the barbiturates, causes proliferation of the smooth endoplasmic reticulum and increases the activity of the cytochrome P450 isoenzymes involved in their metabolism and clearance from the body. Similarly, chronic ingestion of excessive quantities of ethanol causes increased proliferation of the endoplasmic reticulum and induction of these enzymes. This means that a sober alcoholic patient will metabolize and inactivate these drugs very rapidly and may need higher than normal doses for treatment. However, in the drunken alcoholic, ethanol preferentially competes with these drugs for metabolism by the cytochrome P450 isoenzymes. As a result, the inactivation and clearance of the barbiturates is suppressed, with the risk of lethal consequences.

Ethanol-induced fasting hypoglycaemia

This condition develops in chronically malnourished individuals several hours after a heavy drinking binge. This is caused by the inhibition of gluconeogenesis, as described above.

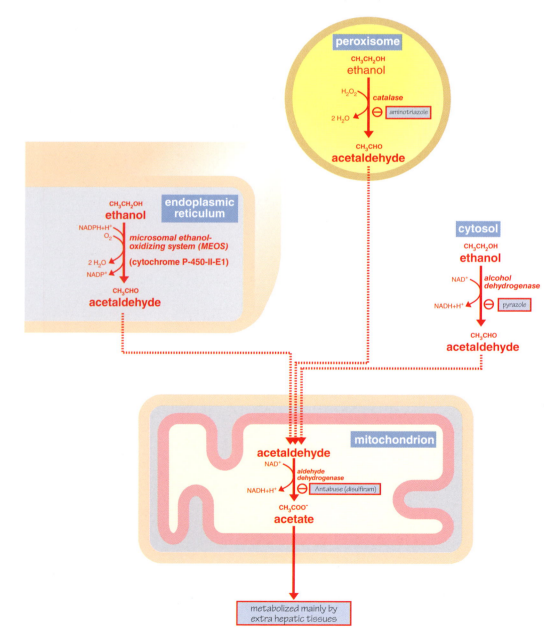

Metabolism at a Glance, Fourth Edition. J. G. Salway. © 2017 John Wiley & Sons Ltd. Published 2017 by John Wiley & Sons Ltd.

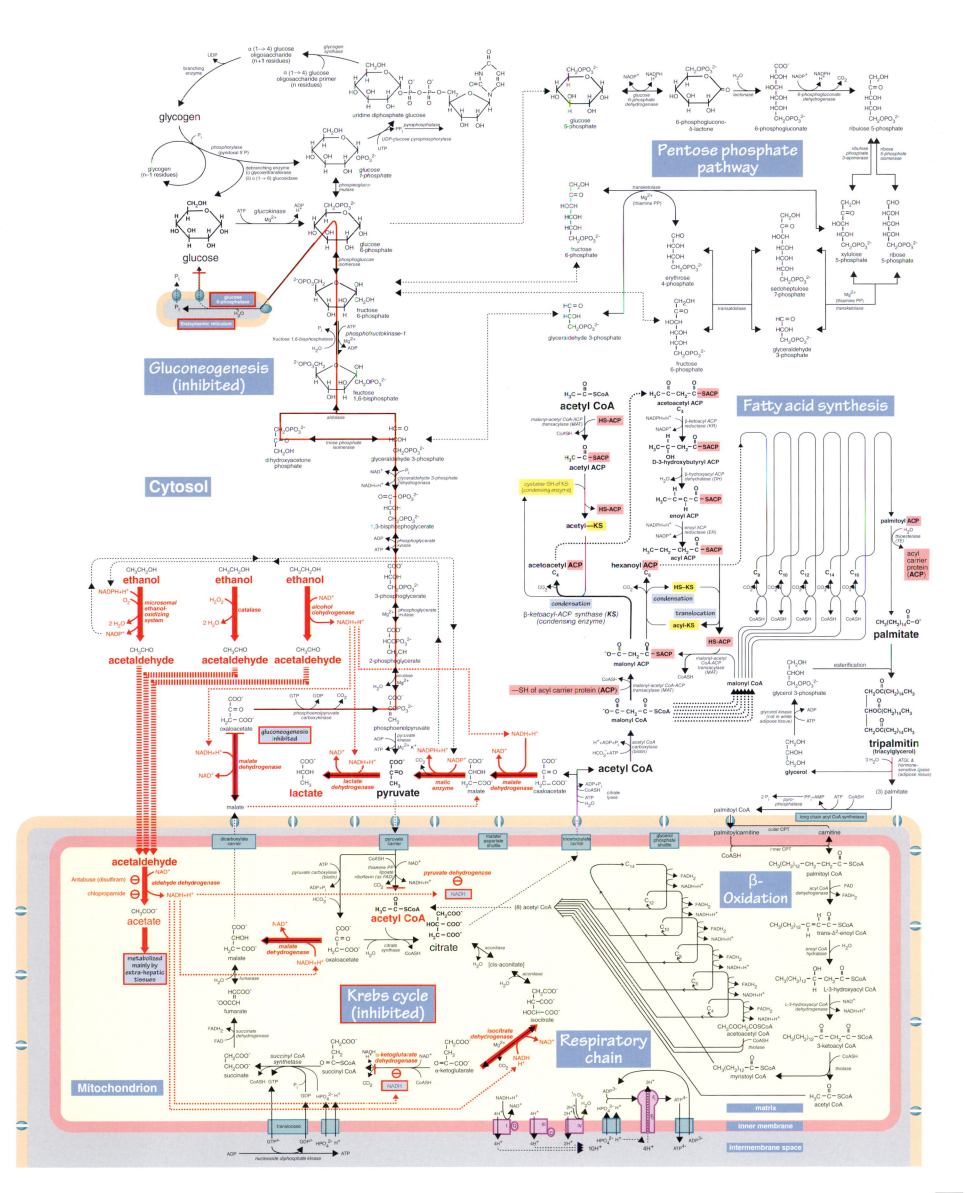

Pyruvate/malate cycle and the production of NADPH

25

The pyruvate/malate cycle has two main functions associated with lipogenesis: (i) it transports acetyl CoA units from the mitochondrion into the cytosol; and (ii) it generates NADPH in the reaction catalysed by the **malic enzyme**.

Chart 25.1: pyruvate/malate cycle

Fatty acid synthesis occurs in the cytosol. However, the carbon source, namely acetyl CoA, is produced by pyruvate dehydrogenase in the mitochondrion. Transport of acetyl CoA from the mitochondrion into the cytosol involves the **pyruvate/malate cycle**. The principal stages are:

1 One molecule of pyruvate is carboxylated by **pyruvate carboxylase** to form **oxaloacetate**.

2 A second pyruvate molecule forms **acetyl CoA** by the **pyruvate dehydrogenase** reaction.

3 The acetyl CoA and oxaloacetate so formed condense to form citrate, which is transported to the cytosol for cleavage by **citrate lyase** to oxaloacetate and **acetyl CoA** for lipogenesis. **Oxaloacetate** is reduced by cytosolic malate dehydrogenase and **malate** is formed. Malate is oxidatively decarboxylated by the **malic enzyme** (malate dehydrogenase, decarboxylating) with the formation of NADPH, CO_2 and pyruvate, thus completing the cycle.

Chart 25.2 Lactate as a substrate for fatty acid synthesis.

Relative contributions of the pentose phosphate pathway and the pyruvate/malate cycle to the provision of NADPH for fatty acid synthesis

For each acetyl unit added to the acyl carrier protein chain (ACP chain) during fatty acid synthesis, two molecules of NADPH are needed (Chapter 27).

Experimental evidence suggests that if glucose is used for fatty acid synthesis, the pentose phosphate pathway supplies 60% of the NADPH needed with 40% produced by the pyruvate/malate cycle.

Fatty acid synthesis is also possible from other precursors, for example amino acids (see Chapter 33) or lactate (Chart 25.2). For instance, if lactate is used for fatty acid synthesis, only 25% of the NADPH needed is provided by the pyruvate/malate cycle.

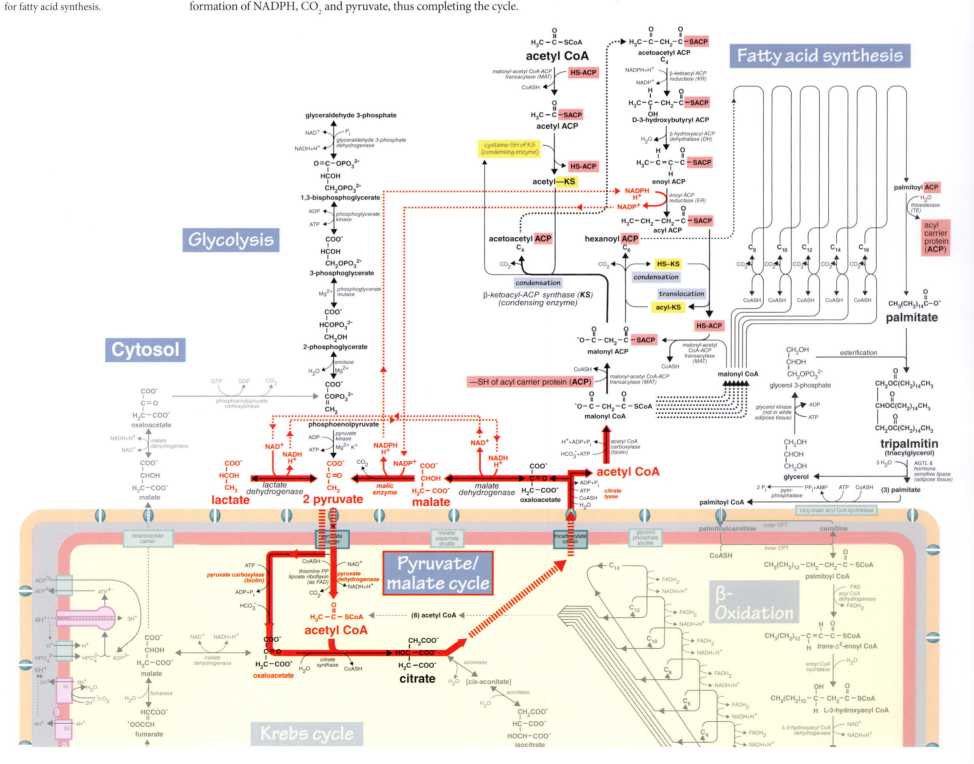

Metabolism at a Glance, Fourth Edition. J. G. Salway. © 2017 John Wiley & Sons Ltd. Published 2017 by John Wiley & Sons Ltd.

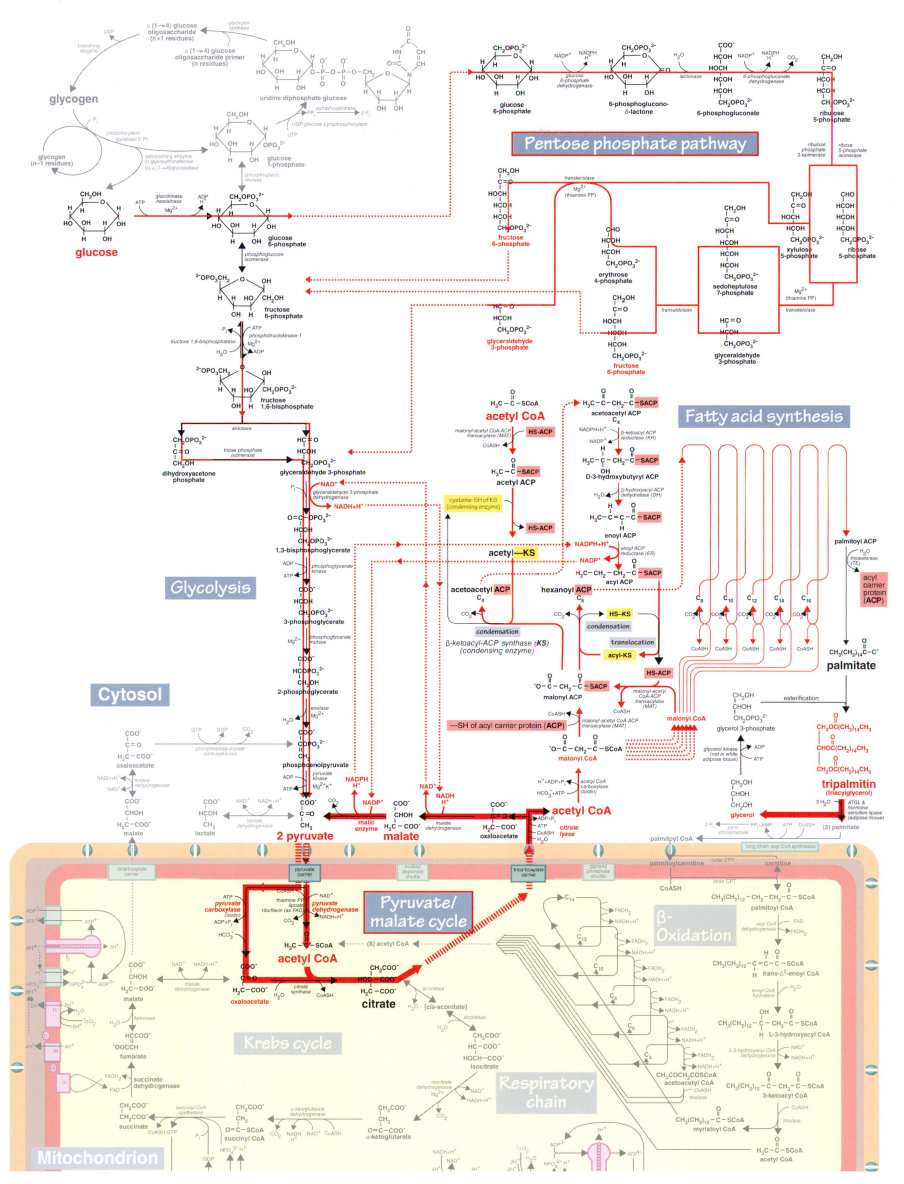

Chart 25.1 The pyruvate/malate cycle.

Metabolism of glucose to fat (triacylglycerol)

26

Importance of fat

The statement 'if you eat too much food, you will become fat' is unlikely to surprise any reader of this book. We know from experience that a surplus of fat in our diet will increase the fat in our body. Furthermore, it is general knowledge that an excess of carbohydrate will be stored as fat. However, a surprising number of people enjoy life under the delusion that they can eat large amounts of protein without the hazard of becoming obese. Sadly, this misconception will be shattered by reality in Chapter 33. Let us turn to the physiological advantages of body fat. Primitive man, like many other carnivorous mammals that hunted for food, was an intermittent feeder. In the days before refrigeration he was unable to store joints from his woolly mammoth in the freezer, to be divided subsequently into a gastronomical routine of breakfast, lunch, dinner and supper. Instead, when food was available the hunters and their families ate all they could, with any surplus to immediate energy requirements being stored in the body, to a certain extent as glycogen but mainly as fat. This fat can provide an energy store for sustenance over periods of starvation lasting several days or even weeks.

Fat provides a very compact store for energy, largely because of its highly reduced and anhydrous nature. In fact, 1 g of fat yields 9 kcal (37 kJ). This compares well with 1 g of carbohydrate, which yields 3.75 kcal (16 kJ), or 1 g of protein, yielding 4 kcal (17 kJ).

Liver cells and fat cells (adipocytes) are both major producers of fat. In addition, with the onset of lactation at the end of pregnancy, the mammary gland develops almost overnight the ability to synthesize prodigious amounts of fat for secretion in the milk.

Chart 26.1: the flow of metabolites when glucose is converted to triacylglycerol

The chart shows the metabolic pathways involved when a surplus of carbohydrate is taken in the diet. We have seen how liver is able to conserve useful, but limited, supplies of energy as glycogen (see Chapter 10). Once these glycogen reserves are full, any additional carbohydrate will be converted to fat as follows: glucose enters the pentose phosphate pathway, the metabolites of which form a temporary diversion from the glycolytic pathway. The metabolites eventually rejoin the main glycolytic route, pass into the mitochondrion and enter Krebs cycle. However, in the fed state the mitochondrial pathways will be working to capacity and generating large amounts of ATP and NADH. Under these circumstances, a control mechanism (see Chapter 19) diverts citrate from Krebs cycle into the cytosol for fatty acid synthesis (see Chapter 27). Although Chart 26.1 shows the formation of **palmitate**, stearate is also formed by this pathway. Both can be esterified with glycerol 3-phosphate to form **triacylglycerols** (see Chapters 29 and 32). **NB:** The vitamin **biotin** is an essential cofactor for the regulatory enzyme **acetyl CoA carboxylase** in the pathway for fatty acid synthesis.

Diagram 26.1: insulin and fat synthesis

Adipocytes are the specialized cells of adipose tissue where triacylglycerols are synthesized and stored. They contain the usual cellular organelles but, because the cell interior is almost completely occupied by a large, spherical fat droplet, the cytosol and organelles are displaced to the periphery. Adipose tissue is widely distributed, being found beneath the skin and especially around the intestines, kidneys and other visceral organs.

Blood capillaries in adipose tissue bring supplies of glucose for fatty acid synthesis. The diagram shows the relationship between adipocytes and a capillary, but is not to scale: in reality, the adipocytes would be much larger. The glucose passes through the capillary wall into the extracellular fluid. After feeding, insulin is released from the pancreas and causes a 30-fold increased rate of transport of glucose into the adipocyte. Insulin causes the translocation of a latent pool of GLUT4 glucose transporters from within the adipocyte cytosol to the plasma membrane. These facilitate the transport of glucose into the cytosol, where it is metabolized to triacylglycerols, which are stored as a spherical droplet as described earlier.

Not all the body's triacylglycerol is made by the adipose tissue. Triacylglycerol is usually available in food and is absorbed from the gut as protein-phospholipid-coated packages known as chylomicrons, whose role is to transport the triacylglycerols from the intestines to the adipocytes for storage. Alternatively, **liver** makes triacylglycerols from glucose for export in a similar package known as a VLDL (very low-density lipoprotein). Likewise, these VLDLs transport triacylglycerol to adipose tissue for storage.

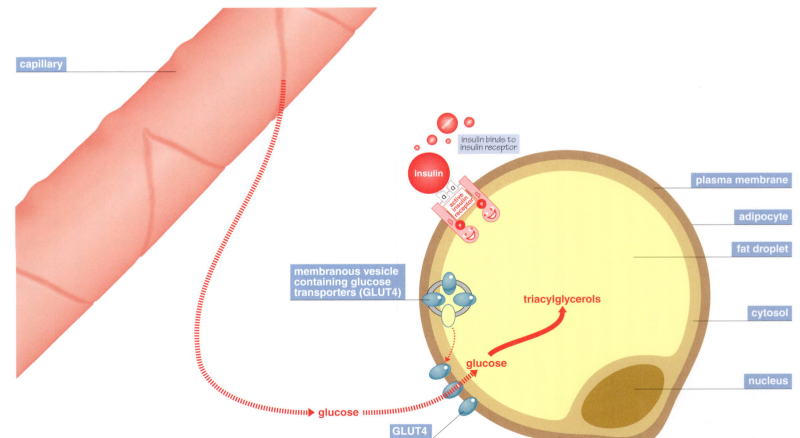

Diagram 26.1 Insulin stimulates the transport of glucose into adipocytes for triacylglycerol synthesis.

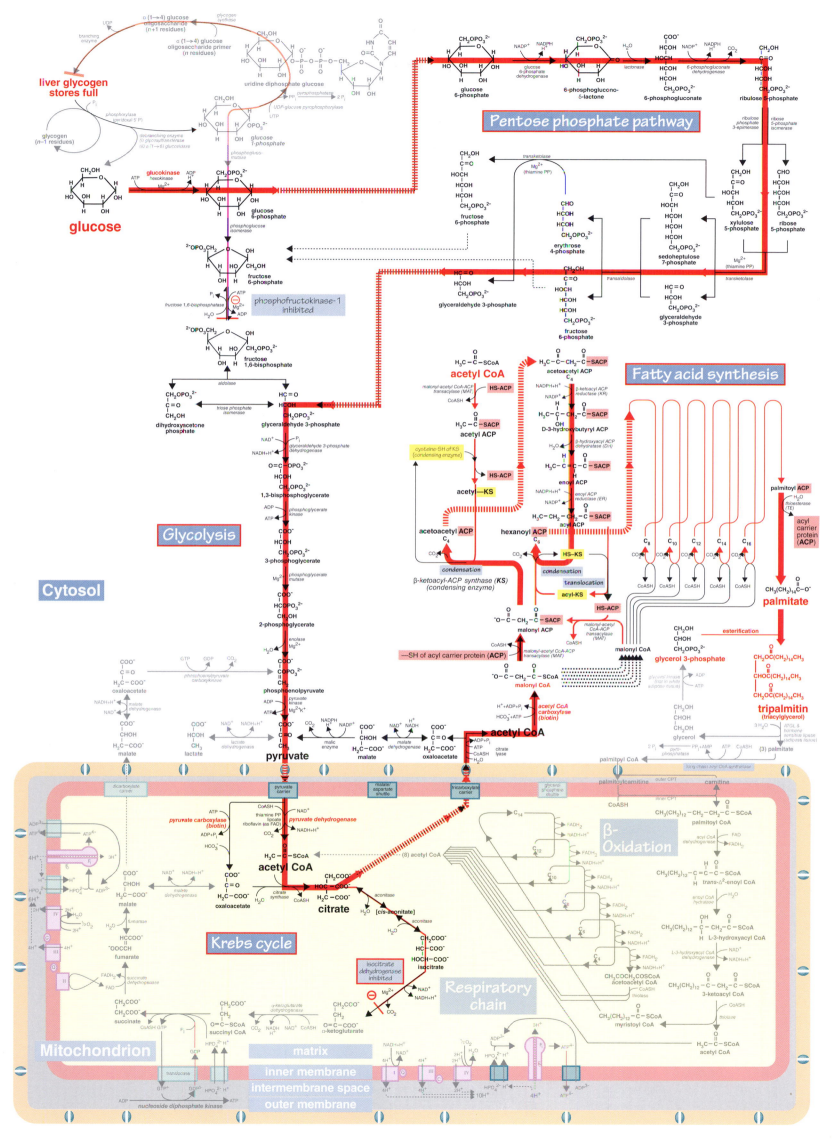

Pentose phosphate pathway

Fatty acid synthesis

Glycolysis

Cytosol

Krebs cycle

Respiratory chain

β-Oxidation

Mitochondrion

glucose

liver glycogen stores full

phosphofructokinase-1 inhibited

isocitrate dehydrogenase inhibited

Chart 26.1
Metabolism of glucose to triacylglycerol.

Metabolism of glucose to fatty acids and triacylglycerol

27

A brief description of how glucose is converted to fat appeared in Chapter 26. It is now time to look at triacylglycerol biosynthesis in more detail.

The liver, adipose tissue and lactating mammary gland are the principal tissues involved in lipogenesis (triacylglycerol synthesis). Liver and adipose tissue make triacylglycerol from glucose under conditions of abundant carbohydrate intake; in other words, when the body has more than enough food to satisfy its immediate needs for energy.

Chart 27.1: synthesis of triacylglycerols from glucose
Importance of citrate in activating fatty acid synthesis

The mitochondrion in the high-energy state has increased amounts of ATP and NADH. These metabolites, both symbols of cellular affluence, reduce the rate of flow of metabolites through Krebs cycle by inhibiting **isocitrate dehydrogenase**. Consequently, the metabolites isocitrate and **citrate** accumulate, and their concentration within the mitochondrion increases. As the concentration of **citrate** rises, it diffuses via the **tricarboxylate carrier** from the mitochondrion into the cytosol, where citrate serves three functions:

1 **Citrate** and ATP are allosteric regulators that reduce the metabolic flux through glycolysis by inhibiting **phosphofructokinase-1**, thereby redirecting metabolites into the pentose phosphate pathway. This pathway produces NADPH, which is an essential coenzyme for fatty acid synthesis.

2 **Citrate** in the cytosol is split by **citrate lyase** (the citrate cleavage enzyme) to form **oxaloacetate** and **acetyl CoA**. The latter is the precursor for fatty acid synthesis.

3 **Citrate** activates **acetyl CoA carboxylase**, which is a regulatory enzyme controlling fatty acid synthesis.

In these three ways, citrate has organized the metabolic pathways of liver or fat cells so that lipogenesis may proceed.

Pentose phosphate pathway generates NADPH for fatty acid synthesis

To reiterate, once the immediate energy demands of the animal have been satisfied, surplus glucose will be stored in the liver as glycogen. When the glycogen stores are full, any surplus glucose molecules will find the glycolytic pathway restricted at the level of phosphofructokinase. Under these circumstances, metabolic flux via the **pentose phosphate pathway** is stimulated.

This is a complex pathway generating **glyceraldehyde 3-phosphate**, which then re-enters glycolysis, thus bypassing the restriction at phosphofructokinase-1. Because of this bypass, the pathway is sometimes referred to as the 'hexose monophosphate shunt' pathway.

One very important feature of the pentose phosphate pathway is that it produces NADPH from NADP+. NADPH is a hydrogen carrier derived from the vitamin niacin, and as such is a phosphorylated form of NAD+, the important functional difference being that, whereas NADH is used for ATP production, NADPH is used for fatty acid synthesis and other biosynthetic reactions.

Fatty acid synthesis and esterification

Starting from glucose, Chart 27.1 shows the metabolic flux via the pentose phosphate pathway and glycolysis to mitochondrial acetyl CoA, and hence via citrate to acetyl CoA in the cytosol. Fatty acid synthesis is catalysed by the fatty acid synthase complex, which requires malonyl CoA. The latter combines with the **acyl carrier protein (ACP)** to form **malonyl ACP**. Fatty acid synthesis proceeds via the cyclical series of reactions as shown in the chart to form **palmitate** (and also stearate, which is not shown). However, fat is stored not as fatty acids but as **triacylglycerols** (triglycerides). These are made by a series of esterification reactions that combine three fatty acid molecules with **glycerol 3-phosphate** (see Chapter 29).

Diagram 27.1: activation of acetyl CoA carboxylase by citrate *in vitro*

Experiments *in vitro* have shown that acetyl CoA carboxylase exists as units (or protomers), which are enzymically inactive. However, citrate causes these protomers to polymerize and form enzymically active filaments that promote fatty acid synthesis. Conversely, the product of the reaction, namely fatty acyl CoA (palmitoyl CoA), causes depolymerization of the filaments. Kinetic studies have shown that, whereas polymerization is very rapid, taking only a few seconds, depolymerization is much slower, with a half-life of approximately 10 minutes. The length of a polymer varies, but on average consists of 20 units, and it has been calculated that a single liver cell contains 50 000 such filaments.

Each of the units contains biotin and is a dimer of two identical polypeptide subunits. The activity is also regulated by hormonally mediated multiple phosphorylation/dephosphorylation reactions (see Chapter 30).

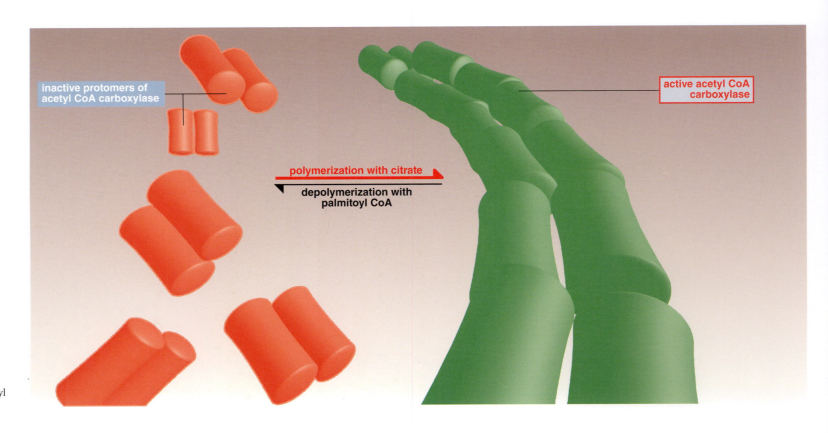

Diagram 27.1 Activation of acetyl CoA carboxylase by citrate.

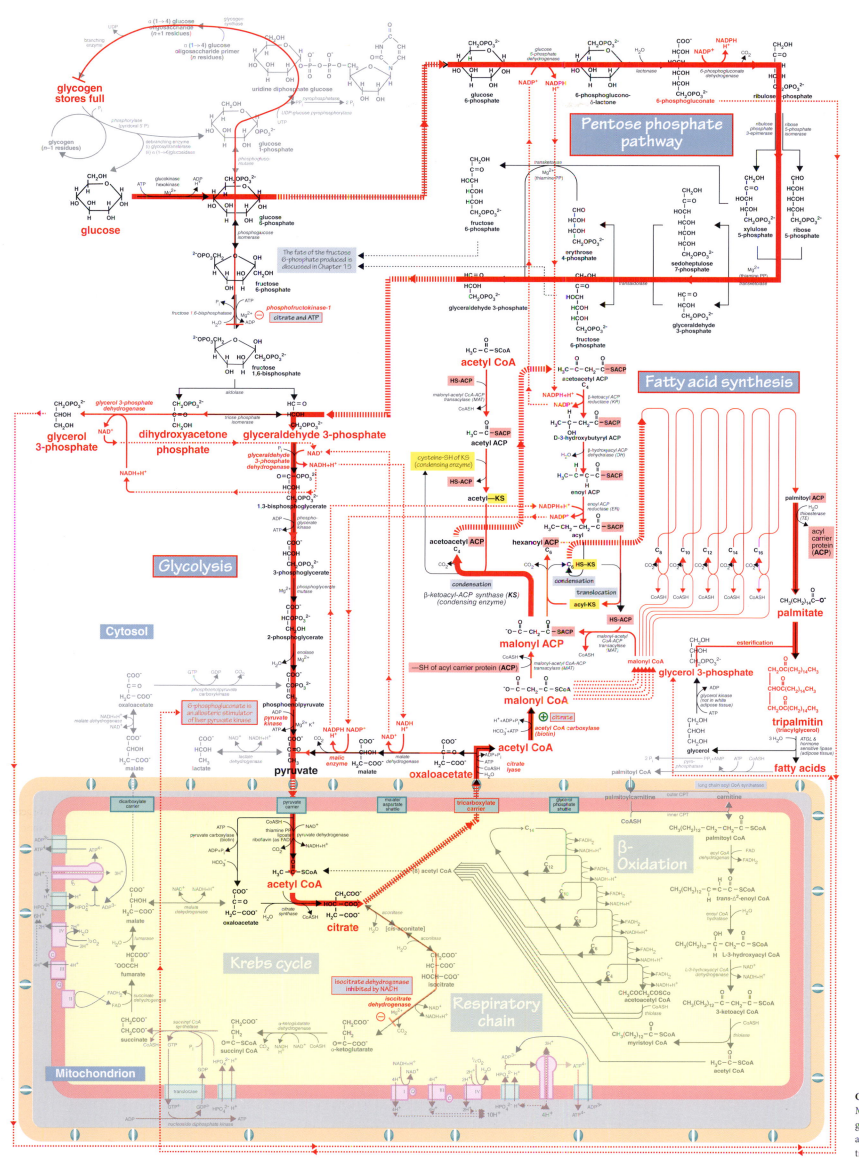

Chart 27.1 Metabolism of glucose to fatty acids and triacylglycerol.

Glycolysis and the pentose phosphate pathway collaborate in liver to make fat

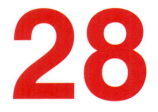

Chart 28.1 (opposite) Metabolism of glucose to fat.

Liver is the biochemical factory of the body

Liver is the great provider and protector and, in metabolic terms, is like Mum, Dad and Grandparents rolled up as one. Its extensive functions include an important role in glucose homeostasis during feeding and fasting. For example, after a meal when abundant glucose is delivered to the liver via the hepatic portal vein, glucose is metabolized to glycogen and is stored in liver. Also, during this feasting, glucose is metabolized to **triacylglycerols** such as **tripalmitin** (Chart 28.1), which are exported to adipose tissue as very low-density lipoproteins (VLDLs) for storage until needed during fasting.

Glycolysis cooperates with the pentose phosphate pathway enabling lipogenesis

Unlike most tissues, for example muscle and nervous tissue, the liver does not use glycolysis for energy metabolism but instead depends on β-oxidation of fatty acids to provide ATP for biosynthetic pathways such as gluconeogenesis and urea synthesis (see Chapter 58). Instead, in liver, glycolysis operates in partnership with the pentose phosphate pathway to produce pyruvate, which is oxidatively decarboxylated to acetyl CoA, the precursor for fatty acid synthesis. However, when glucose is abundant, **ATP and citrate concentrations are increased and these restrict glycolysis at the phosphofructokinase-1 (PFK-1) stage** (see Chapter 27). This obstruction to glycolytic flow means that glucose 6-phosphate is shunted through the pentose phosphate pathway, where it forms **glyceraldehyde 3-phosphate** and **fructose 6-phosphate**. The fate of this fructose 6-phosphate is described in the section on PFK-1 below.

Glucose transport into liver cells

Glucose transport both **into (fed state)** and **out of (fasting)** liver cells is facilitated by the transport protein **GLUT2**, which has a very high K_m for glucose of 20 mmol/l. **Fanconi–Bickel syndrome** is a rare type of glycogen storage disease (type XI) caused by an abnormal GLUT2 expressed in liver, intestinal and renal tubular cells, and pancreatic β-cells. Because of the in–out blockade of glucose transport, patients suffer **hepatorenal glycogen** accumulation and consequent **fasting hypoglycaemia**, while after feeding they experience **transient hyperglycaemia**.

Glucokinase

As mentioned in Chapter 16, **in liver** glucose is phosphorylated to glucose 6-phosphate by **glucokinase** which has a $K_{0.5}$ for glucose of 10 mmol/l. In other words it has a low affinity for glucose and is designed to cope with the enormous surges (up to 15 mmol/l) of glucose arriving in the liver via the hepatic portal vein after feeding. The glucose 6-phosphate so formed can now make glycogen (see Chapters 10 and 11). However, once the liver's glycogen stores are replete, glucose 6-phosphate is metabolized via the **pentose phosphate pathway** (see below). 'Glucokinase activators' (GKAs) are candidate antidiabetic drugs.

Glucokinase is inactivated by sequestration with the glucokinase regulatory protein (GKRP), which is bound within the hepatocyte nucleus (see Chapter 23). Fructose 1-phosphate or high post-prandial concentrations of glucose liberate glucokinase from its regulatory protein and the active glucokinase is translocated into the cytosol where it is stabilized by unphosphorylated phosphofructokinase-2/fructose 2,6-bisphosphatase (PFK-2/F 2,6-bisPase).

Pentose phosphate pathway and triacylglycerol synthesis

The pentose phosphate pathway provides reducing power as NADPH, which is needed for triacylglycerol synthesis (Chart 28.1), biosynthesis of cholesterol (see Chapter 42) and to maintain a supply of reduced glutathione as a defense against oxidative damage (see Chapter 15).

The stoichiometry of the pentose phosphate pathway involving three glucose molecules is shown in Chart 28.1. The three molecules of glucose are phosphorylated by glucokinase to glucose 6-phosphate, which is oxidized by glucose 6-phosphate dehydrogenase to form 3 NADPH and 6-phosphogluconate. This is then oxidized and decarboxylated by 6-phosphogluconate dehydrogenase to form three more NADPH and ribulose 5-phosphate, and three carbons are lost as CO_2. The ribulose 5-phosphate is further metabolized by a series of reactions until the final products are glyceraldehyde 3-phosphate and two molecules of fructose 6-phosphate.

So, the products of the pentose phosphate pathway are **glyceraldehyde 3-phosphate** and **fructose 6-phosphate**. Well clearly, there is no difficulty in the former being metabolized through glycolysis to pyruvate. However, the reader may be puzzled that fructose 6-phosphate is **upstream** of PFK-1 (which is inhibited by ATP and citrate (see Chapter 27)) and thus apparently incapable of further metabolism by glycolysis. The answer to this enigma depends on the regulation of PFK-1, which is explained below.

Phosphofructokinase-1 (PFK-1)

As explained above, the problem is that ATP and citrate inhibit PFK-1, and the fructose 6-phosphate formed by the pentose phosphate pathway is upstream of this blockade. The question is how can this fructose 6-phosphate be metabolized by glycolysis to pyruvate and onwards to fatty acids? The answer to this predicament is **fructose 2,6-bisphosphate (F 2,6-bisP)**, which is produced by the liver isoenzyme of the bifunctional PFK-2/F 2,6-bisPase described in Chapter 16. F 2,6-bisP is a potent allosteric stimulator of PFK-1 and overcomes the inhibition caused by ATP and citrate. The regulation of PFK-2/F 2,6-bisPase is described below.

Furthermore, **ribose 1,5-bisphosphate** (formed from ribulose 5-phosphate in the cooperative pentose phosphate pathway) stimulates PFK-1 and inhibits its opposing enzyme, fructose 1,6-bisphosphatase.

Phosphofructokinase-2/fructose 2,6-bisphosphatase (PFK-2/F 2,6-bisPase)

After feeding with carbohydrate, insulin concentrations are raised and the bifunctional PFK-2/F 2,6-bisPase is dephosphorylated by protein phosphatase-2A (PP-2A). This activates PFK-2 activity, resulting in production of F 2,6-bisP, which stimulates PFK-1 and increases the rate of glycolysis as described above. There is evidence for further cooperation with the pentose phosphate pathway in that **xylulose 5-phosphate (Xu-5P)** activates PP-2A and enhances dephosphorylation of PFK-2/F 2,6-bisPase.

Pyruvate kinase (PK)

During feeding, pyruvate kinase (PK) is allosterically stimulated by **fructose 1,6-bisphosphate** in an example of feed-forward stimulation. This serves to overcome the allosteric inhibition of liver PK caused by alanine that occurs during fasting. Also, insulin activates PP-2A, which dephosphorylates and activates liver PK, reversing its phosphorylated inactive state that prevails during fasting.

Xylulose 5-phosphate (Xu-5P) and ChREBP (carbohydrate response element binding protein)

It is well established that insulin regulates the expression of genes. More recently it has been shown that nutrients such as glucose and fatty acids can also control gene expression. Insulin stimulates the transcription factor **SREBP (sterol response element binding protein)** which regulates transcription not only of the genes involved in the biosynthesis of cholesterol, but also the genes coding enzymes involved in fatty acid synthesis such as **glucokinase**. Glucose can control gene expression through an insulin-independent transcription factor, **ChREBP**, that shuttles between the cytosol and the nucleus. ChREBP, which is constitutively present in liver cells, is phosphorylated and must be dephosphorylated before it can bind to DNA. After feeding with carbohydrate, the concentration of fructose 6-phosphate is increased resulting in an upstream accumulation of pentose phosphate pathway metabolites including **Xu-5P**. This Xu-5P plays an important role in coordinating transcription of the enzymes for *de novo* lipogenesis. Xu-5P activates **PP-2A**, which dephosphorylates **ChREBP** enabling it to diffuse into the nucleus and bind to the **ChoRE** (carbohydrate response element). This promotes transcription of genes resulting in synthesis of enzymes involved in *de novo* lipogenesis: **PFK-1**, **glucose 6-phosphate dehydrogenase**, **pyruvate kinase**, **citrate lyase**, **acetyl CoA carboxylase**, the **enzymes for fatty acid synthesis (fatty acid synthase complex** (see Chapters 27 and 53)) and **acyltransferase**.

Metabolism at a Glance, Fourth Edition. J. G. Salway. © 2017 John Wiley & Sons Ltd. Published 2017 by John Wiley & Sons Ltd.

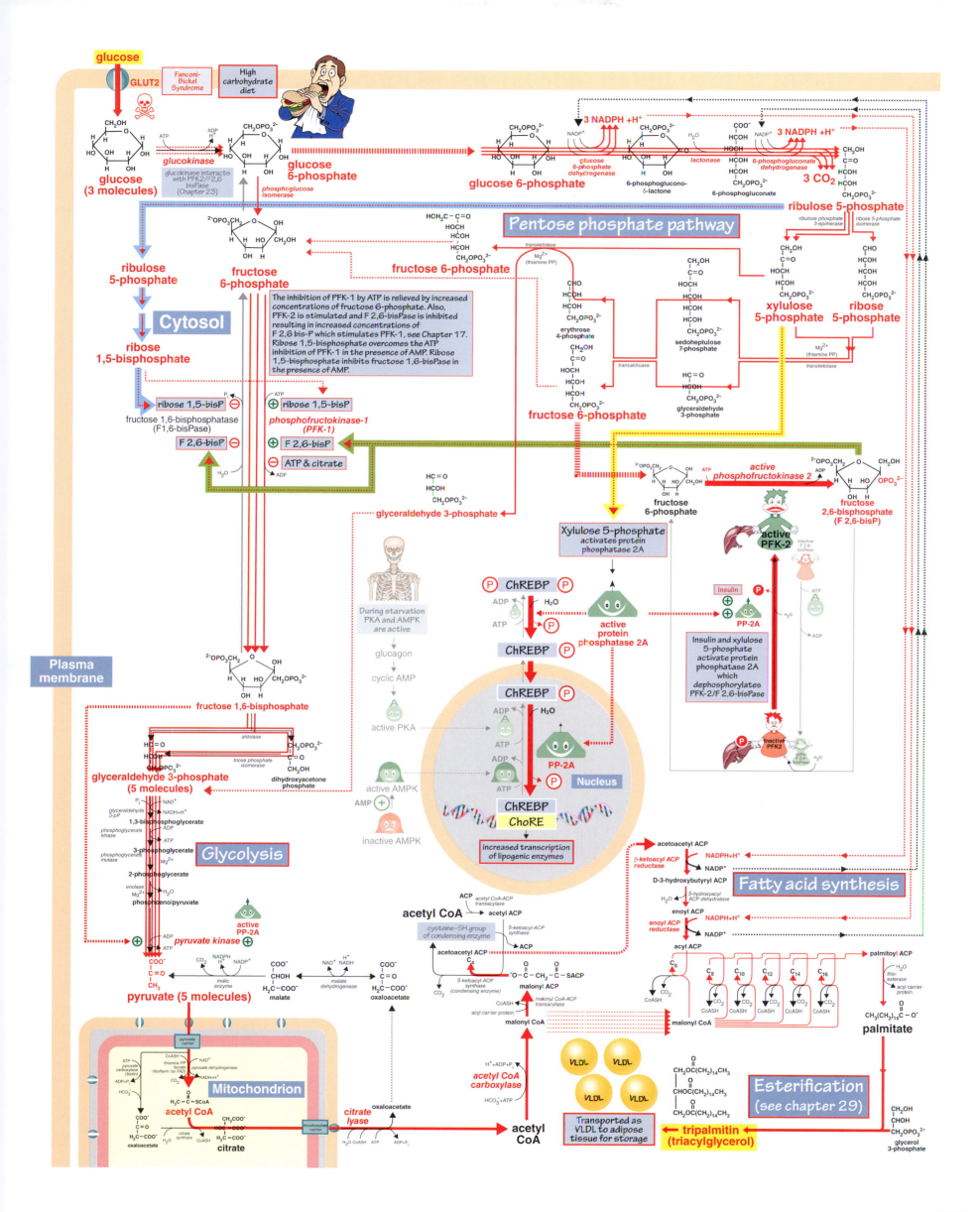

Esterification of fatty acids to triacylglycerol in liver and white adipose tissue

29

Nomenclature comment: 'triacylglycerol' or 'triglyceride'. The term triacylglycerol (TAG) is preferred by chemists and many biochemists, whereas triglyceride is preferred in clinical circles and the USA. Both terms describe the product formed when glycerol is esterified with three fatty acid molecules.

Liver: esterification of fatty acids with glycerol 3-phosphate to form TAG

In Chapter 27 we saw how fatty acids were made from glucose and learned that fatty acids were stored, **not** as fatty acids but that they are esterified with **glycerol 3-phosphate** to form **triacylglycerol**. Thus, the esterification process needs a supply of **fatty acids** and **glycerol 3-phosphate**.

Sources of fatty acids

1 In the **fed state**, fatty acids are synthesised *de novo* from glucose and esterified with **glycerol 3-phosphate** to form **TAG**, which is exported from the liver as VLDL to serve as a fuel for skeletal muscle and heart; and for storage in white adipose tissue (Chart 29.1).

2 An alternative route is *de novo* lipogenesis from amino acids (see Chapter 33).

NB: Liver does not express lipoprotein lipase and so is unable to harvest dietary fatty acids from chylomicrons.

Sources of glycerol 3-phosphate

1 Dietary glucose is metabolized to **glyceraldehyde 3-phosphate**, which is converted to glycerol 3-phosphate (Chart 29.1).

2 Adipose tissue is continually releasing glycerol into the blood **even in the fed state** (see the TAG/fatty acid cycle; Chapter 31). The glycerol goes to the liver where it is phosphorylated to glycerol 3-phosphate by **glycerol kinase** (an enzyme not expressed in adipose tissue).

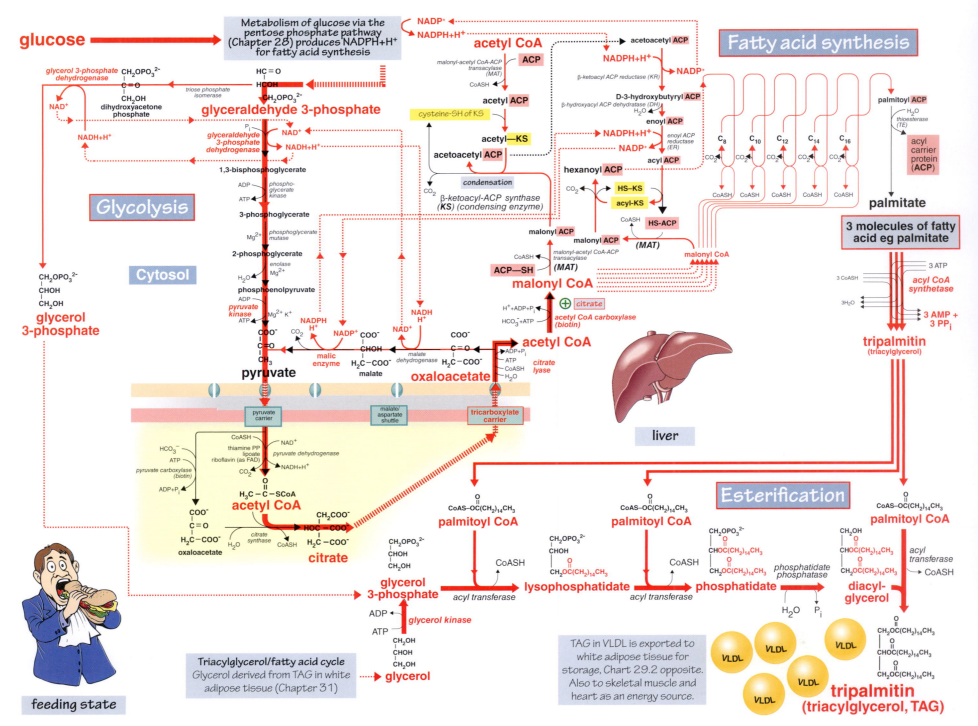

Chart 29.1 *De novo* biosynthesis of fatty acids from glucose, their esterification to TAG and export from liver as VLDL.

Metabolism at a Glance, Fourth Edition. J. G. Salway. © 2017 John Wiley & Sons Ltd. Published 2017 by John Wiley & Sons Ltd.

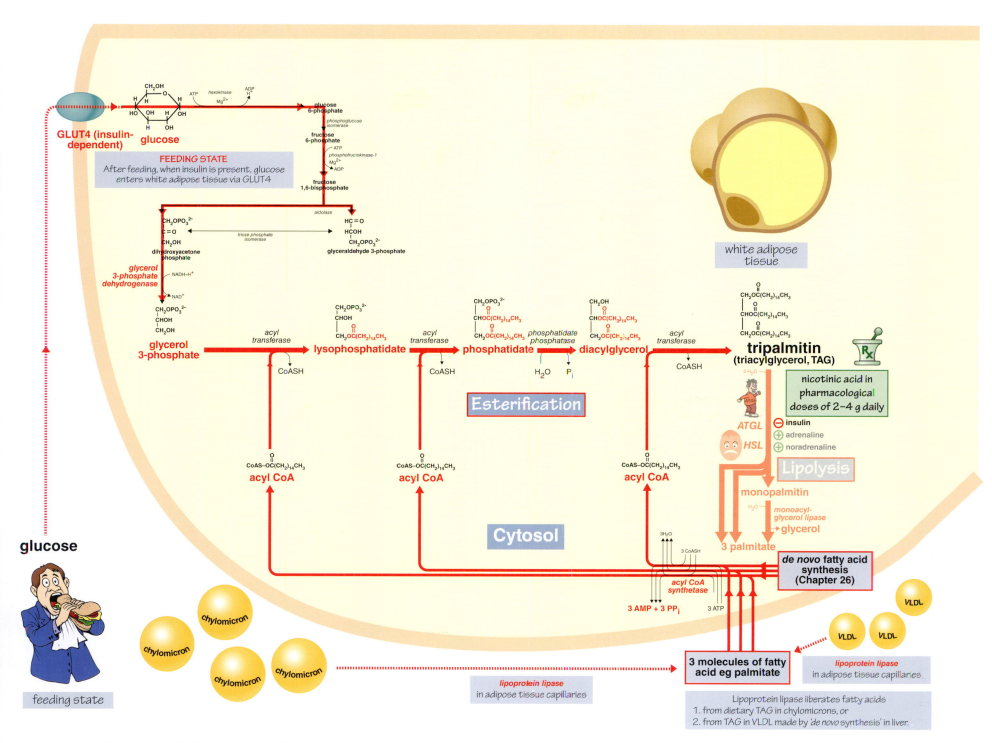

Chart 29.2 Import of dietary fatty acids, their esterification to form TAG and storage in white adipose tissue.

White adipose tissue: esterification and re-esterification of fatty acids with glycerol 3-phosphate to form TAG

Sources of fatty acids

There are four souces of fatty acids:

1 By *de novo* **synthesis** from glucose (not shown in Chart 29.2).

2 From **dietary fatty acids**, which are esterified to TAG in enterocytes and exported from the intestines as **chylomicrons**. In adipose tissue these are hydrolysed by lipoprotein lipase to liberate fatty acids for re-esterification to TAG.

3 From fatty acids made by *de novo* **synthesis** in the liver, esterified and transported as VLDLs to adipose tissue where they are processed by lipoprotein lipase similarly to chylomicrons.

4 Another source of fatty acids is the **triacylglycerol/fatty acid cycle** (see Chapter 31).

Sources of glycerol 3-phosphate

In white adipose tissue there are two sources of glycerol 3-phosphate depending on whether the body is feeding or fasting:

1 **In the fed state** when insulin concentrations are high, adipose tissue is able to take up dietary glucose via the insulin-dependent glucose transporter GLUT4. **Glyceraldehyde 3-phosphate** is produced which is isomerized to dihydroxyacetone phosphate and this is reduced to **glycerol 3-phosphate** (Chart 29.2). **NB:** Glycerol kinase is **not** expressed in white adipose tissue.

2 **During fasting** insulin concentrations are low, so the GLUT4 transporter is not readily available to transport glucose into white adipose tissue for metabolism to glycerol 3-phosphate. Therefore, during fasting, glycerol 3-phosphate is made from amino acids by **glyceroneogenesis** (see Chapter 32).

Mobilization of fatty acids from adipose tissue I: regulation of lipolysis

30

Chart 30.1 (opposite) Regulation of lipolysis in white adipose tissue.

We have seen earlier that when there is an overabundance of fatty acids in the fed state, they are stored as triacylglycerol (TAG) in white adipose tissue (see Chapter 29). During exercise, periods of stress or starvation, the TAG reserves in adipose tissue are mobilized as fatty acids for oxidation as a respiratory fuel. This is analogous to the mobilization of glycogen as glucose units; it occurs under similar circumstances, and is under similar hormonal control.

Fatty acids are a very important energy substrate in red muscle. In liver they are metabolized to the ketone bodies, which can be used as a fuel by muscle and the brain. Because fatty acids are hydrophobic, they are transported in the blood bound to albumin.

Regulation of the utilization of fatty acids occurs at four levels

1 **Lipolysis**, the subject of this chapter, is the hydrolysis of TAG to release free fatty acids and glycerol (Chart 30.1).
2 **Re-esterification.** Recycling of the fatty acids by re-esterification with glycerol 3-phosphate or, alternatively, their mobilization from adipose tissue and release into the blood (see Chapter 31).
3 **Entry into mitochondria.** Transport of the acyl CoA esters into the mitochondrion for β-oxidation (see Chapter 35).
4 **Availability of coenzymes**. The rate of β-oxidation depends on the availability of FAD and NAD⁺ (see Chapter 35).

Lipolysis in white adipose tissue

Lipolysis in adipose tissue involves three lipases acting sequentially (Chart 30.1).
1 First, **adipose triacylglycerol lipase (ATGL)** hydrolyses triacylglycerol to form diacylglycerol.
2 Then, **hormone-sensitive lipase (HSL)** hydrolyses diacylglycerol to form monoacylglycerol.
3 Finally, **monoacylglycerol lipase (MAGL)** hydrolyses monoacylglycerol to form glycerol.

To summarize: hydrolysis of the triacylglycerol tripalmitin produces three molecules of **palmitate** and one molecule of **glycerol**.

Regulation of lipolysis

Lipolysis is stimulated by **adrenaline** during exercise and by **noradrenaline** from noradrenergic nerves (Chart 30.1). The mechanism involves **protein kinase A (PKA)**, as described in Chapter 13, which activates both ATGL and HSL. In addition, in humans, **atrial natriuretic factor (ANF)** released from exercising heart muscle stimulates HSL by a **protein kinase G (PKG)** mediated mechanism (but this does not occur in rodents). Curiously, although **glucagon** stimulates lipolysis *in vitro*, it has no effect *in vivo* in humans.

At the same time, PKA inhibits fatty acid synthesis by phosphorylating serine 77 of acetyl CoA carboxylase-α. Also, **AMP-dependent protein kinase** (Chart 30.1) is activated when it senses the low energy state of the cell prevalent when ATP is hydrolysed to AMP, and phosphorylates serine 79, 1200 and 1215 of acetyl CoA carboxylase.

As a long-term adaptation to prolonged starvation, **cortisol** stimulates the synthesis of HSL, thereby increasing its concentration and activity. Conversely, in the fed state, HSL is inhibited by **insulin**. This occurs when insulin activates cyclic AMP phosphodiesterase-3B which hydrolyses cyclic AMP to AMP.

Regulation of adipose triacylglycerol lipase (ATGL) and hormone-sensitive lipase (HSL)

Fat droplets are globules of TAG surrounded by a protein called **perilipin** (Chart 30.1). Associated with perilipin is a protein, **comparative gene identification 58 (CGI-58)**, which activates **ATGL**. In humans, impaired function of CGI-58 causes the accumulation of TAG (Chanarin–Dorfman syndrome).

As its name suggests, HSL is regulated by hormones. Adrenaline and noradrenaline stimulate the formation of cyclic AMP, which activates **PKA**. PKA polyphosphorylates perilipin, promoting a conformational change that causes CGI-58 to dissociate from perilipin. Then, CGI-58 binds to and thereby activates **ATGL** thus stimulating lipolysis.

In the cytosol, PKA also phosphorylates and activates **HSL**, which facilitates its attachment to the droplet surface for optimal lipolysis. Although phosphorylated HSL is capable of lipolysis by itself, binding to polyphosphorylated perilipin enhances this activity 50-fold, creating **very active HSL**, which is a diacylglycerol lipase (Diagram 30.1).

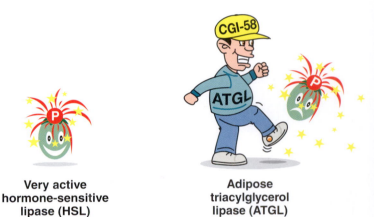

Very active hormone-sensitive lipase (HSL)   **Adipose triacylglycerol lipase (ATGL)**

Diagram 30.1 Adipose triacylglycerol lipase (ATGL): the 'new kid on the block'. Hormone-sensitive lipase (HSL) was first described in adipose tissue in the early 1960s and since then has been the unchallenged principal triacylglycerol lipase in adipose tissue. Consequently, it was a surprise to discover in HSL-knockout mouse models that it was *diacyl*glycerol that accumulated, suggesting HSL is in fact a *diacyl*glycerol lipase. Further research discovered the hitherto unknown **ATGL**. It is now generally accepted that the three lipases **AGTL, HSL and monoacylglycerol lipase (MAGL) work sequentially to liberate fatty acids from triacylglycerol**.

Perilipin and obesity

Perilipin plays an important role in promoting the breakdown and mobilization of fat in adipose tissue. Consequently, an underactive *PERLIPIN* gene has been implicated as a cause of obesity and *PERILIPIN* is one of a few candidates to be dubbed a 'lipodystrophy gene' or 'obesity gene'.

Fatty acid-binding proteins

Fatty acids are detergents. When they are released from TAG as free fatty acids they are toxic and can damage cells. To prevent this they are attached to fatty acid-binding proteins that transport them within the cytosol. Once in the plasma they bind to albumin.

Metabolism at a Glance, Fourth Edition. J. G. Salway. © 2017 John Wiley & Sons Ltd. Published 2017 by John Wiley & Sons Ltd.

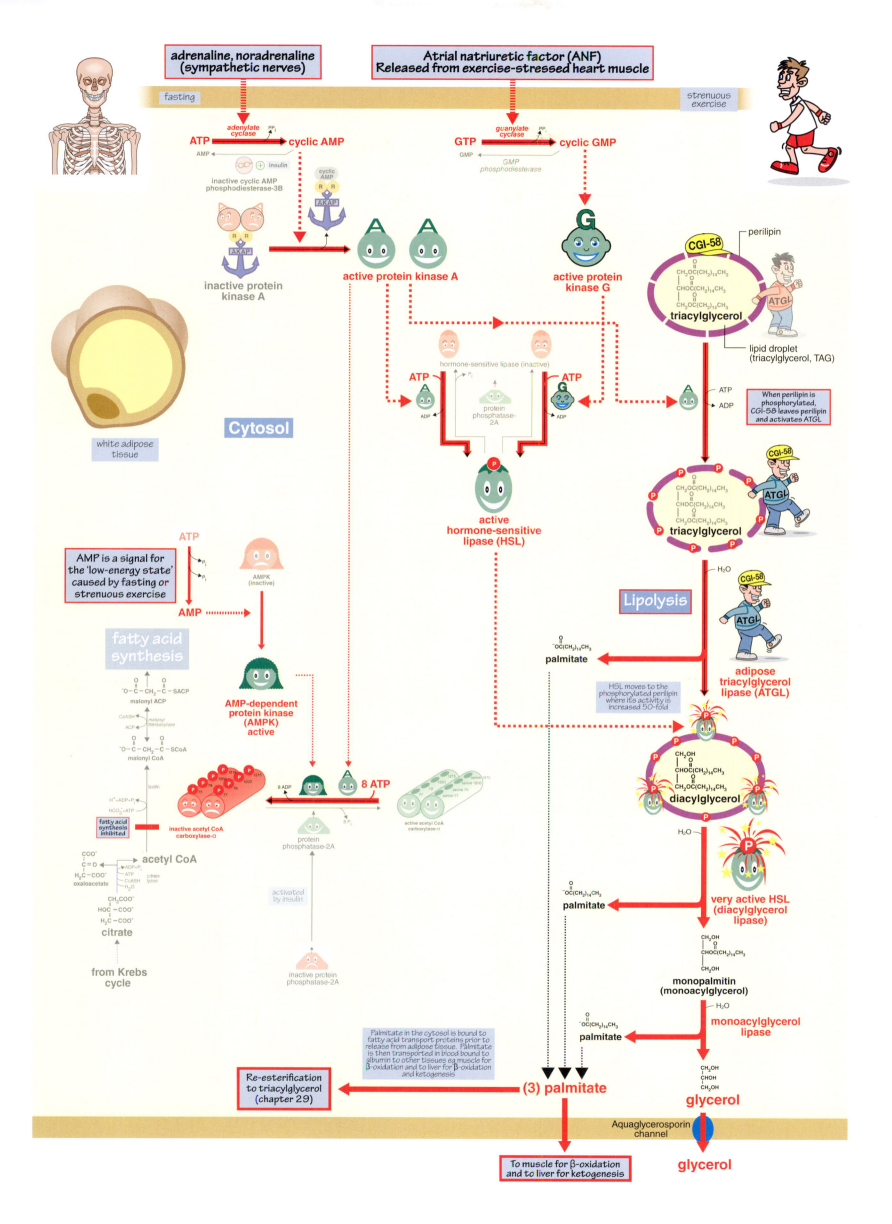

Mobilization of fatty acids from adipose tissue II: triacylglycerol/fatty acid cycle

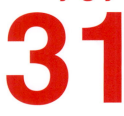

Intuitively, it might be supposed that once fat (**triacylglycerol**) has been deposited in adipose tissue as droplets, it will remain there unchanged until needed as a fuel during starvation or exercise. Surprisingly this is not so. *Triacylglycerol (TAG) molecules are continually hydrolysed to glycerol and fatty acids, only to be re-esterified back to TAGs in what appears to be a futile cycle.* The turnover of TAGs is continuous, irrespective of feeding or fasting. This process has a substantial energy requirement consuming 7 **phosphoanhydride** bonds from four molecules of ATP per cycle.

A futile cycle and waste of ATP? The energy requirement of muscle during strenuous, prolonged exercise can be almost 100-fold greater than at rest. The TAG/fatty acid cycle might appear to be a futile and a profligate waste of energy. However, it ensures a supply of fatty acids is always mobilized and ready-to-go; and this justifies the energy cost.

What is the source of glycerol 3-phosphate in the TAG/fatty acid cycle?

The TAG/fatty acid cycle needs a supply of fatty acids and glycerol 3-phosphate (Chart 31.1). Isotope evidence suggest at least 10% of the fatty acids hydrolysed from TAG are re-esterified to form TAG. However, the extent of re-esterification depends on the nutritional state. **NB: The source of glycerol 3-phosphate also depends on the nutritional state.**

In the fed state, when glucose and insulin are present, glucose uptake into white adipose tissue is facilitated by the insulin-dependent GLUT4 transporters (see Chapter 29) and **glucose is metabolized to form glycerol 3-phosphate**.

During fasting, when insulin levels are low, glucose uptake into cells via GLUT4 transporters is restricted and an alternative pathway for glycerol 3-phosphate production is needed. **Remember, glycerol kinase is not expressed in adipose tissue.** So what is the source of the glycerol 3-phosphate? For decades the answer was fudged (by myself included): for example '*there's sufficient residual insulin activity for glucose uptake to enable glycerol 3-phosphate production by glycolysis*'.

However, back in 1967, Richard Hanson proposed that during fasting, adipose tissue makes glycerol 3-phosphate by a route they called **glyceroneogenesis** in which **amino acids are metabolized to glycerol 3-phosphate**. Incredibly, this pathway has been largely overlooked by biochemists, and this oversight was perpetuated in a debate in the 3rd edition of this book (Diagram 31.1), but is rectified in this new edition (see Chapter 32).

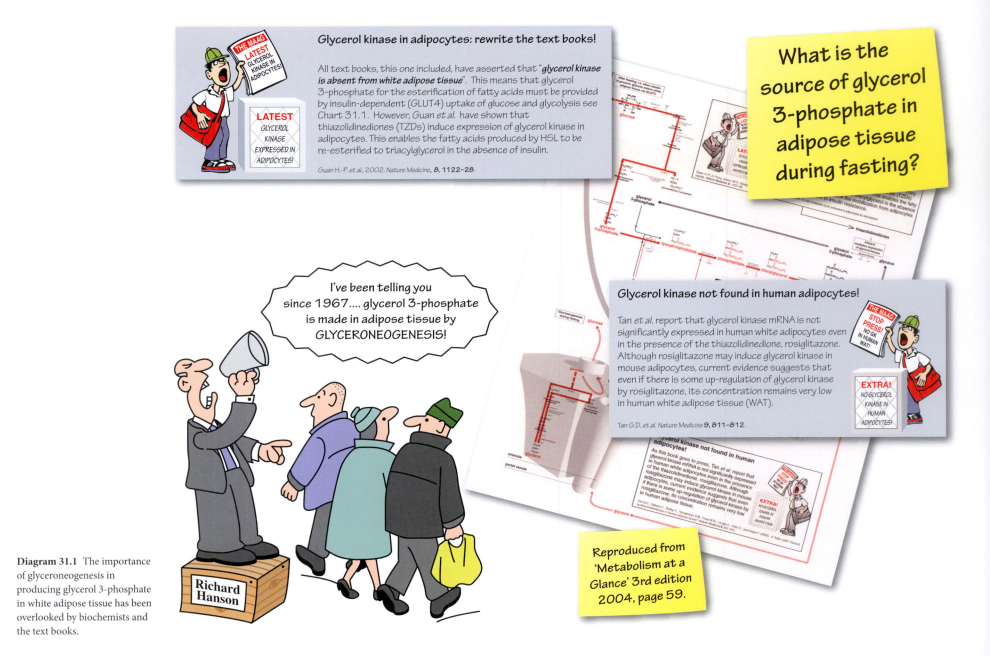

Diagram 31.1 The importance of glyceroneogenesis in producing glycerol 3-phosphate in white adipose tissue has been overlooked by biochemists and the text books.

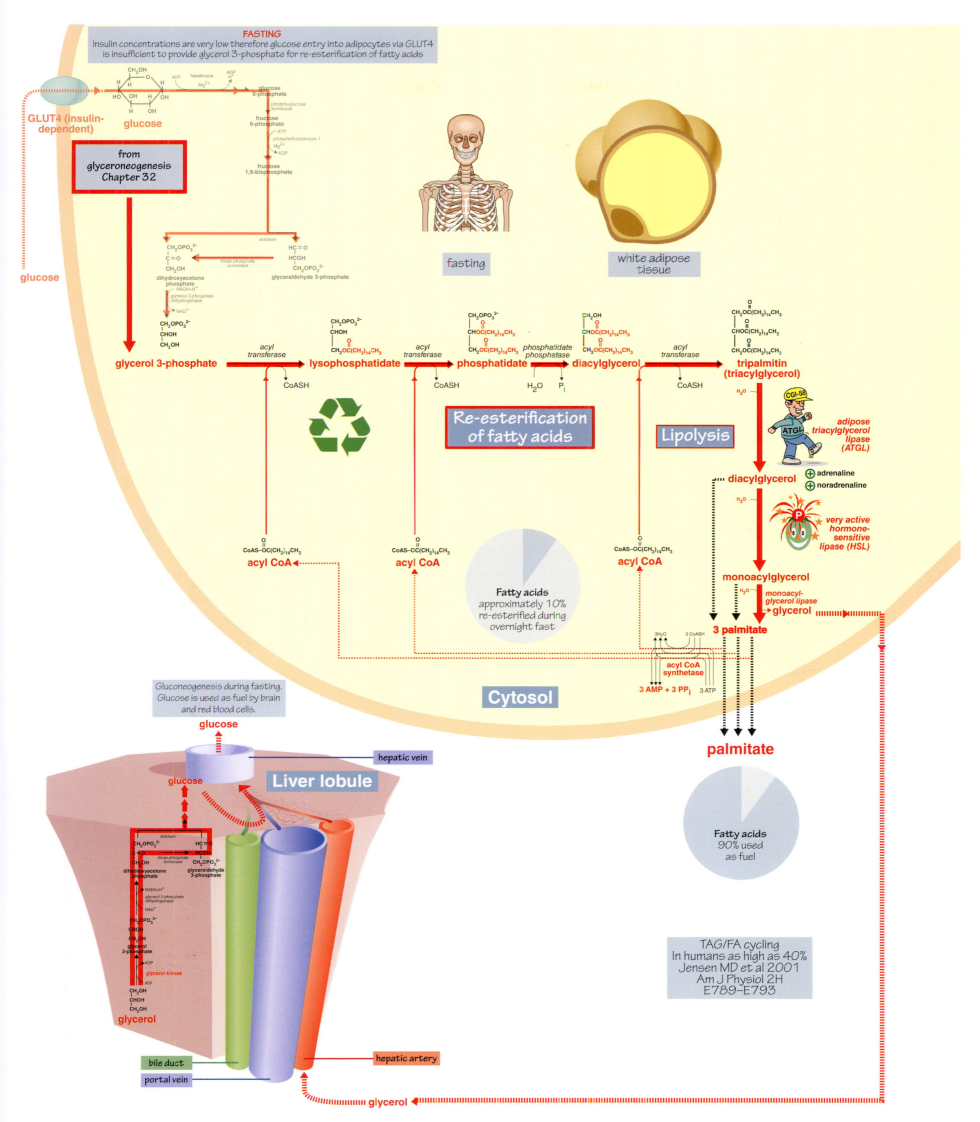

Chart 31.1 The triacylglycerol/fatty acid cycle.

Glyceroneogenesis

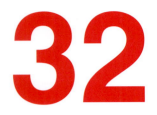

Source of glycerol 3-phosphate for triacylglycerol synthesis

Fatty acids are toxic and must be esterified with **glycerol 3-phosphate** to form triacylglycerol (TAG) (see Chapter 29). **Glycerol 3-phosphate** can be provided in three ways:

1 **Glycerol kinase reaction.** Glycerol kinase can phosphorylate glycerol to form glycerol 3-phosphate. This reaction is restricted to liver and *brown* adipose tissue (see Chapter 29).

2 **From dihydroxyacetone phosphate.** After feeding, glucose metabolism by the **glycolytic pathway** or the **pentose phosphate pathway** forms dihydroxyacetone phosphate, a precursor of glycerol 3-phosphate (see Chapter 29). This process operates in the **fed state** when insulin is available to activate the insulin-dependent glucose transporter GLUT 4.

3 **Glyceroneogenesis**. In contrast to the above, **during fasting**, precursors other than glycerol and glucose can be metabolized by **glyceroneogenesis** to form glycerol 3-phosphate (Chart 32.1).

Glyceroneogenesis is a source of glycerol 3-phosphate

Glyceroneogenesis is the *de novo* biosynthesis of glycerol 3-phosphate from non-glycerol or non-glucose precursors; for example lactate, pyruvate and some of the glucogenic amino acids (see Chapter 33). *Although glyceroneogenesis was first described in 1967 by Richard Hanson and colleagues, its importance has been largely overlooked by the text books.*

The regulatory enzyme for glyceroneogenesis is **phosphoenolpyruvate carboxykinase (PEPCK)**. Most biochemists identify PEPCK exclusively with gluconeogenesis. Indeed, PEPCK plays a crucial role in hepatic and renal gluconeogenesis (see Chapter 18). However, gluconeogenesis does **not** occur in adipose tissue and yet the amount of PEPCK protein expressed in white and brown adipose tissue exceeds that in liver. Why should that be? *It is generally overlooked that PEPCK in adipose tissue provides the glycerol 3-phosphate 'backbone' needed for TAG biosynthesis by the process of glyceroneogenesis.*

Role of glyceroneogenesis in the TAG/fatty acid cycle

In Chapter 31 we saw that TAGs are perpetually being broken down to release fatty acids, with 10% being re-esterified to TAG in a 'futile cycle'. **After feeding**, when insulin concentrations are high, dietary glucose, facilitated by insulin-dependent GLUT4, can be the source of glycerol 3-phosphate (see Chapter 29). However, **during fasting**, when insulin concentrations are very low, glucose entry into adipocytes is restricted and therefore it cannot be the principal precursor of glycerol 3-phosphate. Instead glycerol 3-phosphate is provided by glyceroneogenesis from lactate and glucogenic amino acids (Chart 32.1).

Glyceroneogenesis and type 2 diabetes

White adipose tissue (WAT). In WAT, if PEPCK is experimentally **down-regulated** it may cause type 2 diabetes because the production of glycerol 3-phosphate is decreased, and re-esterification of fatty acids is decreased. Consequently, the TAG/fatty acid cycle is interrupted and the export of fatty acids is increased. Since fatty acids are the preferred fuel for muscle, glucose utilization by muscle is decreased and it accumulates in the blood resulting in hyperglycaemia.

Thiazolidinediones (TZDs). The target for the TZD family of antidiabetic drugs (the 'glitazones', e.g. rosiglitazone) is the peroxisome proliferator-activated receptor, **PPAR-γ**. TZDs are active in WAT and liver where they increase the transcription of PEPCK and stimulate the production of glycerol 3-phosphate. This results in enhanced glyceroneogenesis and increased esterification of fatty acids to TAG. Consequently, the export of fatty acids from WAT into the blood is reduced. Because the blood concentration of fatty acids is decreased, muscle is deprived of fatty acids, which are its preferred fuel. The outcome is that muscle resorts to using glucose as a metabolic fuel and the blood glucose concentration is decreased.

Brown adipose tissue and thermogenesis

Brown adipose tissue (BAT). The expression of PEPCK is much greater in BAT compared with WAT. This is because the primary function of BAT is thermogenesis by uncoupling oxidative phosphorylation (see Chapter 3), which is fuelled by β-oxidation of fatty acids supplied by the TAG/fatty acid cycle. **NB:** The apparently futile cycling of fatty acids by the TAG/fatty acid cycle is an ATP-consuming process that also contributes to thermogenesis.

Effect of cortisol and dexamethasone on PEPCK

NB: In **liver**, PEPCK expression is **increased** by corticosteroids for *gluco*neogenesis (see Chapter 18). Conversely, in **WAT**, corticosteroids **decrease** PEPCK expression, reducing *glycero*neogenesis (Chart 32.1). This *decreases* production of glycerol 3-phosphate, consequently re-esterification of fatty acids is decreased and fatty acids are mobilized from WAT for use as fuel.

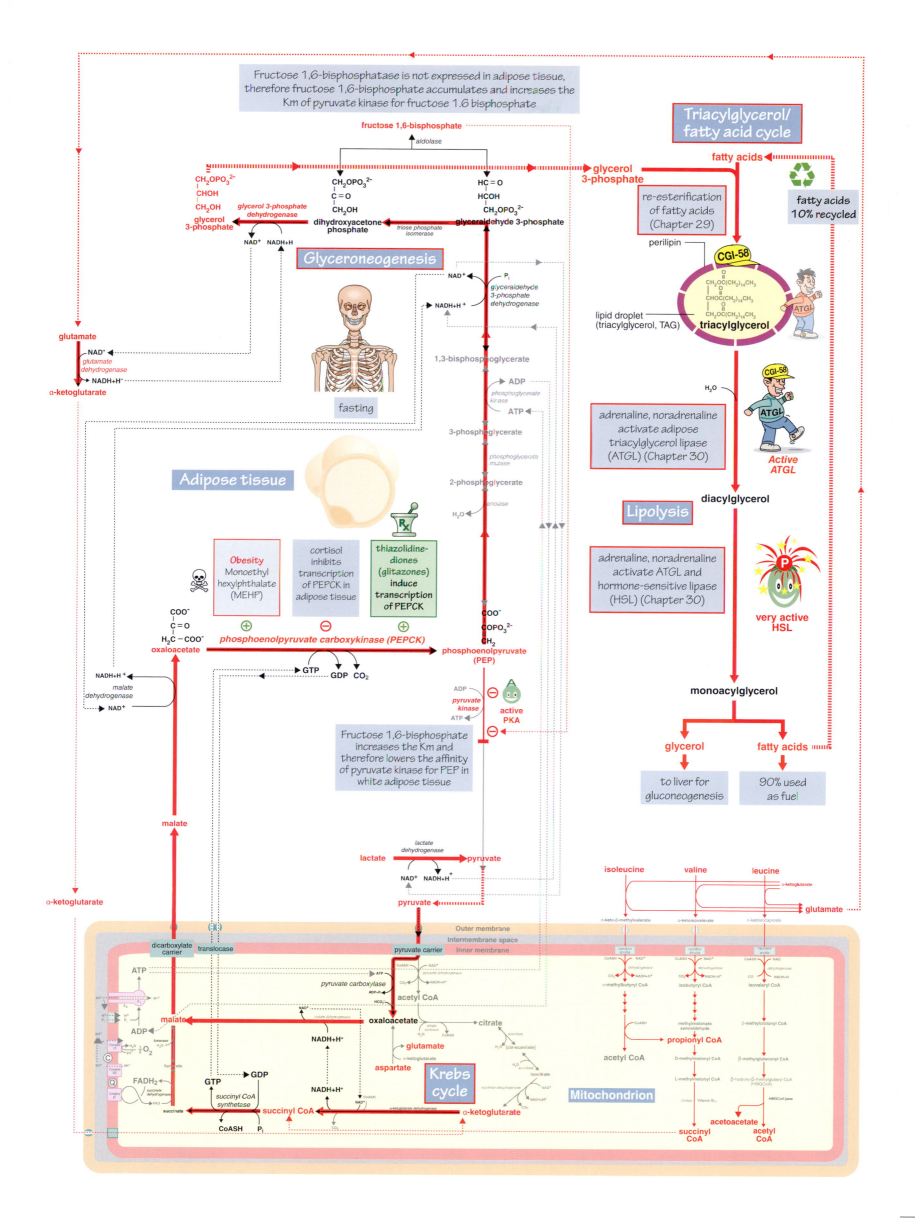

Metabolism of protein to fat after feeding

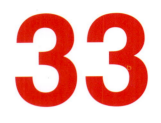
33

In spite of the exhortation by some popular weight-reducing diets to eat large quantities of protein, it should be remembered that surplus dietary protein can be converted to fat. For protein to be converted to **fatty acids** and **triacylglycerols**, the essential precursors for fatty acid synthesis – namely a carbon source, **acetyl CoA**, and biosynthetic reducing power as **NADPH + H⁺** – must be formed. Finally, a source of **glycerol 3-phosphate** is needed to esterify the fatty acids to form triacylglycerol.

Chart 33.1 (opposite) Metabolism of amino acids to fatty acids and triacylglycerol.

Source of acetyl CoA for fatty acid synthesis

Dietary protein is digested by gastric and intestinal proteolytic enzymes to form amino acids. Of these amino acids, glutamine, asparagine, glutamate, aspartate and arginine are to a large extent metabolized within the enterocyte. Glutamine and asparagine are deaminated to glutamate and aspartate, which in turn are transaminated using pyruvate to form alanine and the α-ketoacids: α-ketoglutarate and oxaloacetate. The **alanine** and remaining amino acids are absorbed into the blood and transported to liver.

In liver (with the notable exception of the branched-chain amino acids), transamination with α-ketoglutarate produces glutamate and the corresponding α-ketoacids which are metabolized (see Chart 51.1). The amino nitrogen, carried in the form of glutamate, is detoxified as urea.

The carbon skeletons derived from: alanine, phenylalanine and tyrosine; threonine, cysteine and tryptophan; and proline, histidine and arginine are metabolized eventually to pyruvate (Chart 33.1). Pyruvate enters the mitochondrion and can proceed either via **pyruvate carboxylase** to oxaloacetate, entering the pyruvate/malate cycle (see Chapter 25), or it can be decarboxylated to acetyl CoA by **pyruvate dehydrogenase**.

The ketogenic amino acids (and fragments of the dual glucogenic/ketogenic amino acids), namely threonine, lysine and tryptophan are metabolized to acetyl CoA. **NB:** Although phenylalanine and tyrosine when degraded yield acetoacetate, this cannot be metabolized by the liver and so is likely to be exported for use as fuel (see Chapter 37). Since fatty acid synthesis occurs in the cytosol, acetyl CoA is transported from the mitochondrion to the cytosol by the **pyruvate/malate cycle** (see Chapter 25). Citrate is transported to the cytosol, where it is cleaved by **citrate lyase** to form oxaloacetate and **acetyl CoA**. The **acetyl CoA** is now available for fatty acid synthesis.

Sources of NADPH + H⁺ for fatty acid synthesis

There are three possible sources of NADPH + H⁺. By far the most important is the **cytosolic isocitrate pathway** (Chart 33.1). In rat liver the activity of **cytosolic isocitrate dehydrogenase (ICDH)** is much greater than other sources of NADPH + H⁺. It is 24-fold more active than the **malic enzyme** (pyruvate/malate cycle) and 13 times more active than **glucose 6-phosphate dehydrogenase** (pentose phosphate pathway).

Cytosolic isocitrate pathway

Cytosolic NADP⁺-dependent ICDH is a major producer of NADPH + H⁺ for fatty acid biosynthesis. Transgenic mice that overexpressed cytosolic ICDH developed a fatty liver and became both hyperlipidaemic and obese. It is proposed in Chart 33.1 that whereas citrate must be cleaved by citrate lyase to form acetyl CoA in the cytosol, some of the cytosolic citrate is metabolized by cytosolic aconitase to isocitrate. Then NADP⁺-dependent cytosolic ICDH oxidizes isocitrate to form α-ketoglutarate and NADPH + H⁺ is made available for lipogenesis. The α-ketoglutarate is transaminated to glutamate that enters the mitochondrion for deamination to α-ketoglutarate for metabolism in Krebs cycle. Excess glutamate generated by amino acid transamination is metabolized by glutamate dehydrogenase, liberating the amino group as ammonia, which is detoxified by forming urea.

Pyruvate/malate cycle

Chapter 47 describes the metabolism of amino acids to glucose in the starved state. Furthermore, it is explained that, following refeeding, there is a transitional period during which liver remains in gluconeogenic mode, notwithstanding the fact that it now has an abundant supply of glucose for glycolysis. Moreover, lipolysis and β-oxidation of fatty acids continue during this transition period. However, in due course following refeeding, insulin, which is secreted by the pancreas, gains hormonal dominance, β-oxidation ceases, fatty acids are formed and triacylglycerols are exported as VLDLs.

Insulin activates pyruvate dehydrogenase promoting the oxidative decarboxylation of pyruvate to acetyl CoA and providing a carbon source for lipogenesis. Insulin also inhibits transcription of the **cytosolic PEPCK-C** gene. This leads to decreased cytosolic phosphoenolpyruvate carboxykinase (PEPCK-C) activity, and malate from amino acid precursors cannot be metabolized via **cytosolic** oxaloacetate to phosphoenolpyruvate. Malate takes an alternative route and is oxidatively decarboxylated by the **malic enzyme** to form pyruvate and **NADPH + H⁺**.

Pentose phosphate pathway

In normal diets glucose or fructose are produced as precursors for the pentose phosphate pathway, which can generate NADPH + H⁺ for fatty acid synthesis (see Chapter 15). In real life, it is inconceivable that a diet would be completely devoid of carbohydrates as a source of substrates for the pentose phosphate pathway. *However, in Chart 33.1 the hypothetical scenario of a total lack of glucose and fructose is presumed, consequently the pentose phosphate pathway would not operate and is not shown.*

Sources of glycerol 3-phosphate for the esterification of fatty acids to triacylglycerols

Glyceroneogenesis

In the absence of glucose, glycerol 3-phosphate can be made from nonglucose precursors such as serine, glycine and some of the glucogenic amino acids by **glyceroneogenesis** (Chart 33.1). As mentioned earlier, after feeding, expression of PEPCK-C is inhibited by insulin. An alternative pathway is provided by mitochondrial PEPCK (PEPCK-M) that takes oxaloacetate generated from some glucogenic amino acids and produces phosphoenolpyruvate as a precursor for glycerol 3-phosphate formation.

Glyceraldehyde 3-phosphate

Under typical circumstances when dietary glucose is available, glycolysis and the pentose phosphate pathway will form glyceraldehyde 3-phosphate. This is a precursor of dihydroxyacetone phosphate, which is oxidized to glycerol 3-phosphate. *However, in the unlikely and hypothetical scenario envisaged here of a total lack of glucose and fructose, glycolysis and the pentose phosphate pathway would not operate.*

Glycerol kinase

Glycerol kinase is expressed in liver. However, since its substrate glycerol is supplied from lipolysis of triacylglycerols in white adipose tissue, it is not relevant to lipogenesis from a protein source in the current context.

Reference

Koh H-J., Lee S-M., Son B-J., *et al.* (2004) Cytosolic NADP⁺-dependent isocitrate dehydrogenase plays a key role in lipid metabolism. *J Biol Chem*, **279**, 39968–74.

Metabolism at a Glance, Fourth Edition. J. G. Salway. © 2017 John Wiley & Sons Ltd. Published 2017 by John Wiley & Sons Ltd.

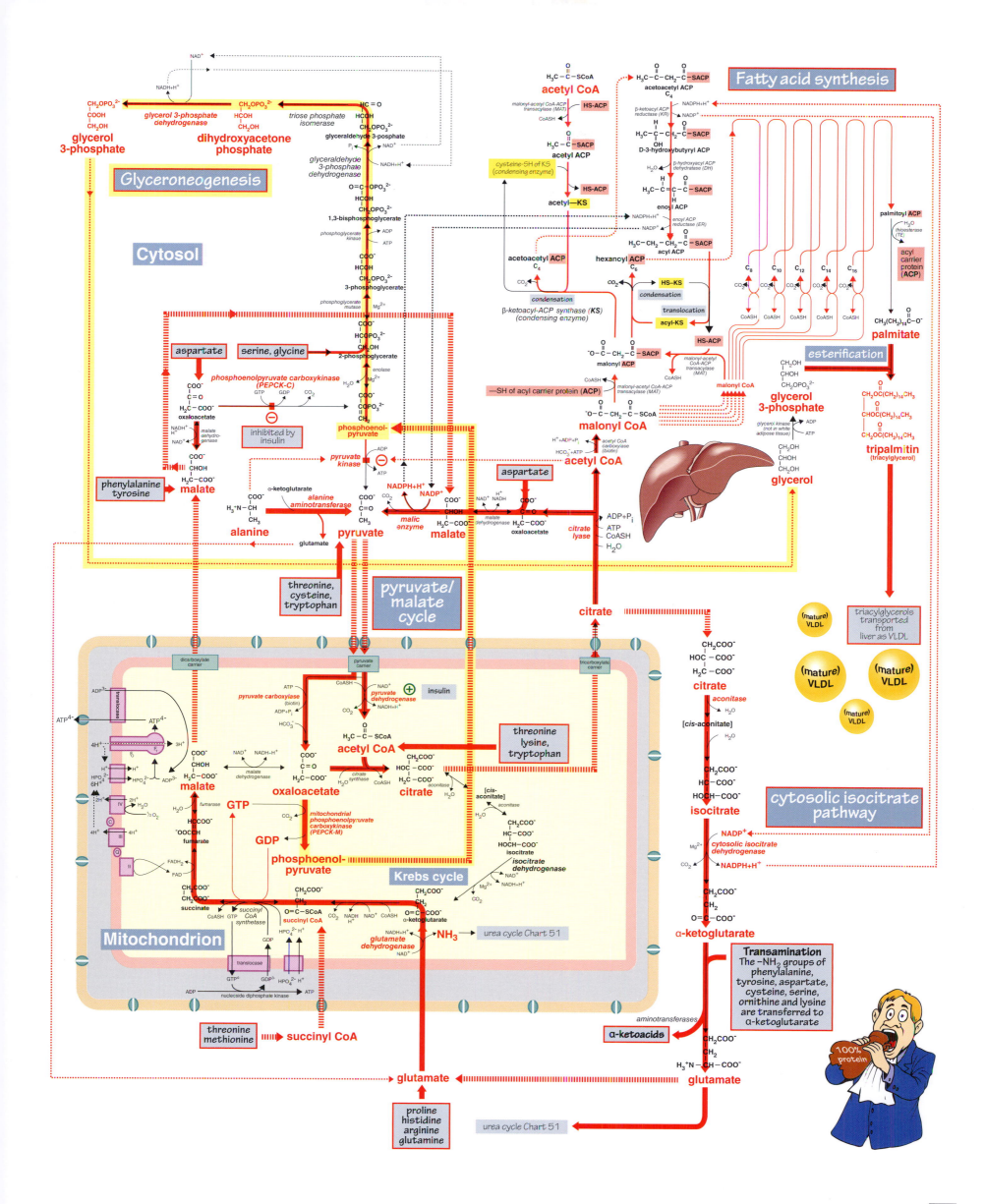

Elongation and desaturation of fatty acids

34

We have seen in Chapter 27 how ($C_{16:0}$) palmitate and ($C_{18:0}$) stearate are formed by the fatty acid synthase complex. These products can be modified in various ways. Additional carbon atoms can be added to form long-chain fatty acids. Alternatively, or as well, fatty acids can be desaturated to yield products with one or more double bonds. The long-chain polyunsaturated fatty acids so formed are used for synthesizing membrane phospholipids and the prostaglandins.

Elongation of fatty acids by the endoplasmic reticulum pathway

An example of chain elongation followed by desaturation is shown in Chart 34.1. Here ($C_{18:3}$) γ-**linolenic acid** is initially lengthened to ($C_{20:3}$) **dihomo-γ-linolenoyl CoA**, which is desaturated to ($C_{20:4}$) **arachidonoyl CoA**.

The endoplasmic reticulum pathway by which fatty acids are elongated is similar to the pathway for fatty acid synthesis described in Chapter 27. The principal differences are:

1 For chain elongation, the two NADPH-dependent **reductase** enzymes and the **dehydratase** are located on the cytosolic surface of the smooth endoplasmic reticulum.
2 Instead of acyl carrier protein (ACP), the intermediates for chain elongation are bound to CoA.
3 The 2-carbon donor is **malonyl CoA** (not malonyl ACP).

Desaturation of fatty acids

Mammals have three desaturases: $Δ^5$-, $Δ^6$- and $Δ^9$-fatty acyl CoA desaturases. These enzymes have a broad chain-length specificity and occur mainly in liver. **NB:** Previous reports of $Δ^4$-desaturase activity are now in doubt (see opposite).

A wide range of different fatty acids can be produced by a combination of the elongation and desaturase reactions. For example, in the chart opposite, $Δ^5$-**desaturase** is used to form **arachidonic acid**, whereas in Diagram 34.1, the $Δ^9$-**desaturase** is shown oxidizing ($C_{16:0}$) palmitoyl CoA to ($C_{16:1}$) palmitoleoyl CoA.

The desaturase system, which is located in the membrane of the smooth endoplasmic reticulum, consists of the **desaturase(s)**, **cytochrome b_5** and **cytochrome b_5 reductase**.

Diagram 34.1 Desaturation of palmitoyl CoA to form palmitoleoyl CoA.

Diagram 34.1: desaturation of palmitoyl CoA to form palmitoleoyl CoA

When palmitoyl CoA is desaturated to palmitoleoyl CoA it should be noted that molecular oxygen is the terminal electron acceptor and that it receives **two** pairs of electrons: one originating from the 9,10 double bond of palmitoyl CoA and the second donated by NADH.

Let us first consider the electrons derived from the 9,10 C–H bond of palmitoyl CoA in the reaction catalysed by $Δ^9$-**desaturase**. The desaturases are enzymes that contain non-haem ferric iron (Fe^{3+}). The electrons reduce two atoms of this to the ferrous (Fe^{2+}) state prior to the electrons being passed on to oxygen, which combines with $2H^+$ to form water.

Next, consider the electrons provided by NADH. A pair of electrons is donated to the FAD prosthetic group of **cytochrome b_5 reductase**, which is consequently reduced to $FADH_2$. The electrons are then accepted by **cytochrome b_5**, which in turn donates the electrons to oxygen, which combines with $2H^+$ to form water.

Elongation of short-chain fatty acids occurs in mitochondria

The mitochondrial pathway for chain elongation is essentially a reversal of β-oxidation with one exception. The last step in elongation, i.e. the reaction catalysed by **enoyl CoA reductase**, requires NADPH for elongation (Chart 34.1), whereas the corresponding enzyme for β-oxidation, acyl CoA dehydrogenase, requires FAD (see Chapter 9). The mitochondrial pathway appears to be important for elongating fatty acids containing 14 or fewer carbon atoms. In Chart 34.1, this is exemplified by the elongation of ($C_{14:0}$) myristoyl CoA to form ($C_{16:0}$) palmitoyl CoA.

Essential fatty acids

As mentioned earlier, higher mammals, including humans, have enzymes capable of desaturating fatty acids at the $Δ^5$, $Δ^6$ and $Δ^9$ positions. However, they are incapable of desaturation beyond the C_9 carbon atom. Nevertheless, certain polyunsaturated fatty acids are vital for maintaining health, in particular the 'n-6 family' members, dihomo-γ-linolenic acid and arachidonic acid. These are 20-carbon chain fatty acids that are precursors of the eicosanoid hormones (Greek *eikosi*: twenty), i.e. the prostaglandins, thromboxanes and leukotrienes, which contain 20 carbon atoms. Accordingly, the n-6 family precursor linoleic acid ($C_{18:2}$, all *cis*-$Δ^{9,12}$), for example, is essential in the diet and is known as an 'essential fatty acid'. After sequential $Δ^6$-desaturation, 2-carbon chain elongation and $Δ^5$-desaturation, linoleic acid is transformed to arachidonic acid.

Evening primrose and starflower oils: 'the elixir of life'?

Normally, given a healthy diet, linoleic acid is an adequate precursor of its family of polyunsaturated fatty acids. There are circumstances, however, possibly including diabetes mellitus, where $Δ^6$-desaturase activity is relatively inactive, which limits the conversion of linoleic acid to dihomo-γ-linolenic acid and arachidonic acid. Although controversial, clinical trials suggest that dietary supplementation with γ-linolenic acid ($C_{18:3}$, all *cis*-$Δ^{6,9,12}$) is beneficial in preventing and minimizing many of the complications of diabetes. Indeed, evening primrose and starflower oils, which are rich in γ-linolenic acid, are currently enjoying a reputation for a wide range of health benefits. As illustrated in Chart 34.1, γ-linolenic acid is independent of $Δ^6$-desaturase in forming the polyunsaturated products, since it requires only elongation and $Δ^5$-desaturation.

Therapeutic benefits of evening primrose oil, starflower oil and fish oils

The γ-linolenic acid in evening primrose oil and starflower oil is, via dihomo-γ-linolenic acid, a precursor of the series 1 prostaglandins. Fish oils are rich in the n-3 fatty acid eicosapentanoic acid (EPA) which is a precursor of the series 3 prostaglandins. It is known that, out of the different prostaglandins, the series 2 prostaglandins have the most potent inflammatory

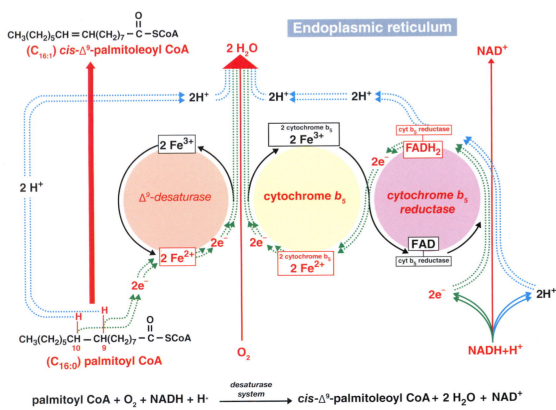

Endoplasmic reticulum

$CH_3(CH_2)_5CH = CH(CH_2)_7 - C - SCoA$
($C_{16:1}$) *cis*-$Δ^9$-palmitoleoyl CoA

$CH_3(CH_2)_5CH - CH(CH_2)_7 - C - SCoA$
($C_{16:0}$) palmitoyl CoA

palmitoyl CoA + O_2 + NADH + H^+ $\xrightarrow{\text{desaturase system}}$ *cis*-$Δ^9$-palmitoleoyl CoA + 2 H_2O + NAD^+

Metabolism at a Glance, Fourth Edition. J. G. Salway. © 2017 John Wiley & Sons Ltd. Published 2017 by John Wiley & Sons Ltd.

effects, sometimes with pathological consequences. Dietary supplementation with γ-linolenic acid or EPA causes proportionally enhanced production of the benign series 1 and 3 prostaglandins, thereby displacing the potent inflammatory effects of the 2 series. Clinical trials with these oils have shown beneficial effects in the treatment of inflammatory diseases such as psoriasis and rheumatoid arthritis.

Is there a Δ⁴-desaturase?

Recent evidence suggests that, contrary to previous dogma, microsomes do not possess Δ^4-desaturase activity. However, Δ^4-desaturation can occur by mystical molecular manoeuvering, meritworthy of a magician. This involves the cooperation of the endoplasmic reticulum and, probably, the peroxisomes. First of all the long-chain fatty acid designated for Δ^4-desaturation is **chain-lengthened by 2-carbon groups**. Cunningly, Δ^6-desaturation then occurs and the Δ^6 very-long-chain fatty acid is exported for partial chain-shortening (2-carbon groups) by peroxisomal β-oxidation. Thus, abracadabra, the resulting fatty acid, having been reduced by two carbons, is now a Δ^4-desaturated fatty acid that is returned to the endoplasmic reticulum for phospholipid synthesis.

Reference

Mohammed B.S., Luthria D.L., Bakousheva S.P., and Sprecher H. (1997) Regulation of the biosynthesis of 4,7,10,13,16-docosapentaenoic acid. *J Biochem*, **326**, 425–30.

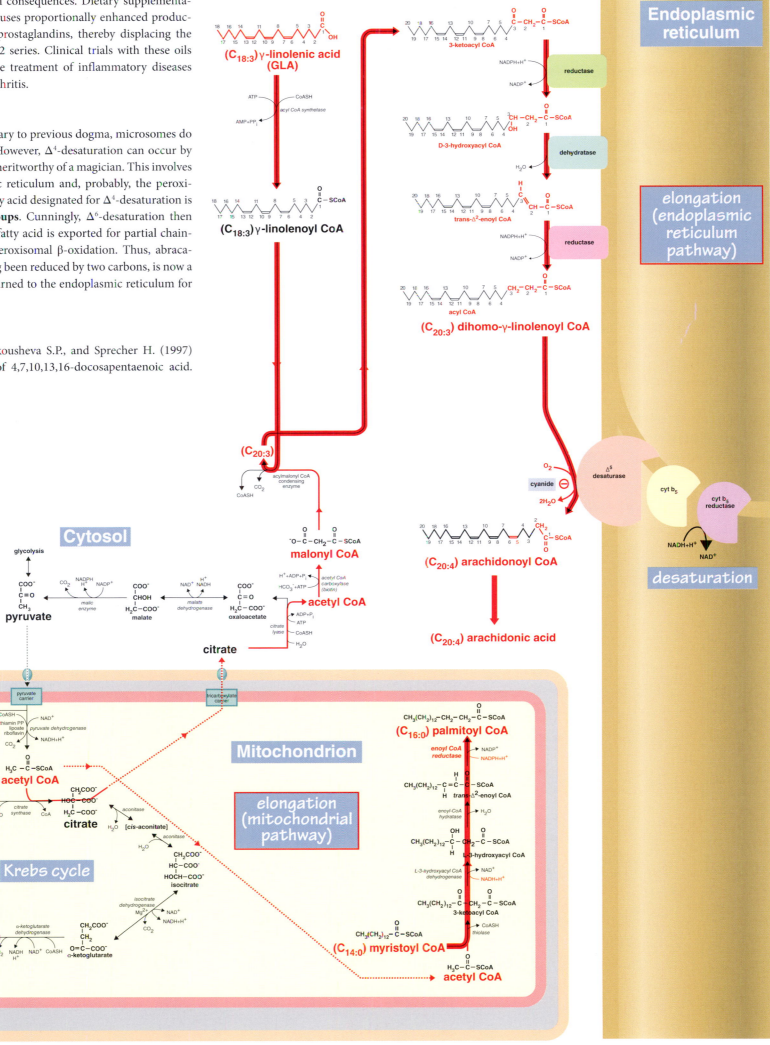

Chart 34.1 Elongation and desaturation of fatty acids.

Fatty acid oxidation and the carnitine shuttle

35

The release of fatty acids from triacylglycerols in adipose tissue is regulated by adipose triacylglycerol lipase and hormone-sensitive lipase (see Chapter 30). The fatty acids, bound to albumin, are then transported to the liver and muscles for utilization. The rate of uptake by these tissues of the fatty acids is proportional to the concentration of the latter in the blood. In all tissues, the rate of β-oxidation is regulated by the availability of coenzyme A, which is regenerated following the utilization of acetyl CoA for ketogenesis in liver, and by citrate synthase in muscle. In liver, β-oxidation is regulated by controlling mitochondrial uptake of fatty acids by the carnitine shuttle. In muscle, an additional regulatory factor is the availability of the coenzymes NAD$^+$ and FAD, which are regenerated from their reduced forms when ATP is produced by oxidative phosphorylation in exercising muscle.

Transport of activated fatty acids into the mitochondrial matrix by the carnitine shuttle is inhibited by malonyl CoA in liver

Fatty acids are activated by long-chain acyl CoA synthetase to form acyl CoA, for example **palmitoyl CoA** (Chart 35.1). A transport system, the **carnitine shuttle**, is needed to enable long-chain fatty acids to cross the inner mitochondrial membrane. **In liver**, this transport is inhibited by **malonyl CoA** (and there is some evidence this may be significant in skeletal muscle and pancreatic β-cells). Since malonyl CoA is produced in liver during fatty acid synthesis, this ensures that the newly formed fatty acids are not immediately transported into the mitochondrion for degradation by β-oxidation.

The carnitine shuttle consists of **carnitine/acylcarnitine translocase** and two **carnitine-palmitoyl transferases (CPTs)**: an outer **CPT I** and an inner **CPT II**. Although not shown in the chart, it is possible that *in vivo* CPT II and membrane-bound very-long-chain acyl CoA dehydrogenase (VLCAD) are contiguous to facilitate substrate channelling.

Availability of the coenzymes FAD and NAD$^+$ for β-oxidation

The various acyl CoA dehydrogenases (see below) need a supply of FAD, which must be regenerated from FADH$_2$ by oxidation via the **electron-transfer flavoprotein (ETF)** and respiratory chain. Likewise, the **3-hydroxyacyl CoA dehydrogenases** of β-oxidation require NAD$^+$ as the coenzyme. However, they have to compete with the three NAD$^+$-dependent dehydrogenases of Krebs cycle for the limited NAD$^+$ available. In exercising muscle when both pathways are highly active, β-oxidation may be limited by the supply of NAD$^+$.

Acyl CoA dehydrogenases

Mitochondria contain four FAD-dependent, acyl CoA dehydrogenases, which act on very-long-, long-, medium- and short-chain fatty acids, although there is some overlap of specificities. These are located in both the matrix and the inner membrane of the mitochondrion.

Very-long-chain acyl CoA dehydrogenase (VLCAD, active with C$_{12}$–C$_{24}$ fatty acids) is situated in the inner membrane. It has an FAD prosthetic group, which is reduced to FADH$_2$ and the electrons transferred to another FAD prosthetic group of the **ETF**, which is a soluble matrix protein (Chart 35.1). The electrons now pass to **ETF:ubiquinone oxidoreductase (ETF:QO)** – an iron-sulphur flavoprotein located in the inner membrane – before passing to ubiquinone (Q) and entering the respiratory chain. *NB: The carnitine shuttle is unable to transport **very-long-chain fatty acids** and so, confusingly, the principal substrates for VLCAD in mitochondria are **long**-chain fatty acids. Oxidation of very-long-chain fatty acids occurs in the peroxisomes* (see Chapter 39).

The other three acyl CoA dehydrogenases, which are located in the matrix, are: **long-chain acyl CoA dehydrogenase (LCAD, C$_8$–C$_{20}$), medium-chain acyl CoA dehydrogenase (MCAD, C$_4$–C$_{12}$)** and **short-chain acyl CoA dehydrogenase (SCAD, C$_4$ and C$_6$)**. **NB**: In humans the function of LCAD is not understood and so it has not been shown in Chart 35.1.

Δ²-Enoyl CoA hydratases

The long-chain hydratase is part of the membrane-bound **trifunctional enzyme**, which is a hetero-octamer of four α- and four β-subunits. The short-chain hydratase (also active with substrates up to C$_{16}$) is located in the matrix.

3-Hydroxyacyl CoA dehydrogenases

There is considerable overlap of specificity between the membrane-bound **long-chain 3-hydroxyacyl CoA dehydrogenase (LCHAD)**, which is part of the α-subunit of the **trifunctional enzyme**, and the matrix **short-chain hydroxyacyl CoA dehydrogenase (SCHAD)**.

3-Oxoacyl CoA thiolases (ketothiolases)

There are three thiolases: (i) a component of the β-subunit of the **trifunctional enzyme**; (ii) a '**general' thiolase** or **medium-chain 3-ketoacylthiolase (MCKAT)** found in the matrix with broad activity covering C$_6$ to C$_{16}$; and (iii) a specific acetoacetyl CoA thiolase.

MCAD and LCHAD deficiency
Sudden infant death syndrome

It is thought up to 3% of cases of sudden infant death syndrome (SIDS) are caused by β-oxidation disorders such as a deficiency of MCAD or LCHAD. In this condition, β-oxidation is restricted and so there is increased oxidation of glucose as a respiratory fuel to meet the demands for energy (see Chapter 6). If the reserves of glycogen become exhausted, this may result in fatal hypoglycaemia.

MCAD deficiency, carnitine deficiency and abnormal metabolites

In MCAD deficiency, there is a tendency for the (C$_{10}$) acyl CoA, (C$_8$) acyl CoA and (C$_6$) acyl CoA intermediates to accumulate. Accordingly, they are diverted in three directions:

1 They can be metabolized by ω-oxidation to form the dicarboxylic acids, sebacic acid, suberic acid and adipic acid.
2 They can be conjugated with carnitine to form carnitine conjugates, which are excreted in the urine. This urinary loss of carnitine conjugates can cause carnitine deficiency. In turn, this impairs fatty acid transport into the mitochondrion thereby further restricting β-oxidation.
3 Suberic acid and hexanoyl CoA can conjugate with glycine to form suberylglycine and hexanoylglycine.

Also, β-oxidation of the unsaturated fatty acid, linoleic acid, produces *cis*-Δ⁴-decenoate, which accumulates in MCAD deficiency (see Chapter 38) and is used diagnostically.

Glutaric acidurias

It is convenient to mention these disorders of amino acid metabolism here because of their link with fatty acid metabolism.

Glutaric aciduria I

This condition is due to a deficiency of glutaryl CoA dehydrogenase causing an increased excretion of glutarate in the urine.

Glutaric aciduria II (multiple acyl CoA dehydrogenase deficiency, MADD)

In this condition, although glutaryl CoA dehydrogenase is normal, the defect is downstream in the flow of reducing equivalents at the level of ETF or ETF:QO. Because these components are essential for the oxidation of numerous acyl CoA intermediates involved in both amino acid and fatty acid metabolism, this condition has also been called multiple acyl CoA dehydrogenase deficiency (MADD). In particular, glutaryl CoA formed from lysine and tryptophan metabolism accumulates if ETF or ETF:QO are deficient, causing glutarate to appear in the urine (Chart 35.1).

Reference

Eaton S., Bartlett K., Pourfarzam M. (1996) Review article: Mammalian β-oxidation. *Biochem J*, **320**, 345–57.

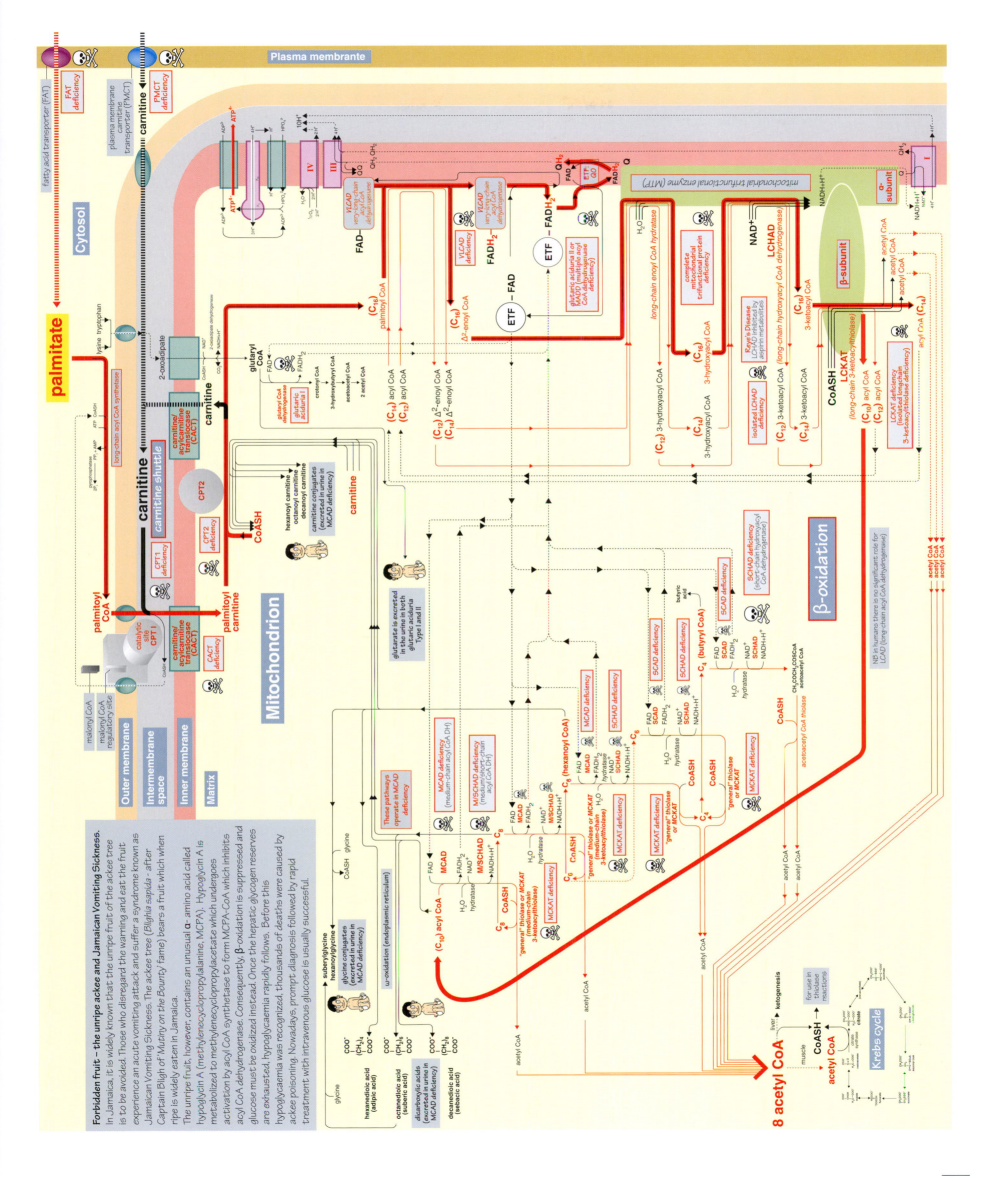

Ketone bodies

36

The misunderstood 'villains' of metabolism

Diabetic patients know that the detection of 'ketone bodies' (namely D-3-hydroxybutyrate, acetoacetate and acetone) in their urine is a danger signal that their diabetes is poorly controlled. Indeed, in severely uncontrolled diabetes, if ketone bodies are produced in massive supranormal quantities they are associated with ketoacidosis. In this life-threatening complication of diabetes mellitus, the acids D-3-hydroxybutyric acid and acetoacetic acid are produced rapidly, causing high concentrations of protons that overwhelm the body's acid–base buffering system, with a consequential dangerous decrease in blood pH. It is this low pH due to the protons that is so harmful, and not the ketone bodies themselves.

Until the mid-1960s, it was thought that ketone bodies were 'metabolic garbage' with no beneficial physiological role. However, it is now realized that, during starvation, the brain uses the ketone bodies as a fuel in addition to its usual fuel glucose. This **regulated and controlled** production of ketone bodies causes a state known as **ketosis**. In ketosis, the blood pH remains buffered within normal limits. This is a very important glucose-sparing (and therefore tissue-protein-conserving) adaptation to starvation that compensates for exhaustion of the glycogen reserves. (It should be remembered that the brain cannot use fatty acids as a fuel.)

Chart 36.1: ketogenesis

During starvation, prolonged severe exercise or uncontrolled diabetes, the rate of production of ketone bodies is increased. The most important precursors for ketogenesis are fatty acids derived from triacylglycerols. However, certain amino acids (leucine, isoleucine, lysine, phenylalanine, tyrosine and tryptophan) are also ketogenic.

Ketogenesis from triacylglycerols

The ketone bodies are produced in liver mitochondria from **fatty acids**, which in turn are produced by the action of **hormone-sensitive lipase** on **triacylglycerols** stored in adipose tissue. The fatty acids are subjected to β-oxidation to form **acetyl CoA**. The interdependent relationship between the pathways for β-oxidation and gluconeogenesis is emphasized in Chapter 18 and illustrated in Chart 36.1, which shows how mitochondrial **oxaloacetate** is diverted towards gluconeogenesis. Hence, oxaloacetate, which is needed by the **citrate synthase** reaction for acetyl CoA to enter Krebs cycle, is directed away from the mitochondrion to the cytosol for gluconeogenesis. Consequently, there is an increased flux of acetyl CoA through **acetoacetyl CoA thiolase** towards ketogenesis.

Ketogenesis involves the **acetoacetyl CoA thiolase** reaction, which combines two molecules of acetyl CoA to form **acetoacetyl CoA**. This in turn is condensed with a third acetyl CoA by **HMG CoA synthase** to form 3-hydroxy 3-methylglutaryl CoA (**HMG CoA**) (Chart 36.1). Finally, HMG CoA is cleaved by **HMG CoA lyase** to form **acetoacetate** and acetyl CoA. The NADH formed by the L-3-hydroxyacyl CoA dehydrogenase reaction of β-oxidation could be coupled to the reduction of acetoacetate to **D-3-hydroxybutyrate**, thereby regenerating NAD+. Acetone is produced by non-enzymic decarboxylation of acetoacetate, and is formed in relatively small proportions compared with the acids.

The rate of ketogenesis is coupled to the supply of fatty acids and the regulation of β-oxidation, as described in Chapters 30 and 35.

The ketone bodies are thought to leave the mitochondrion by a carrier mechanism in exchange for pyruvate.

Ketogenesis from amino acids

Certain amino acids can wholly or partially be used for ketogenesis. The details of these pathways are shown in Chapters 45 and 46. Entry to ketogenesis is at acetyl CoA (isoleucine), acetoacetate (phenylalanine and tyrosine), HMG CoA (leucine) or acetoacetyl CoA (lysine and tryptophan), as outlined in Chart 36.1.

Diagram 36.1: fatty acids are mobilized from adipose tissue for ketogenesis in the liver

In the ketotic state, hormone-sensitive lipase is active and triacylglycerols are hydrolysed to glycerol and fatty acids. The liberated fatty acids leave the adipocyte and diffuse into the blood, where they are bound to albumin and transported to the liver. In the liver, β-oxidation and ketogenesis occur. The 'ketone bodies' acetoacetate and D-3-hydroxybutyrate that are produced are exported as fuel for tissue oxidation, especially by muscle and the brain.

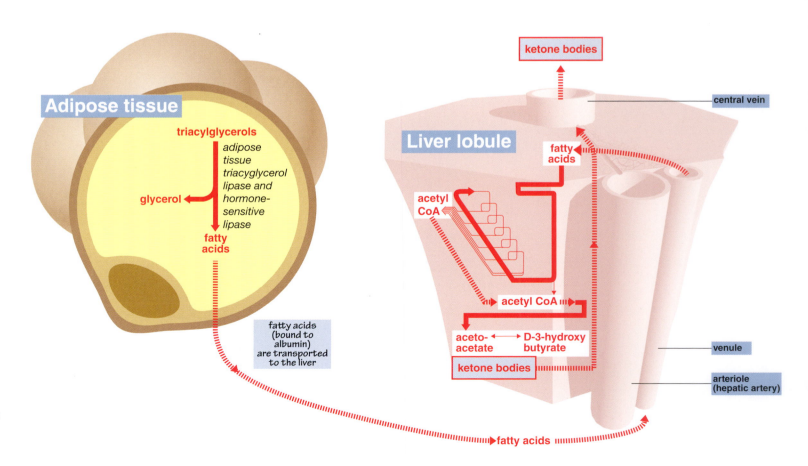

Diagram 36.1 Fatty acid mobilization from adipose tissue for ketogenesis in the liver.

Metabolism at a Glance, Fourth Edition. J. G. Salway. © 2017 John Wiley & Sons Ltd. Published 2017 by John Wiley & Sons Ltd.

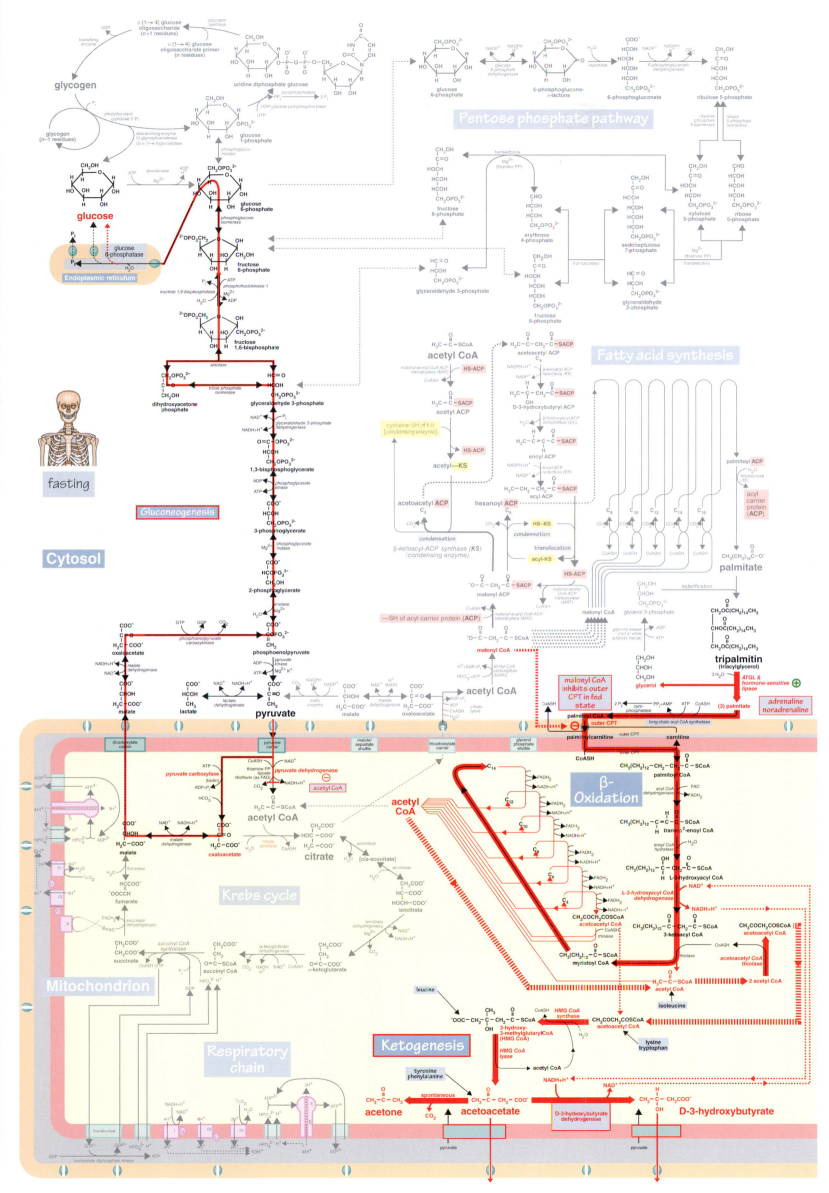

Chart 36.1 Ketogenesis.

Ketone body utilization

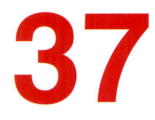

Chart 37.1 (opposite) Ketone body utilization.

Ketone bodies are an important fuel for the brain during starvation

The brain has an enormous need for respiratory fuel, each day requiring approximately 140 g of glucose, which is equivalent to nearly 600 kcal (2510 kJ) (it should be remembered that the brain cannot use fatty acids as a fuel). The large quantities of ATP produced are needed by the sodium pump mechanism, maintaining the membrane potentials, which in turn are essential for the conduction of nerve impulses. Clearly, to stay alive, the brain must be supplied with respiratory fuel at all times!

During starvation, once the glycogen reserves are exhausted, the rate at which ketone bodies are produced from fatty acids by the liver is increased so they can be used by tissues, but particularly the brain, to generate ATP. Consequently, the use of glucose as a fuel by the brain is considerably reduced. The advantage of switching to ketone bodies for energy is because, during starvation, glucose is obtained by gluconeogenesis from muscle protein. This causes wasting of the muscles and so the 'glucose-sparing' effect of the ketone bodies is an important adaptation to the stress of starvation.

Chart 37.1: utilization of ketone bodies

The ketone bodies are first converted to acetyl CoA, which can then be oxidized by Krebs cycle. The enzymes needed are **D-3-hydroxybutyrate dehydrogenase, 3-ketoacyl CoA transferase** and **acetoacetyl CoA thiolase**. It should be noted that the 3-ketoacyl CoA transferase is not found in liver. Consequently, liver is unable to use the ketone bodies as respiratory fuel. On the other hand, although several tissues are capable of ketone utilization – notably muscle and kidney – ketone bodies are particularly important as a fuel for brain and other nerve cells during starvation.

As illustrated in Chart 37.1, D-3-hydroxybutyrate dehydrogenase is bound to the inner mitochondrial membrane, where it catalyses the formation of acetoacetate from D-3-hydroxybutyrate. Then, in the presence of 3-ketoacyl CoA transferase, CoA is transferred from succinyl CoA to form acetoacetyl CoA. Subsequently, in the presence of CoA and acetoacetyl CoA thiolase,

acetoacetyl CoA is cleaved to yield two molecules of acetyl CoA for oxidation in Krebs cycle.

ATP yield from the complete oxidation of D-3-hydroxybutyrate

NB: The calculation below uses the 'non-integral' values for P/O ratios (see Chapter 3). The oxidation of D-3-hydroxybutyrate generates two molecules of acetyl CoA, which yield a net total equivalent to 21.25 molecules of ATP as follows:

	ATP yield
D-3-hydroxybutyrate dehydrogenase	
1 NADH	2.5
Krebs cycle	
6 NADH	15
2 FADH$_2$	3
Succinyl CoA synthetase (via GTP)	1
But 1 H$^+$ is used by the phosphate carrier	
This is equivalent to loss of 0.25 ATP	−0.25
Total	**21.25 ATP**

Similarly, acetoacetate can generate a total equivalent to 18.75 molecules of ATP.

It should be noted that one of the pair of succinyl CoA molecules is temporarily diverted from Krebs cycle for the 3-ketoacyl CoA transferase reaction, where it 'activates' acetoacetate. This energy is therefore not available for ATP synthesis. The succinate liberated is, however, free to return to Krebs cycle for further oxidation.

In comparison with glucose, the ketone bodies are a very good respiratory fuel. Whereas 100 g of glucose generates 8.7 kg of ATP, 100 g of D-3-hydroxybutyrate can yield 10.5 kg ATP, and 100 g of acetoacetate produces 9.4 kg of ATP.

Diagram 37.1 Generalized scheme representing the delivery of glucose and ketone bodies to nerve cells. The relationship of a capillary to a non-myelinated and a myelinated axon are shown. Electron microscopy has demonstrated that, in myelinated axons, small clusters of mitochondria occur at the node of Ranvier. It is most probable that in myelinated axons the glucose transporters will also be located at these nodes, which are very metabolically active. On the other hand, in non-myelinated axons, mitochondria and glucose transporters are probably distributed uniformly along the length of the axon. In both types of axon, glucose and the ketone bodies diffuse from the capillary, through the axolemma (via the GLUT3 glucose transporter) and into the axoplasm for metabolism.

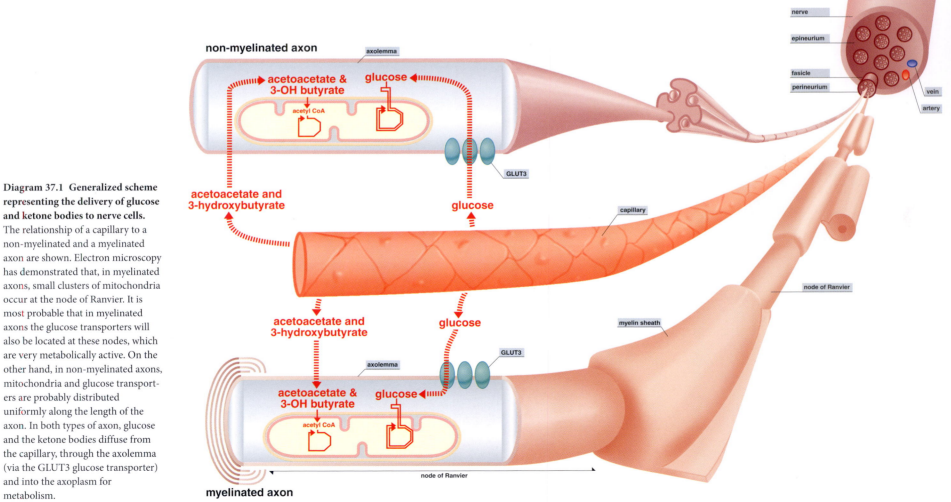

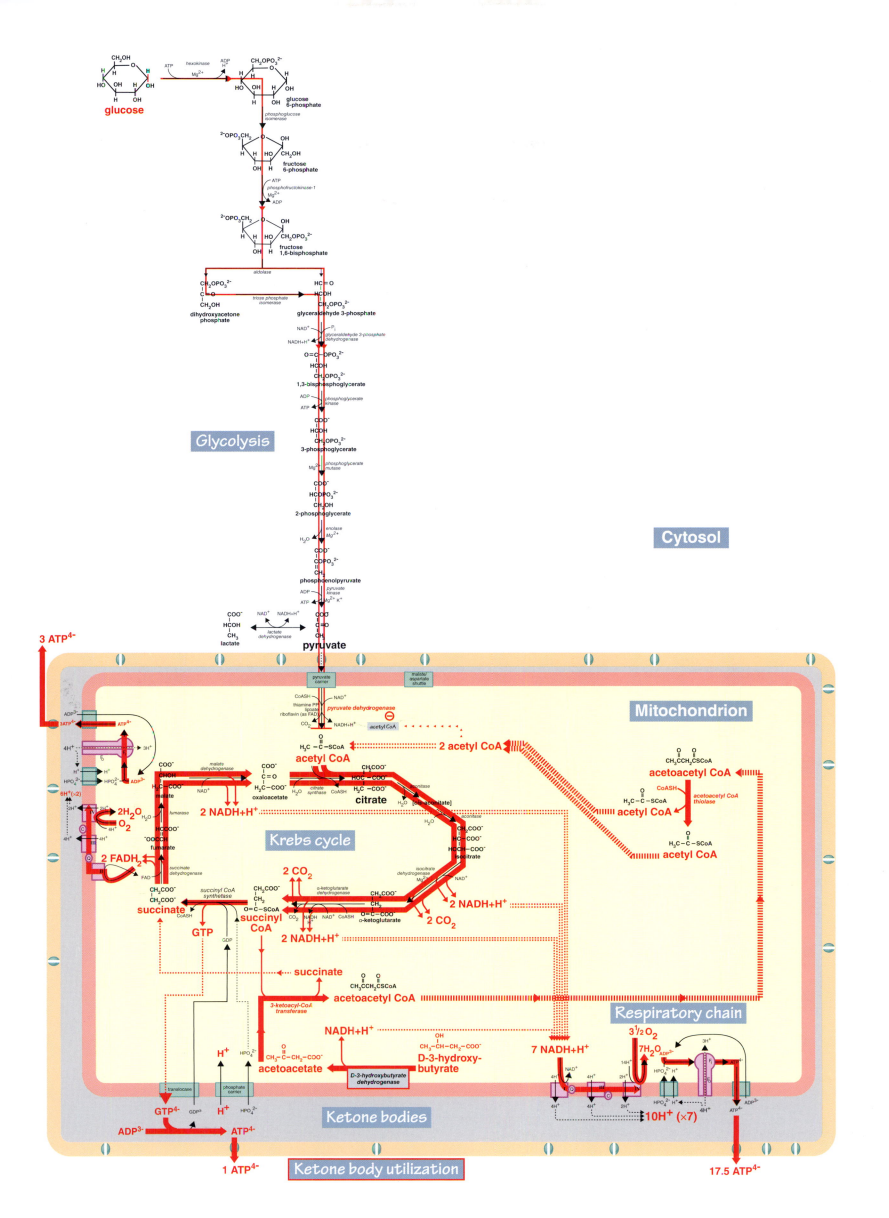

β-Oxidation of unsaturated fatty acids

38

The naturally occurring unsaturated fatty acids have double bonds in the ***cis***-configuration, but β-oxidation, as described in Chapter 9, produces intermediates with the ***trans***-configuration. This stereoisomeric complication means that β-oxidation of unsaturated fatty acids requires two additional enzymes: **3,2-enoyl CoA isomerase** and **2,4-dienoyl CoA reductase**.

Chart 38.1: β-oxidation of linoleic acid

The β-oxidation of the polyunsaturated fatty acid linoleic acid is illustrated in Chart 38.1, which demonstrates the similarities and differences in comparison with the saturated fatty acid derivative palmitoyl CoA (see Chart 9.1 and Chapter 35). The oxidation of unsaturated fatty acids is relatively slow compared with saturated fatty acids because the former are transported slowly into mitochondria by the **carnitine shuttle** (see Chapter 35).

Cycles 1–3

The first three cycles of β-oxidation, whereby linoleate ($C_{18:2}$) is shortened to dodecadienoyl CoA ($C_{12:2}$) via $C_{16:2}$ and $C_{14:2}$, are identical to the reactions for saturated fatty acids described in Chapters 9 and 35.

Cycle 4 requires 3,2-enoyl CoA isomerase (*cis*-Δ^3 [or *trans*-Δ^3] → *trans*-Δ^2-enoyl CoA isomerase)

The all *cis*-$C_{12:2}$ product (*cis*-Δ^3-*cis*-Δ^6-dodecadienoyl CoA) is not a substrate for enoyl CoA hydratase. The enzyme 3,2-enoyl CoA isomerase catalyses conversion of the *cis*-Δ^3 double bond to a *trans*-Δ^2 double bond. The hydration of the resulting *trans*-Δ^2-enoyl CoA is mediated by enoyl CoA hydratase. The dehydrogenase and thiolase reactions subsequently produce ($C_{10:1}$) *cis*-Δ^4-decenoyl CoA and acetyl CoA.

Cycle 5 requires both a 'novel' reductase and the isomerase

Cycle 5 begins with ($C_{10:1}$) *cis*-Δ^4-decenoyl CoA, which is oxidized as usual by acyl CoA dehydrogenase. However, the *cis*-Δ^4 double bond of the *trans*-Δ^2-*cis*-Δ^4 product inhibits the hydratase reaction. The enzyme **2,4-dienoyl CoA reductase** catalyses the reduction of this metabolite by NADPH to form the *trans*-Δ^3-enoyl CoA intermediate. This is then isomerized by the versatile 3,2-isomerase, which changes the *trans*-Δ^3- to the *trans*-Δ^2-enoyl CoA form, which is a substrate for enoyl CoA hydratase. The usual sequence of β-oxidation reactions catalysed by the dehydrogenase and thiolase then produce ($C_{8:0}$) octanoyl CoA.

Cycles 6–8

Since ($C_{8:0}$) octanoyl CoA is fully saturated, it is oxidized by the familiar β-oxidation pathway to yield acetyl CoA.

What about the epimerase reaction?

Several textbooks describe the need for a '3-hydroxyacyl CoA epimerase' in the pathway for the β-oxidation of unsaturated fatty acids. This is because it used to be thought that enoyl CoA hydratase added water across a *cis*-Δ^2 double bond to form the D-isomer of hydroxyacyl CoA, i.e. not the L-isomer

Diagram 38.1 Fatty acid nomenclature. NB: Although the compounds shown could exist in theory, relatively few are known to occur in nature except as metabolic intermediates.

		Prefix											Suffix
Number of carbon atoms present		C_6	C_8	C_{10}	C_{12}	C_{14}	C_{16}	C_{18}	C_{20}	C_{22}	C_{24}	C_{26}	
	nil	hexan...	octan...	decan...	dodecan...	tetradecan...	hexadecan...	octadecan...	eicosan...	docosan...	tetracosan...	hexacosan...	**...oic**
	1	hexen...	octen...	decen...	dodecen...	tetradecen...	hexadecen...	octadecen...	eicosen...	docosen...	tetracosen...	hexacosen...	**...oic**
Number of carbon-to-carbon double-bonds present	2	hexa...	octa...	deca...	dodeca...	tetradeca...	hexadeca...	octadeca...	eicosa...	docosa...	tetracosa...	hexacosa...	**...dienoic**
	3		octa...	deca...	dodeca...	tetradeca...	hexadeca...	octadeca...	eicosa...	docosa...	tetracosa...	hexacosa...	**...trienoic**
	4			deca...	dodeca...	tetradeca...	hexadeca...	octadeca...	eicosa...	docosa...	tetracosa...	hexacosa...	**...tetraenoic**
	5				dodeca...	tetradeca...	hexadeca...	octadeca...	eicosa...	docosa...	tetracosa...	hexacosa...	**...pentaenoic**
	6					tetradeca...	hexadeca...	octadeca...	eicosa...	docosa...	tetracosa...	hexacosa...	**...hexaenoic**

Identification of carbon atoms

Numbering from carboxyl carbon atom	10	9	8	7	6	5	4	3	2	1
Greek letters	ω				ε	δ	γ	β	α	
Numbering from ω carbon atom	ω1	ω2	ω3	ω4	ω5	ω6				
Numbering from n carbon atom (methyl group)	n-1	n-2	n-3	n-4	n-5	n-6				

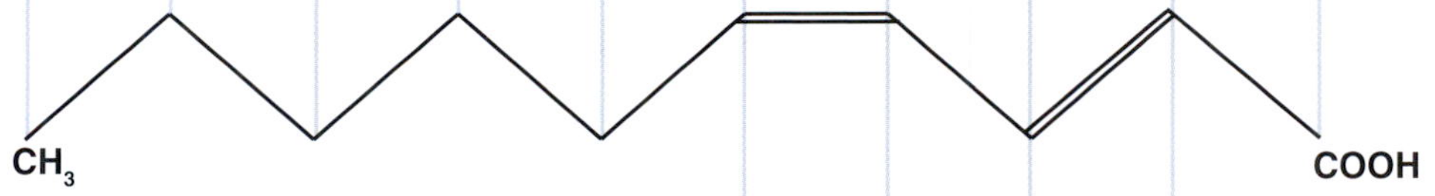

Identification of double bonds

Double bonds. Symbolized by Δ and superscript representing position		Δ^4-		Δ^2-
ω-family. Indicates position of double bond from the methyl end	ω6			
n-family. Indentical to above — a more modern convention	n-6			
Isomeric form. *cis-* or *trans-* (the convention preferred by biochemists)	*cis-*		*trans-*	
or, *Z* or *E* (the convention preferred by chemists)	*Z*		*E*	

Summary

The fatty acid shown above is named as follows:
Length of carbon chain is **10** carbon atoms, $C_{10:}$
There are two **2** carbon-to-carbon double-bonds present. $C_{10:2}$
Hence the above example is a $C_{10:2}$ unsaturated fatty acid, namely ***trans*-Δ^2-, *cis*-Δ^4-decadienoic acid**
which is a **n-6** (or alternatively **ω6**) unsaturated fatty acid.
NB: This is not a common, naturally occurring fatty acid. However, its thioester with CoA is formed during the β-oxidation of linoleic acid (see Chart opposite)

Confusion! *The* α*- and* γ*- prefixes of* α*- and* γ*-linolenate are* ***not*** *based on the above conventions.*

Metabolism at a Glance, Fourth Edition. J. G. Salway. © 2017 John Wiley & Sons Ltd. Published 2017 by John Wiley & Sons Ltd.

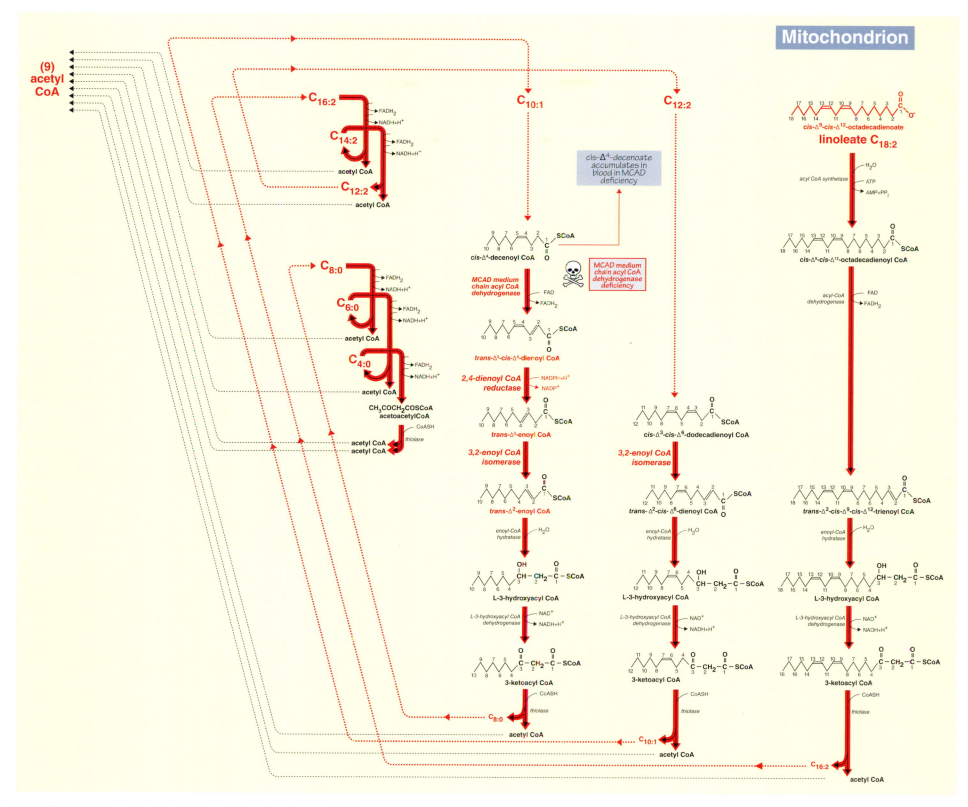

Chart 38.1 β-Oxidation of linoleic acid (C$_{18:2}$n-6). In medium-chain acyl CoA dehydrogenase (MCAD) deficiency, *cis*-Δ^4-**decenoate** accumulates in the blood, and the finding of increased levels in a patient is used in the diagnosis of this condition (see Chapter 35).

needed for L-3-hydroxyacyl CoA dehydrogenase. The epimerase was thought to be needed to invert the configuration of the hydroxyl group at C$_3$ from the D-isomer to the L-isomer, thereby providing a suitable substrate for the L-3-hydroxyacyl CoA dehydrogenase.

Current opinion is that the epimerase is not in the mitochondria but is instead found in the peroxisomes. Indeed, this 'epimerase' activity

is due to the reactions of two distinct 2-enoyl CoA hydratases in peroxisomes.

Fatty acid nomenclature

This is complicated and a knowledge of Greek helps. The various elements involved in the naming of fatty acids are summarized in Diagram 38.1.

Peroxisomal β-oxidation

39

Mitochondria are not the only location for β-oxidation

The pathway for the β-oxidation of fatty acids was once thought to be restricted exclusively to mitochondria. However, mammalian peroxisomal β-oxidation of fatty acids was confirmed in 1976 by Lazarow and de Duve. Peroxisomal β-oxidation occurs in both liver and the kidney. It is now thought that approximately 90% of short- and medium-chain fatty acids are oxidized in the mitochondria, whilst approximately 10% are oxidized in the peroxisomes in the basal state. However, under conditions of induced proliferation of the peroxisomes, whether by drugs (e.g. clofibrate) or a high-fat diet, the relative importance of peroxisomal β-oxidation is substantially increased.

Whereas the structural changes in the metabolic intermediates formed during β-oxidation are chemically identical in both the peroxisomes and mitochondria, different and distinct enzymes are involved in the two organelles. Peroxisomal β-oxidation is more versatile than the mitochondrial pathway. It can metabolize a wide variety of fatty acid analogues, notably dicarboxylic acids and branched-chain fatty acids (see Chapters 40 and 41), also bile acid precursors and prostaglandins. An important function of peroxisomal β-oxidation is for chain-shortening of very-long-chain fatty acids (VLCFAs) (i.e. C_{22} and longer) in preparation for their subsequent oxidation by mitochondria. It should be noted that VLCFAs cannot enter mitochondria by the carnitine shuttle.

Chart 39.1: chain-shortening of very-long-chain fatty acids by peroxisomal β-oxidation

The distinguishing features of peroxisomal β-oxidation can be seen in the chart, using $C_{26:0}$ **cerotate** as an example:

1 **Activation.** A **very-long-chain acyl CoA synthetase**, which is located on the cytosolic side of the peroxisomal membrane, activates the fatty acid to form **cerotoyl CoA**.
2 **Transport across the peroxisomal membrane.** The peroxisomal membrane contains a **transporter protein ABCD1**, which enables the ceratoyl CoA to cross it by active transport.
3 **Oxidation of fatty acids.** In peroxisomes, the first oxidation step is catalysed by the FAD-containing enzyme **acyl CoA oxidase**. NB: This reaction, in which the electrons are passed directly to oxygen, is insensitive

to the respiratory chain inhibitor, cyanide (see Chapter 3). The hydrogen peroxide formed is broken down to water and oxygen in the presence of **catalase**. Note also that, in contrast to mitochondrial β-oxidation which employs FAD-dependent acyl CoA dehydrogenase, ATP is not formed in peroxisomes at this stage and instead the energy is dissipated as heat.
4 **Bifunctional enzyme.** The bifunctional enzyme has both **enoyl CoA hydratase** and **L-3-hydroxyacyl CoA dehydrogenase** activity. The dehydrogenase forms NADH which, unlike in the mitochondrial situation, is not used for ATP synthesis. Instead it is oxidized by **monodehydroascorbate reductase**, a transmembrane cytochrome b561 haem-containing protein, and NAD⁺ is regenerated.
5 **Peroxisomal β-ketothiolase.** This enzyme forms the chain-shortened fatty acyl CoAs and acetyl CoA.

Products of peroxisomal β-oxidation

The products of chain-shortening are **acetyl CoA** and the newly formed acyl CoA (i.e. palmitoyl CoA, as shown in Chart 39.1). The precise details of their subsequent fate are not yet clear. In principle, both of these could leave the peroxisome unchanged, or they could be hydrolysed by peroxisomal hydrolase to acetate, or to their free acyl derivatives. Another possibility is that acylcarnitine might be formed in the peroxisome prior to export to the mitochondria for further β-oxidation. Because of this uncertainty, the representation in the chart should be regarded as a simplification.

Peroxisomal β-oxidation of unsaturated fatty acids

The mitochondrial β-oxidation of unsaturated fatty acids is described in Chapter 38. However, there is now evidence that suggests that some unsaturated fatty acids are readily metabolized by peroxisomal β-oxidation. Accordingly, peroxisomes have a **2,4-dienoyl CoA reductase**. They also have **3,2-enoyl CoA isomerase** and $\Delta^{3,5}, \Delta^{2,4}$ **dienoyl CoA isomerase** activities.

X-linked adrenoleukodystrophy and Lorenzo's oil

X-linked adrenoleukodystrophy (X-ALD) is a degenerative neurological disease caused by mutations of the *ABCD1* gene that codes the **peroxisomal**

Diagram 39.1 Nomenclature of some naturally occurring fatty acids.

Saturated

Notional name	Systematic name	Common name	
$C_{6:0}$	hexanoic acid	caproic acid	Latin *caper* goat
$C_{8:0}$	octanoic acid	caprylic acid	Latin *caper* goat
$C_{10:0}$	decanoic acid	capric acid	Found in butter, coconut oil etc
$C_{12:0}$	dodecanoic acid	lauric acid	Found in berries of laurel
$C_{14:0}$	tetradecanoic acid	myristic acid	*Myristica* : nutmeg tree (found in nutmeg oil etc.)
$C_{16:0}$	hexadecanoic acid	palmitic acid	Found in palm oil
$C_{18:0}$	octodecanoic acid	stearic acid	Greek *stear* fat
$C_{20:0}$	eicosanoic acid	arachidic acid	Arachis : peanut
$C_{22:0}$	docosanoic acid	behenic acid	In oil of ben, seed oil of the horse-radish tree, *Moringa pterygospermum*
$C_{24:0}$	tetracosanoic acid	lignoceric acid	Latin *lignum* wood (found in beech-wood tar)
$C_{26:0}$	hexacosanoic acid	cerotic acid	Greek *keros* wax
$C_{28:0}$	octacosanoic acid	montanic acid	In montan wax (extracted from lignite)

Unsaturated

Notional name	Systematic name	Common name	
$C_{4:1}$	*trans*-Δ^2-tetraenoic acid	crotonic acid	Greek *kroton* castor-oil plant
$C_{16:1}$ n−7	*cis*-Δ^9-hexadecenoic acid	palmitoleic acid	Palm oil
$C_{18:1}$ n−9	*cis*-Δ^9-octadecenoic acid	oleic acid	Latin *oleum* oil
$C_{18:1}$ n−7	*cis*-Δ^{11}-octadecenoic acid	vaccenic acid	Latin *vacca* cow (in beef fat)
$C_{18:2}$ n−6	all *cis*-$\Delta^{9,12}$-octadecadienoate	linoleic acid	Latin *linum* flax, and *oleum* oil (in linseed oil etc)
$C_{18:3}$ n−3	all *cis*-$\Delta^{9,12,15}$-octadecatrienoic acid	α-linolenic acid	
$C_{18:3}$ n−6	all *cis*-$\Delta^{6,9,12}$-octadecatrienoic acid	GLA (γ-linolenic acid)	GLA (Found in evening primrose oil)
$C_{20:1}$ n−9	*cis*-Δ^{11}-eicosenoic acid	gondoic acid	
$C_{20:4}$ n−6	all *cis*-$\Delta^{5,8,11,14}$-eicosatetraenoic acid	arachidonic acid	*Arachis* : peanut
$C_{20:5}$ n−3	all *cis*-$\Delta^{5,8,11,14,17}$-eicosapentaenoic acid	EPA (timnodonic acid)	Eicosapentaenoic acid (found in fish oil)
$C_{22:1}$ n−9	*cis*-Δ^{13}-docosenoic acid	erucic acid	Latin *eruca* cabbage (in seed oil of *Cruciferae* : mustard, rape etc)
$C_{22:5}$ n−3	all *cis*-$\Delta^{7,10,13,16,19}$-docosapentaenoic acid	clupanodonic acid	*Clupeidae* herring (found in fish oil)
$C_{22:6}$ n−3	all *cis*-$\Delta^{4,7,10,13,16,19}$-docosahexaenoic acid	DHA (cervonic acid)	Docosahexaenoic acid (found in fish oil)

Metabolism at a Glance, Fourth Edition. J. G. Salway. © 2017 John Wiley & Sons Ltd. Published 2017 by John Wiley & Sons Ltd.

ATP-binding cassette transporter (ABCD1). The ABCD1 transporter is a protein dimer located in the peroxisomal outer membrane that actively transports the CoA thioesters of VLCFAs ($C_{22:0}$–$C_{26:0}$) into the matrix of the peroxisome for β-oxidation. ATP is consumed in the process. ABCD1 was previously called the adrenal leucodystrophy protein, (ALDP). A dysfunctional ABCD1 transporter results in accumulation of VLCFAs especially $C_{26:0}$ (cerotic acid) in the tissues and plasma.

ABCD3, another member of the transporter family, transports VLCFAs but at only 2% of the rate of ABCD1 and so is unable to compensate in X-ALD.

X-ALD attracted public attention when Lorenzo Odone featured in the film *Lorenzo's Oil* released in 1993 by Universal Studios. The remarkable perseverance of his parents, Augusto and Michaela Odone, led to the formulation of 'Lorenzo's oil' which is a 4:1 mixture of glyceryl trioleate ($C_{18:1}$) and glyceryl trierucate ($C_{22:1}$). Lorenzo's oil has been used to treat X-ALD since the early 1990s but has never been subjected to investigation by rigorous clinical trials. Consequently, although Lorenzo's oil is not the treatment of choice for X-ALD, its potential therapeutic benefits for some patients can neither be confirmed nor disproved.

When X-ALD patients were given a diet low in VLCFAs, surprisingly plasma $C_{26:0}$ fatty acids did not decrease. This was due to a compensatory increase in *de novo* synthesis via chain-elongation (see Chapter 34) which probably explains why $C_{22:0}$ (behenic acid) does not accumulate in X-ALD.

It is now known that VLCFA can be metabolized by the **ω-oxidation pathway** (see Chapter 41). The initial reactions are catalysed by cytochrome P450 enzymes. The dicarboxyl VLCFAs so formed are readily oxidized by β-oxidation. Pharmacological intervention by inducing the cytochrome P450 enzymes offers a therapeutic strategy by stimulating the catabolism of VLCFAs by ω-oxidation, which serves as a rescue pathway (see Chapter 41).

Reference

Wanders R.J.A., Komen J., Kemp S. (2010) Fatty acid ω-oxidation as a rescue pathway for fatty acid oxidation disorders in humans. *FEBS J*, 278, **182**–94.

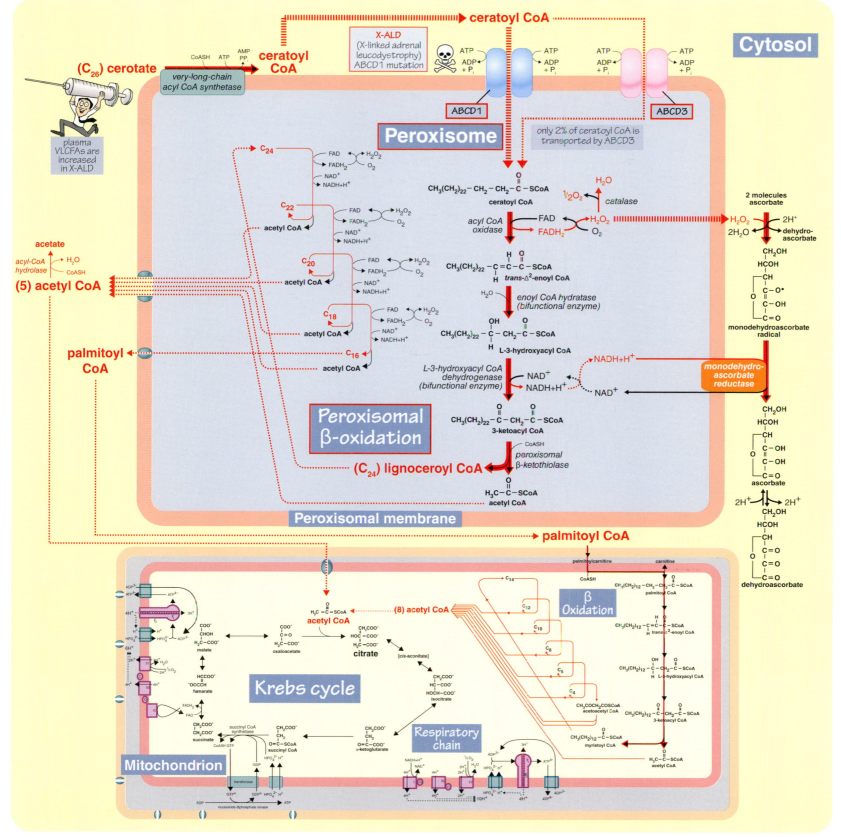

Chart 39.1
Peroxisomal β-oxidation of cerotic acid.

α- and β-oxidation

40

Phytol metabolism

Phytol is a component of the chlorophyll molecule. Bacterial action in the rumen of ruminants liberates phytol from chlorophyll and this is metabolized to phytanic acid. However, in the human intestines, phytol remains attached to chlorophyll and cannot be absorbed. The human diet contains some phytol but its contribution to the production of phytanic acid is not known.

Dietary phytanic acid (3,7,11,15-tetramethylhexadecanoic acid)

In humans, the daily consumption of phytanic acid is about 50–100 mg. Dairy products and fats derived from grazing animals, especially cows fed silage, are rich in phytanic acid. Other significant sources are fish, fish oils and vegetable oils.

α-Oxidation of phytanic acid to pristanic acid

Phytanic acid cannot be oxidized by the **fatty acid β-oxidation pathway** because of a methyl group on the β- (i.e. 3-) carbon atom. Accordingly, prior to β-oxidation, the terminal carbon (C1) must be removed by **α-oxidation** in the **peroxisomes** to form **pristanic acid**, 2,6,10,14-tetramethylhexadecanoic acid. The result is that a methyl group is now on carbon **2** so the 3- (i.e. β-) position is free for the β-oxidation of **pristanoyl CoA** to proceed.

Phytanic acid combines with CoASH to form phytanoyl CoA, which is 2-hydroxylated by **phytanoyl CoA 2-hydroxylase (PAHX)** to form **2-hydroxyphytanoyl CoA**. The C1 terminal carbon is removed as formic acid by **2-hydroxyphytanoyl CoA lyase**. The resulting **pristanal** is dehydrogenated to **pristanic acid** by what is thought to be an $NAD(P)^+$-dependent **fatty aldehyde dehydrogenase (FALDH)**, but this is controversial.

α-Methylacyl CoA racemase

Pristanic acid is activated to **pristanoyl CoA**, which is a racemic mixture of the (**2S**)- and (**2R**)-epimers (Chart 40.1). The (2R)-epimer cannot be used for β-oxidation and is converted to the (2S)-epimer by **α-methylacyl CoA racemase (AMACR)**, which is located in both peroxisomes and mitochondria.

AMACR overexpression. AMACR (known to oncologists as **P504S**) is overexpressed in tumours, especially prostatic carcinoma. Antibodies to AMACR are used to reveal prostatic carcinoma in biopsy tissue.

AMACR deficiency. A deficiency of AMACR in humans is associated with adult-onset sensory motor neuropathy and with liver dysfunction in infants. AMACR also converts C27 bile acyl CoAs between their (2R)- and (2S)-stereoisomers during the metabolism of bile salts.

β-Oxidation of fatty acids

Most β-oxidation of long-chain fatty acids occurs in the mitochondria. However, the **peroxisomes** have a vital function in the β-oxidation of: (i) **very-long-chain fatty acids** (see Chapter 39); (ii) **branched-chain fatty acids** such as the CoASH thioester of pristanic acid; and (iii) **fatty dicarboxylic acids** (formed by ω-oxidation, see Chart 41.1). In both mitochondria and peroxisomes, β-oxidation of fatty acids is a long, complicated metabolic pathway involving numerous specific enzymes. Nevertheless, each oxidative cycle involves the following reactions: (i) FAD-linked dehydrogenation; (ii) hydration; (iii) NAD^+-linked dehydrogenation; and (iv) thiolytic cleavage.

β-Oxidation of pristanoyl CoA. The first three β-oxidation cycles occur in the **peroxisome**. The medium-chain fatty acyl CoA so formed, **4,8-dimethylnonanoyl CoA**, leaves the **peroxisome** and is transported to the **mitochondria** for a further three cycles of β-oxidation.

The process of β-oxidation in both the peroxisomes and the mitochondria produces a total of **3 acetyl CoA**, **3 propionyl CoA** and one molecule of **isobutyryl CoA**.

Refsum's disease (also known as adult Refsum's disease (ARD))

Deficiency of **phytanoyl CoA 2-hydroxylase** results in **Refsum's disease**, which is characterized by the accumulation of phytanic acid. Phytanic acid also accumulates, albeit to a lesser extent, in peroxisome biogenesis disorders such as neonatal adrenoleukodystrophy, infantile Refsum's disease, rhizomelic chondrodysplasia punctata type 1 and Zellweger's syndrome, in which peroxisomes are absent.

A potential treatment for Refsum's disease (and other disorders of fatty acid metabolism such as X-linked adrenoleukodystrophy, see Chapter 39) is by stimulating the **ω-oxidation pathway** to remove phytanic acid in an alternative catabolic route described as a 'rescue pathway' (see Chapter 41).

Metabolism at a Glance, Fourth Edition. J. G. Salway. © 2017 John Wiley & Sons Ltd. Published 2017 by John Wiley & Sons Ltd.

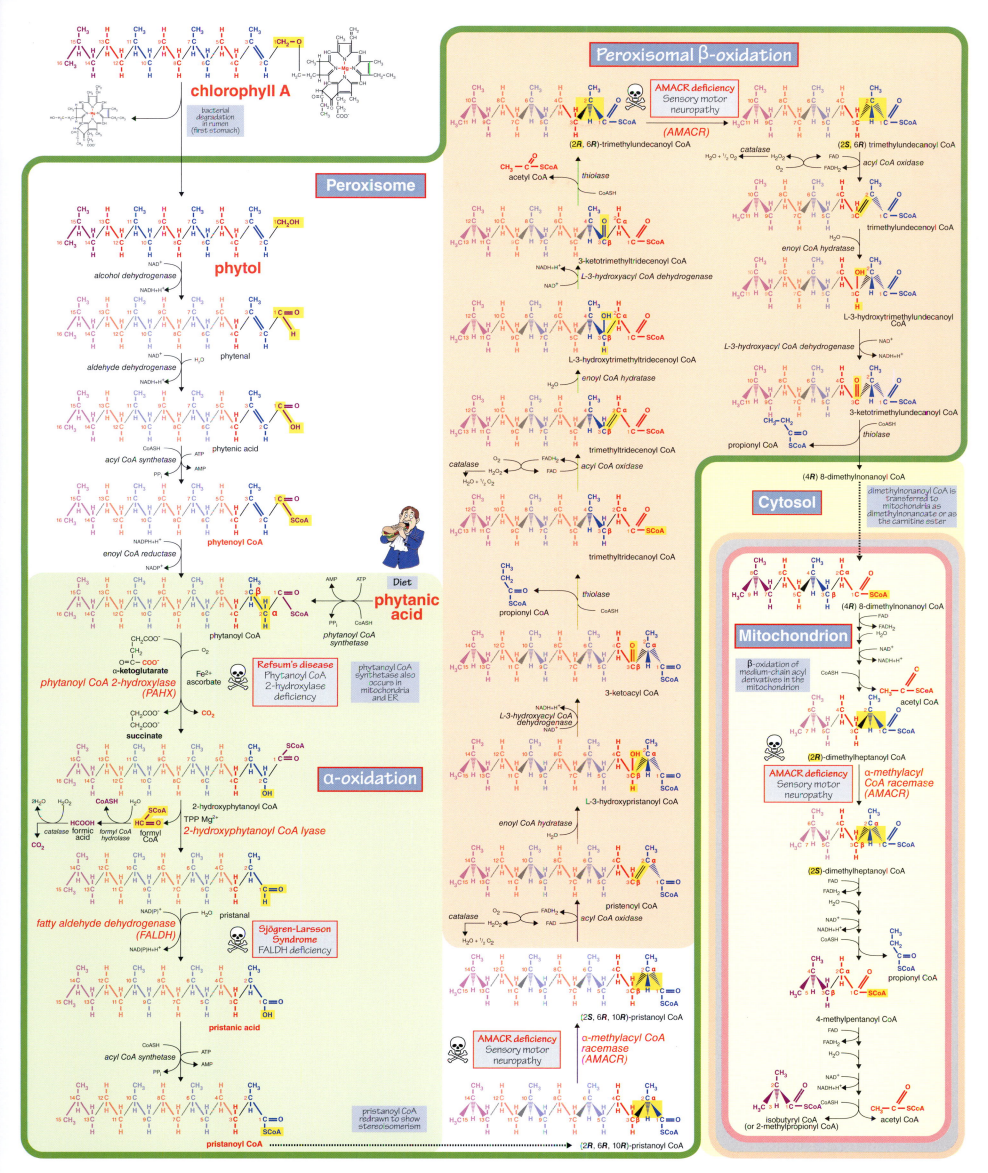

Chart 40.1 Catabolism of phytol and phytanic acid by the sequence of α-oxidation, peroxisomal β-oxidation and mitochondrial β-oxidation.

ω-Oxidation

41

Metabolism of phytanic acid by α-oxidation followed by β-oxidation

The preferred pathway for oxidation of **phytanic acid** is by preliminary **α-oxidation** followed by **β-oxidation**. However, studies using microsomes from human liver reveal a minor pathway, namely that of **ω-oxidation**. Although ω-oxidation is usually insignificant, it is possible it could function as a 'rescue pathway' in disorders of fatty acid metabolism such as Refsum's disease (see Chapter 40) and X-linked adrenoleukodystrophy (see Chapter 39).

ω-Oxidation pathway for phytanoate

The ω-oxidation oxidation pathway involves three stages: (i) ω-oxidation; (ii) the α-methylacyl CoA racemase (AMACR) reaction; and (iii) β-oxidation in both the peroxisomes and mitochondria.

ω-Oxidation

Phytanic acid (3,7,11,15-tetramethylhexadecanoic acid) is hydroxylated on the terminal carbon 16 (i.e. the **ω-carbon** atom, Chart 41.1) in a reaction catalysed by the cytochrome P450 enzymes, either **CYP 4A11** or **CYP 4F2** to form **16-hydroxyphytanic acid**. After subsequent dehydrogenase and hydroxylation reactions, the product 16-carboxyphytanic acid is formed. This combines with CoASH to form 16-carboxyphytanoyl CoA.

NB: The numbering of the carbon atoms might be confusing. This is because the addition of a new CoASH to what was originally the terminal carbon, that is ω- or C16 carbon, has changed the priority for numbering so what was originally carbon 16 is now carbon 1.

α-Methylacyl CoA racemase (AMACR)

AMACR is a racemase located in both peroxisomes and mitochondria. **NB:** 16-Carboxyphytanoyl CoA exists as a racemic mixture of 2*R*- and 2*S*-epimers and must be converted to the **2*S*-epimer** by **AMACR** because **only the *S*-epimers can enter the β-oxidation pathway**.

NB: The term β-oxidation might be confusing: *remember as explained earlier, what originally was the **ω-carbon** atom is now **carbon 1**; and what*

*originally was the **ω-3 carbon** atom is the new **β-carbon** (carbon 3) and is a candidate for β-oxidation.*

AMACR and disease. Excessive activity of AMACR is associated with cancer. Decreased activity of AMACR is associated with sensory motor neuropathy.

β-Oxidation

Following the AMACR reaction, the methyl group on the α-carbon is the 2*S*-epimer and β-oxidation can proceed. Peroxisomal β-oxidation has been described in Chapter 39. β-Oxidation starts in the **peroxisomes** where they are reduced in length to shorter molecules that can be catabolized in the **mitochondria**.

The products of ω-oxidation followed by β-oxidation are: three molecules of **propionyl CoA**, two molecules of **acetyl CoA** and one molecule of **4-methyladipoyl CoA**, which can be hydrolysed to **3-methyladipic acid (3-MAA)**.

ω-Oxidation of phytanic acid in adult Refsum's disease (ARD): a potential 'rescue pathway'?

Phytanic acid is normally catabolized by **α-oxidation followed by β-oxidation** (see Chapter 40). In patients with ARD, the α-oxidation pathway is compromised and phytanic acid accumulates. However, in such patients, excretion of 3-MAA occurs, indicating the ω-oxidation pathway is unusually active and provides a 'rescue pathway' for the disposal of phytanic acid. Indeed, in patients with ARD on a low phytanic acid diet, the ω-oxidation pathway can metabolize all the phytanic acid consumed. Since the activity of the cytochrome P450 enzymes needed for ω-oxidation can be induced several-fold, this offers a potential therapeutic strategy to reduce phytanic acid concentrations in ARD.

Reference

Wanders R.J.A., Komen J., Kemp S. (2011) Fatty acid ω-oxidation as a rescue pathway for fatty acid oxidation disorders in humans. *FEBS J*, **278**, 182–94.

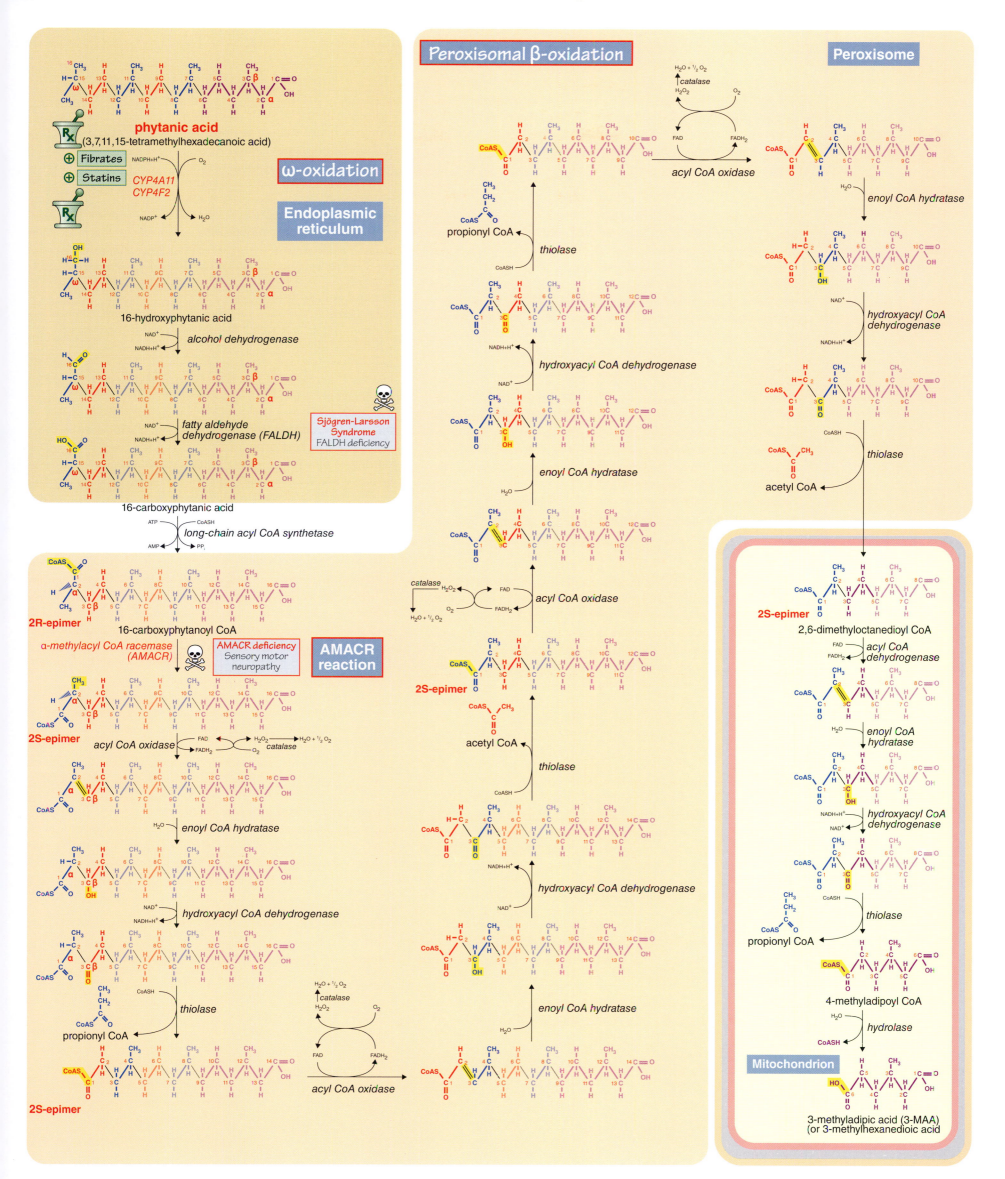

Chart 41.1 Catabolism of phytanic acid by the sequence of ω-oxidation, peroxisomal β-oxidation and mitochondrial β-oxidation.

Cholesterol

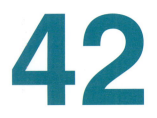

42

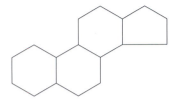

Diagram 42.1 Gonane: the parent nucleus of steroids.

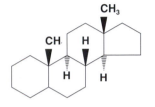

α-projection (below plane of paper) |||||⋯
β-projection (above plane of paper) ▬▶

Diagram 42.2 Orientation of projection formulae.

Cholesterol: friend or foe?

Despite cholesterol's notorious reputation as a major cause of cardiovascular disease, this much maligned molecule has many useful functions. It is a major component of membranes, particularly myelin in the nervous system. Cholesterol is the precursor of the **bile salts** and **steroid hormones**. Intermediates involved in cholesterol biosynthesis are precursors of **ubiquinone**, **dolichol**, **vitamin D** and the **geranyl and farnesyl isoprenoid** groups, which anchor proteins to membranes.

Steroids: nomenclature

Diagram 42.1. The parent nucleus of the steroids is gonane.

Diagram 42.2. When groups such as methyl groups are substituted into the steroid nucleus, they can be orientated below or above the plane of the paper. If below the plane of the paper, they are in the α-projection. If above the plane, they are in the β-projection.

Diagram 42.3. The gonane nucleus is described by the letters A, B, C and D. The addition of a methyl group at C18 of the gonane nucleus forms estrane. The addition of another methyl group at C19 forms androstane. If the nucleus is extended beyond C17, numbering is as shown.

Diagram 42.4. The number of carbon atoms involved determines the name of the modified nucleus, for example cholane, the nucleus of cholic acid, and derived bile salts, has 24 carbon atoms.

Diagram 42.5. Steroid nomenclature can be confusing especially when synonyms are used, e.g. see 14-norlanosterol.

Biosynthesis of cholesterol

Cholesterol is normally available in the diet, but it can also be synthesized from acetyl CoA derived from **glucose** as shown in Chart 42.1. The enzyme controlling cholesterol synthesis is **3-hydroxy 3-methylglutaryl CoA (HMG CoA) reductase**, the regulation of which is complex. However, it can be inhibited by the 'statin' drugs, which are used to treat hypercholesterolaemia. The biosynthesis of cholesterol needs numerous molecules of $NADPH + H^+$ which are produced by the pentose phosphate pathway. Important early intermediates are **squalene** and **lanosterol**.

Metabolism of lanosterol to cholesterol

The intermediate **lanosterol** can be metabolized to cholesterol by two pathways. Usually the **Bloch pathway** is the major route but sometimes the **Kandutsch and Russell pathway** is significant. For the Kandutsch and Russell pathway to operate, lanosterol must be reduced to **24,25-dihydrolanosterol** by sterol Δ^{24}-reductase. Note that at several stages in the Bloch pathway, sterol Δ^{24}-reductase can reduce Bloch pathway intermediates to their equivalent intermediates in the Kandutsch and Russell pathway. However, at the beginning of both pathways, three methyl groups must be removed from lanosterol (or 24,25-dihydrolanosterol).

Demethylation of lanosterol and 24,25-dihydrolanosterol

Removal of the α-methyl group at C14 on lanosterol as formic acid (HCOOH), and the α- and β-methyl groups on C4 of lanosterol as carbon dioxide, is a priority. The former is achieved by **CYP 51A1 (lanosterol 14-α-demethylase)** and the latter by the **C-4 demethylation complex**. The same applies to **24,25-dihydrolanosterol** in the Kandutsch and Russell pathway.

Kandutsch and Russell pathway for the biosynthesis of cholesterol from lanosterol

An alternative to the Bloch pathway was described by Kandutsch and Russell in preputial gland tumours. Here, the **primary reaction** is the reduction of lanosterol by **sterol Δ^{24}-reductase** to 24,25-dihydrolanosterol. This is then converted to cholesterol by a pathway that parallels the Bloch pathway. By contrast, in the Bloch pathway, the **final reaction** is the reduction of desmosterol by **sterol Δ^{24}-reductase** to cholesterol. Although there is evidence the Kandutsch and Russell pathway operates in liver, it is probably a minor pathway.

Bae and Paik shunt

The preferred link between the Bloch and the Kandutsch pathways was proposed by Bae and Paik. The membrane-bound enzyme sterol Δ^{24}-reductase can reduce the C24(25) double bond in **any** of the 19 sterol intermediates formed during cholesterol biosynthesis. However, Bae and Paik suggested the principal location is the reduction of **cholesta-7,24-dien-3β-ol** to **lathosterol** (Chart 42.1).

Disorders of cholesterol metabolism: Smith–Lemli–Opitz (SLO) syndrome

Although originally classified in 1964, the chemical pathology of SLO syndrome was not determined until 1993 when Tint *et al.* demonstrated a deficiency of **7-dehydrocholesterol reductase** (Chart 42.1). SLO syndrome is an autosomal recessive disorder in which **7-dehydrocholesterol** (5,7-cholesta-dien-3β-ol) accumulates in the plasma and tissue. Other products have been reported in patients with SLO syndrome, namely **8-dehydrocholesterol** (5,8-cholestadien-3β-ol). Also the B ring is aromatized by oxygen radicals to form **19-nor-5,7,9,(10)-cholestrien-3β-ol**, and similarly **5,7,9(11)-cholestatrien-3β-ol** is produced. The condition is characterized by multiple malformations, impaired brain development with abnormal myelination, and hypocholesterolaemia. In the past, SLO syndrome was frequently not diagnosed and probably designated as 'multiple congenital abnormality syndrome of unknown aetiology'. However, SLO syndrome is better diagnosed today using modern screening procedures.

Other disorders of cholesterol biosynthesis are much less common. For example **desmosterolosis** to date has only had nine cases described, of which four are from one family with five independent cases. However, as analytical techniques improve for identifying the precursors of cholesterol, it is likely that other disorders of cholesterol metabolism will be discovered.

NB: 7-Dehydrocholesterol is a precursor of vitamin D (see Chapter 43).

Cholesterol metabolism and cancer

Cancer cells proliferate rapidly in an excessive and uncontrolled manner. Cholesterol is a vital component of cell membranes and so the rapid growth of these cancer cells needs a commensurate supply of cholesterol.

References

Bae S.H., Paik Y.K. (1997) *Biochem J*, **326**, 609–16.

Herman G.E., Kratz L. (2012) *Am J Med Genet Part C Semin Med Genet*, **160C**, 301–21.

Kandutsch A.A., Russell A.E. (1960) *J Biol Chem*, **235**, 2256–61.

Diagram 42.3 Numbering and ring letters.

Class	Number of carbon atoms	Example
Gonane	17	(parent nucleus of steroids)
Estrane	18	œstradiol (estradiol)
Androstane	19	testosterone
Pregnane	21	Progesterone, glucocorticoids, aldosterone
Cholane	24	cholic acid (bile salts)
Cholestane	27	cholesterol

Diagram 42.4 Nomenclature according to the number of carbon atoms in the steroid.

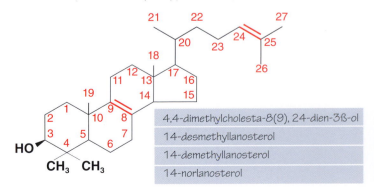

4,4-dimethylcholesta-8(9), 24-dien-3ß-ol
14-desmethyllanosterol
14-demethyllanosterol
14-norlanosterol

Diagram 42.5 Nomenclature: synonyms for 14-norlanosterol ('nor' means without a methyl).

Metabolism at a Glance, Fourth Edition. J. G. Salway. © 2017 John Wiley & Sons Ltd. Published 2017 by John Wiley & Sons Ltd.

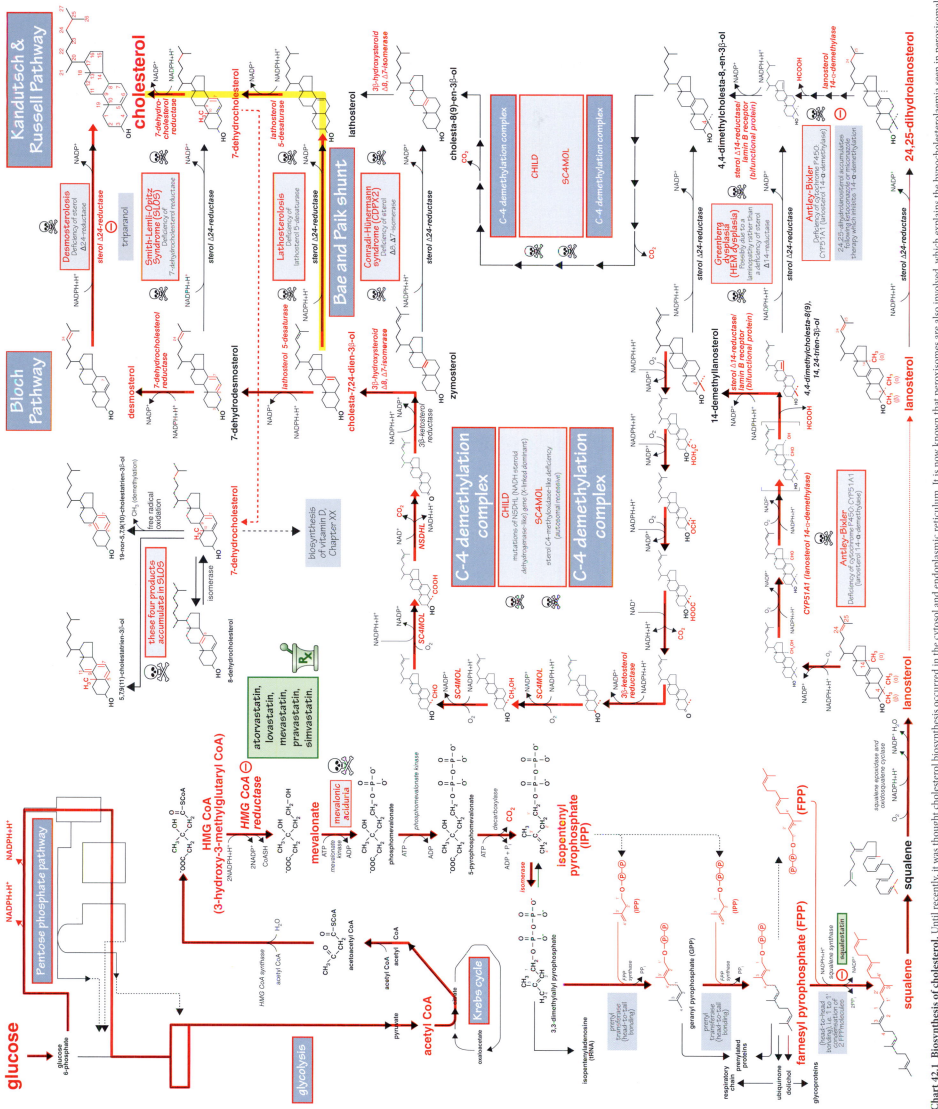

Chart 42.1 Biosynthesis of cholesterol. Until recently, it was thought cholesterol biosynthesis occurred in the cytosol and endoplasmic reticulum. It is now known that peroxisomes are also involved, which explains the hypocholesterolaemia seen in peroxisomal deficiency disorders such as Zellweger's syndrome.

Steroid hormones and bile salts

43

Steroid hormones

The principal steroid hormones are **aldosterone** (mineralocorticoid), **cortisol** (glucocorticoid), **testosterone** and **dihydrotestosterone** (androgens) and **oestradiol** (oestrogen) (Chart 43.1). Aldosterone is synthesized in the region of the adrenal cortex called the zona glomerulosa, whereas cortisol is made in both the zona fasciculata and zona reticularis. Similarly, the sex hormones testosterone and oestradiol are synthesized *de novo* from acetyl CoA precursors or from cholesterol in the testes and ovaries respectively.

The steroid hormones are synthesized from cholesterol by pathways with a common point of control. It is thought that the translocation of cholesterol into the mitochondrion is regulated by the **st**eroid **a**cute **r**egulatory (**StAR**) protein, which may be governed by the trophic hormones. (**NB:** The mitochondrial peripheral benzodiazepine receptor (PBR), which is not shown in the chart, may also be involved in cholesterol uptake.) Here **cholesterol desmolase** cleaves the side chain to form **pregnenolone**, which is the precursor of all the steroid hormones. A series of cytochrome P450-dependent reactions follow that consume NADPH, making substantial energy demands on the cell.

Bile acids (salts)

Biosynthesis of the bile salts **cholate** and **chenodeoxycholate** from **cholesterol** is regulated by **7-α-hydroxylase** (Diagram 43.1). The bile salts are conjugated with glycine or taurine to form the glycine- or taurine-conjugates.

Ursodeoxycholic acid (UDCA) is an example of a bile acid that is used to treat itching in obstetric cholestasis. It is also used to treat gall stones and primary biliary cirrhosis. Recent research suggests that UDCA and its taurine-conjugate tauroursodeoxycholic acid improve the function of substantia nigral transplants in animal studies and might benefit patients with Parkinson's disease. However, this awaits clinical trials. UDCA is named from *Ursa* (Latin: 'bear') and was traditionally 'harvested' from the cannulated gall bladders of captive bears. Its systematic name is: 3α,7β-dihydroxy-5β-cholan-24-oic acid (Diagram 43.2).

Ursodeoxycholic acid
Systematic (IUPAC) name
3α, 7β-dihydroxy-5β-cholan-24-oic acid

Diagram 43.2 Ursodeoxycholic acid (3α,7β-dihydroxy-5β-cholan-24-oic acid).

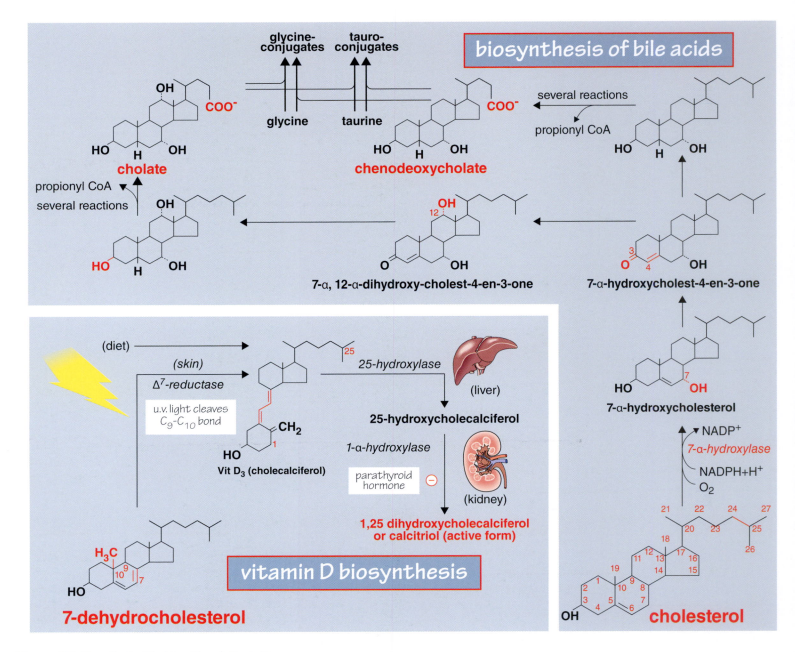

Diagram 43.1 Biosynthesis of the bile acids and vitamin D.

Metabolism at a Glance, Fourth Edition. J. G. Salway. © 2017 John Wiley & Sons Ltd. Published 2017 by John Wiley & Sons Ltd.

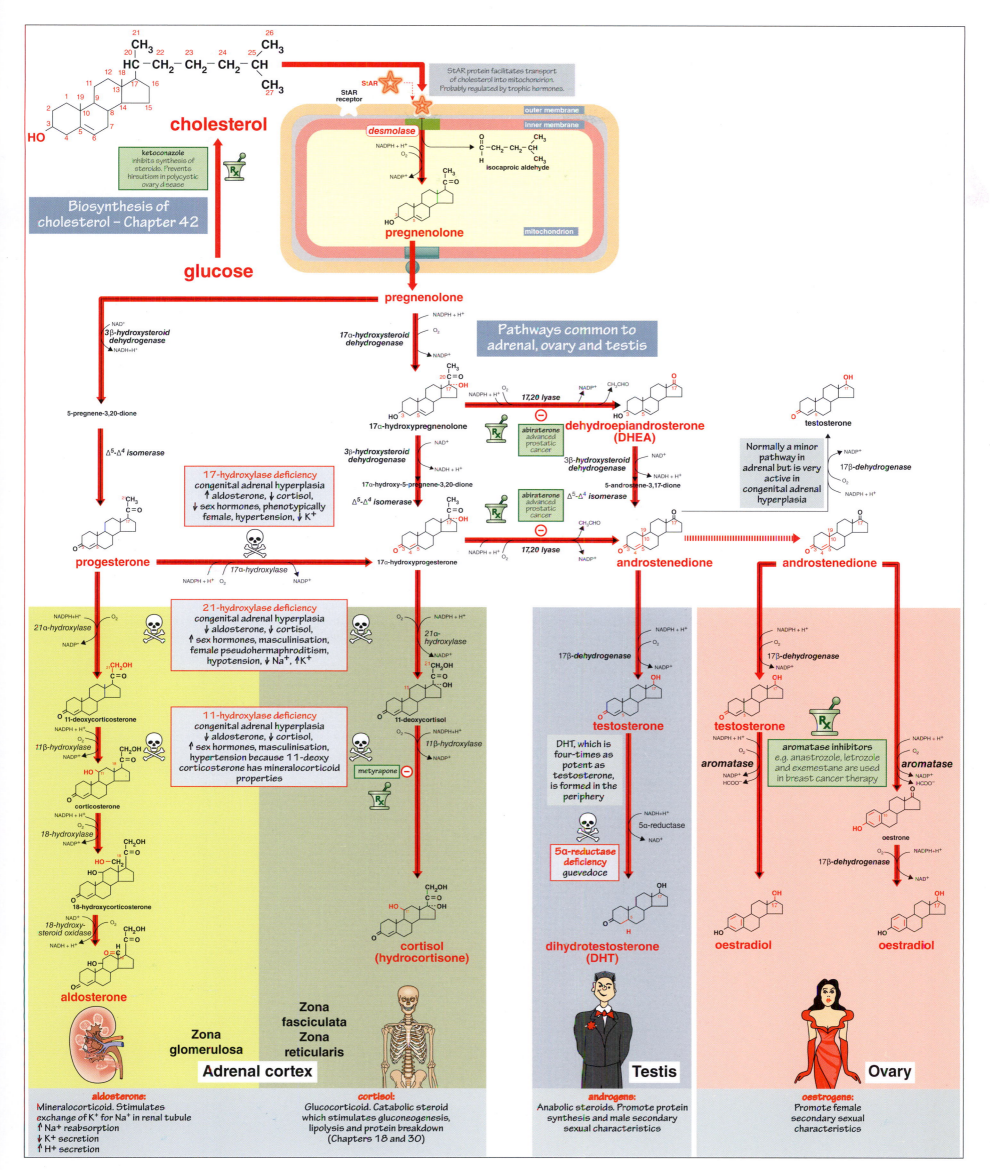

Chart 43.1 Biosynthesis of the steroid hormones.

Biosynthesis of the non-essential amino acids

44

Whereas plants and some bacteria are capable of synthesizing all of the amino acids necessary for the formation of cellular proteins and other vital molecules, this is not the case in mammals. Mammals, including humans, can synthesize only 11 of these amino acids, namely tyrosine, aspartate, asparagine, alanine, serine, glycine, cysteine, glutamate, glutamine, proline and arginine. These are known as the **non-essential amino acids**, and their biosynthesis is shown in Chart 44.1. The other nine amino acids – phenylalanine, threonine, methionine, lysine, tryptophan, leucine, isoleucine, valine and histidine – cannot be synthesized. They are known as the **essential amino acids**.

Tyrosine

Biosynthesis of tyrosine. Tyrosine is formed from the essential amino acid phenylalanine in the presence of phenylalanine monooxygenase.

Uses of tyrosine. Tyrosine is a precursor in the synthesis of adrenaline, noradrenaline, thyroxine and the pigment, melanin.

Serine, glycine and cysteine

These amino acids are made from intermediates formed by glycolysis.

Biosynthesis of serine. Serine is synthesized by a pathway commonly known as the 'phosphorylated pathway'. First, 3-phosphoglycerate is oxidized to 3-phosphohydroxypyruvate, which is then transaminated to 3-phosphoserine. Finally, hydrolysis by a specific phosphatase yields serine. This phosphoserine phosphatase is inhibited by serine providing feedback regulation of the pathway. **NB**: The so-called 'non-phosphorylated pathway' for serine metabolism is important in the gluconeogenic state (see Chapter 47).

Uses of serine. Serine is a component of the phospholipid, phosphatidylserine. Also, serine is a very important source of 1-carbon precursors for biosynthesis (see Chapters 54 and 55).

Biosynthesis of glycine. Glycine can be formed by two routes, both of which involve serine. Glycine is formed from serine by a reversible reaction catalysed by **serine hydroxymethyltransferase**, which is a pyridoxal phosphate-dependent enzyme existing as both cytosolic and mitochondrial isoforms. This enzyme uses the coenzyme tetrahydrofolate (THF), which is formed by reduction of the vitamin folic acid (see Chapter 54). It accepts a 1-carbon fragment from serine to form N^5,N^{10}-methylene tetrahydrofolate, and glycine is formed.

An alternative route for glycine synthesis uses CO_2 and NH_4^+ in a reaction catalysed by the mitochondrial enzyme **glycine synthase** (also known as the glycine cleavage enzyme when working in the reverse direction; see Chapter 46). The second carbon atom is derived from N^5,N^{10}-methylene THF obtained from serine in the previously mentioned reaction catalysed by serine hydroxymethyltransferase.

Uses of glycine. The demand for **glycine** by the body is considerable, and it has been estimated that the requirement for endogenous synthesis of glycine is between 10 and 50 times the dietary intake. Apart from its contribution to cellular proteins, glycine is required for the synthesis of purines, collagen, porphyrins, creatine and glutathione and conjugation with bile salts. Glycine can also be conjugated with certain drugs and toxic substances to facilitate their excretion in the urine. Finally, glycine is made by mitochondria in brain cells, where it acts as an inhibitory neurotransmitter. Hypotheses have implicated a deficiency of serine hydroxymethyltransferase with schizophrenia.

Biosynthesis of cysteine. Cysteine can be formed from serine provided that the essential amino acid methionine is available to donate a sulphur atom. When there is a metabolic demand for cysteine, homocysteine condenses with serine to yield cystathionine in a reaction catalysed by cystathionine synthase. Cystathionine is then cleaved by cystathionase to release cysteine.

Uses of cysteine. Cysteine is a component of the tripeptide glutathione (γ-glutamylcysteinylglycine).

Aspartate and asparagine

Biosynthesis of aspartate. Aspartate is readily formed by the transamination of oxaloacetate by glutamate in the presence of aspartate aminotransferase (AST).

Uses of aspartate. Aspartate is an amino donor in urea synthesis, and in both pyrimidine and purine synthesis.

Biosynthesis of asparagine. Asparagine is synthesized by amide transfer from glutamine in the presence of asparagine synthetase.

Uses of asparagine. Asparagine is incorporated into cellular proteins but appears to have no other role in mammals.

Glutamate, glutamine, proline and arginine

These amino acids are formed from the Krebs cycle intermediate α-ketoglutarate.

Biosynthesis of glutamate. Glutamate is formed by the reductive amination of α-ketoglutarate by glutamate dehydrogenase.

Biosynthesis of glutamine. Glutamine is formed from glutamate and NH_4^+ in an ATP-requiring reaction catalysed by glutamine synthetase (see Chapters 45 and 51).

Uses of glutamine. Glutamine is a very important source of nitrogen for purine and pyrimidine (and hence nucleic acid) synthesis (see Chapters 54 and 55). Glutamine is also important in regulating pH in acidotic conditions.

Biosynthesis of proline. In the presence of pyrroline 5-carboxylate synthetase, glutamate is converted to glutamate γ-semialdehyde, which spontaneously cyclizes to pyrroline 5-carboxylate. This can then be reduced to proline.

Biosynthesis of arginine. Pyrroline 5-carboxylate is in equilibrium with glutamate γ-semialdehyde, which can be transaminated by ornithine transaminase to yield ornithine. Ornithine can then enter the urea cycle and so form arginine (see Chapter 51).

Uses of arginine. Arginine is an intermediate in the urea cycle and is the precursor of creatine. It is also the source of the vasodilator nitric oxide.

Metabolism at a Glance, Fourth Edition. J. G. Salway. © 2017 John Wiley & Sons Ltd. Published 2017 by John Wiley & Sons Ltd.

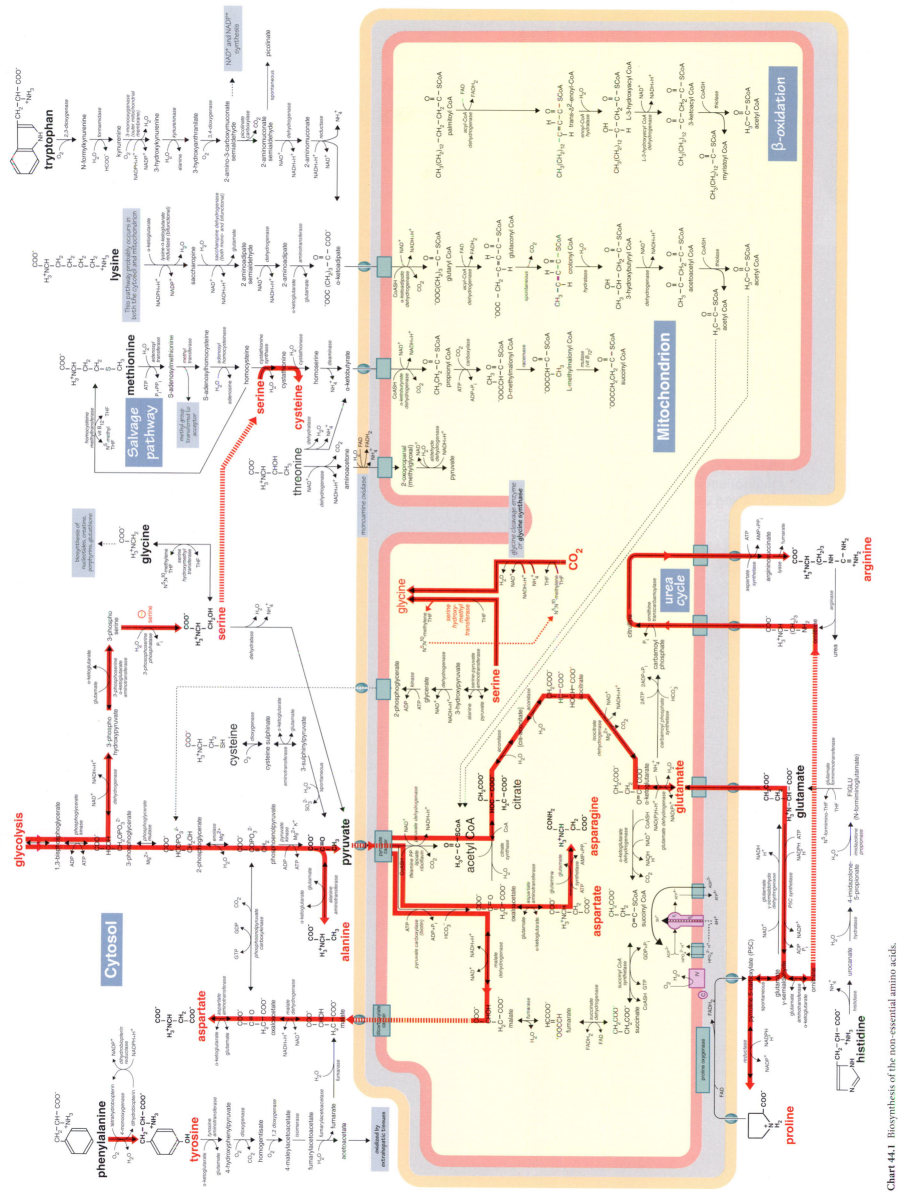

Chart 44.1 Biosynthesis of the non-essential amino acids.

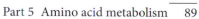

Catabolism of amino acids I

45

Proteins, whether of dietary origin in the fed state or derived from muscle protein in starvation, can be degraded to amino acids for direct oxidation as a respiratory fuel with the generation of ATP. However, it is also possible that, in the fed state, amino acids may first be converted to glycogen or triacylglycerol for fuel storage prior to energy metabolism. Alternatively, in starvation, certain glucogenic amino acids are initially converted in muscle to alanine, which is subsequently converted by the liver to glucose to provide fuel for the brain and red blood cells. Finally, the ketogenic amino acids form the ketone bodies, which are a valuable fuel for the brain in starvation.

The catabolism of aspartate and the branched-chain amino acids (BCAAs) will be emphasized here, and catabolism of the remaining amino acids will be described in Chapter 46.

Dietary protein as a source of energy in the fed state

Protein is digested in the gastrointestinal tract to release its 20 constituent amino acids. If they are surplus to the body's requirement for incorporation into proteins or other essential molecules derived from amino acids, they may be metabolized to glycogen or fat (see Chapters 33 and 47) and subsequently used for energy metabolism. Alternatively, they can be oxidized directly as a metabolic fuel. However, different tissues have different abilities to catabolize the various amino acids.

Metabolism of muscle protein during starvation or prolonged exercise

In the fed state, muscle uses glucose and fatty acids for energy metabolism. However, during fasting, starvation or prolonged exercise, protein from muscle plays an important role in glucose homeostasis. For example, during an overnight fast the hepatic glycogen reserves can be depleted and life-threatening hypoglycaemia must be prevented. Remember that fat cannot be converted to glucose (see Chapter 20), apart from the glycerol derived from triacylglycerol metabolism. Consequently, muscle tissue remains as the only glucogenic source and must be 'sacrificed' to maintain blood glucose concentrations and thus ensure a vital supply of energy for the red blood cells and brain.

During starvation, muscle protein must first be broken down into its constituent amino acids, but the details of intracellular proteolysis are still not fully understood. It was once thought that, following proteolysis, all of the different amino acids were released from the muscle into the blood in proportion to their composition in muscle proteins. Research has shown that this idea is more complicated than originally supposed. During fasting, the blood draining from muscle is especially enriched with alanine and glutamine, which can each constitute up to 30% of the total amino acids released by muscle, a proportion greatly in excess of their relative abundance in muscle proteins. Alanine released from muscle is taken up by the liver in a process known as the **glucose alanine cycle**. Glutamine is not taken up by the liver, but is used by the intestines as a fuel and by the kidney for gluconeogenesis and pH homeostasis.

Catabolism of the branched-chain amino acids (BCAAs)

The oxidation of the BCAAs (leucine, isoleucine and valine) is shown in Chart 45.1. The branched-chain α-ketoacid dehydrogenase (BCKADH) resembles pyruvate dehydrogenase. Moreover, the oxidation of the acyl CoA derivatives formed by this reaction has many similarities with the β-oxidation of fatty acids, which is included in Chart 45.1 for the purpose of comparison. **NB:** Not all tissues can oxidize the BCAAs. Whereas muscle has BCAA aminotransferase activity, liver lacks this enzyme. However, liver has BCKADH activity and can oxidize the branched-chain ketoacids.

It should be noted that, in starvation and diabetes, the activity of muscle BCKADH is increased up to five-fold, thereby promoting oxidation of the BCAAs in muscle.

Chart 45.1: formation of alanine and glutamine by muscle

Alanine and the glucose alanine cycle

The glucose alanine cycle was proposed by Felig, who demonstrated increased production of alanine by muscle during starvation. The BCAAs are the major donors of amino groups for alanine synthesis. Pyruvate, for transamination to alanine, can be formed from isoleucine and valine (via succinyl CoA), from certain other amino acids (e.g. aspartate) or, alternatively, from glycolysis. The alanine so formed is exported from muscle and is transported via the hepatic artery to the liver, where it is used for gluconeogenesis (Diagram 45.1).

Glutamine

Glutamine is the most abundant amino acid in the blood. As shown in Chart 45.1 (and Chart 51.1), BCAAs are major donors of the amino groups used to form glutamate, which is further aminated by glutamine synthetase to form glutamine.

Ketogenic amino acids leucine and isoleucine as an energy source

As shown in Chart 45.1, the entire carbon skeleton of leucine and carbon fragments from isoleucine are converted to acetoacetate or acetyl CoA, which can be converted into acetoacetate in liver (see Chapter 36). The ketone bodies can then be oxidized as a respiratory fuel by extrahepatic tissues, as described in Chapter 37.

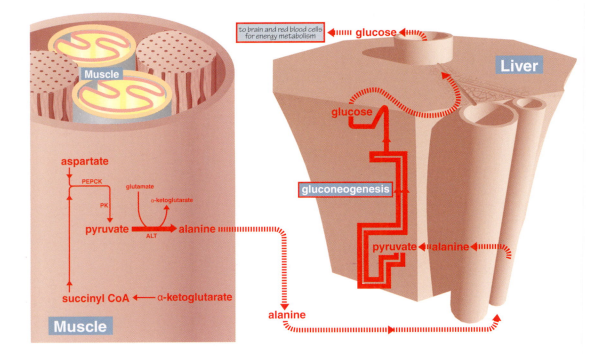

Diagram 45.1 Formation of alanine from muscle protein. In starvation, the amino acids derived from muscle protein are degraded to ketoacids. Some of the carbon skeletons from these ketoacids enter Krebs cycle and are metabolized via phospho-enolpyruvate carboxykinase (PEPCK) and pyruvate kinase (PK) to pyruvate. Alanine aminotransferase (ALT) is very active in muscle and so much of the pyruvate produced is transaminated to alanine, which leaves the muscle and is transported in the blood to the liver.
Gluconeogenesis from alanine in liver. In liver, alanine is reconverted to pyruvate, which is used for gluconeogenesis. **NB:** Pyruvate kinase in liver is inhibited in the gluconeogenic state both by protein kinase A phosphorylation and directly by alanine (see Chapter 18). This prevents the futile recycling of pyruvate which would otherwise happen. The glucose formed can be used for energy metabolism, especially by the brain and red blood cells.

Metabolism at a Glance, Fourth Edition. J. G. Salway. © 2017 John Wiley & Sons Ltd. Published 2017 by John Wiley & Sons Ltd.

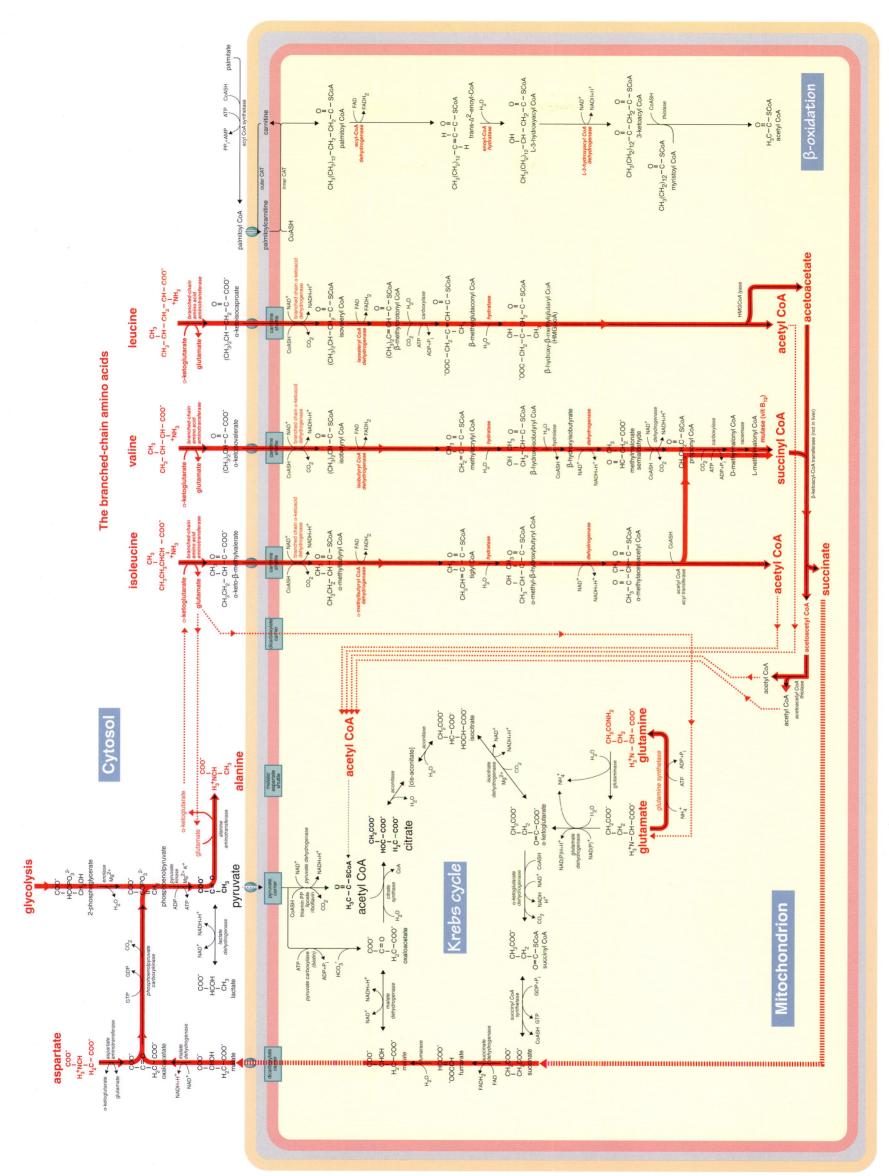

Chart 45.1 Formation of alanine and glutamine by muscle.

Catabolism of amino acids II

46

Alanine. Alanine is in equilibrium with pyruvate, which is oxidatively decarboxylated to CO_2 and acetyl CoA. The latter can then be oxidized in Krebs cycle (Chart 46.1).

Glycine. Although there are several possible routes for glycine catabolism, the mitochondrial **glycine cleavage system** is probably the most important in mammals. This enzyme complex is loosely bound to the mitochondrial inner membrane and has several similarities to the pyruvate dehydrogenase complex. It oxidatively decarboxylates glycine to carbon dioxide and N^5,N^{10}-methylene-tetrahydrofolate.

Serine. When needed as a respiratory fuel, serine undergoes deamination by serine dehydratase to form pyruvate.

Threonine. The most important route for the catabolism of threonine in humans is via the **threonine dehydratase pathway** to form **α-ketobutyrate**. This is metabolized to succinyl CoA, as outlined for methionine metabolism. In experimental animals the **aminoacetone pathway** is the major pathway for threonine catabolism. Threonine dehydrogenase forms the unstable intermediate 2-amino-3-oxobutyrate, which is spontaneously decarboxylated to aminoacetone for further catabolism to pyruvate.

Cysteine. There are several possible pathways for cysteine degradation but the most important in mammals is oxidation by cysteine dioxygenase to cysteine sulphinate. This is then transaminated to form 3-sulphinylpyruvate (also known as β-mercaptopyruvate or thiopyruvate), which is converted to pyruvate in a spontaneous reaction.

Methionine. Methionine is activated in an ATP-dependent reaction to form S-adenosylmethionine (SAM), which is the major carrier of methyl groups, beating tetrahydrofolate (THF) into second place as a donor in biosynthetic methylations. For example, SAM is used in the methylation of noradrenaline to adrenaline by noradrenaline N-methyltransferase. Consequently, the original methionine molecule is demethylated to form S-adenosylhomocysteine, then the adenosyl group is removed to homocysteine. This intermediate can be metabolized in two ways:

1 It can be recycled to methionine in a salvage pathway where the methyl donor is N^5-methyl-THF, using a vitamin B_{12}-dependent reaction catalysed by homocysteine methyltransferase. This is an important pathway that helps to conserve this essential amino acid.

2 It can be degraded to succinyl CoA, which can be further metabolized to pyruvate for energy metabolism.

Lysine. Lysine is unusual in that it cannot be formed from its corresponding α-ketoacid, α-keto-ε-aminocaproic acid, which cyclizes to form Δ^1-piperidine-2-carboxylic acid. Degradation of lysine occurs via saccharopine, a compound in which lysine and α-ketoglutarate are bonded as a secondary amine formed with the carbonyl group of α-ketoglutarate and the ε-amino group of lysine. Following two further dehydrogenase reactions, α-ketoadipate is formed by transamination. This enters the mitochondrion and is oxidized by a pathway with many similarities to the β-oxidation pathway. Acetoacetyl CoA is formed, thus lysine is classified as a ketogenic amino acid (see Chapter 36).

Tryptophan. Although tryptophan can be oxidized as a respiratory fuel, it is also an important precursor for the synthesis of NAD^+ and $NADP^+$ (see Chapter 50). The regulatory mechanisms involved in the first step of tryptophan catabolism catalysed by tryptophan dioxygenase (also known as tryptophan pyrrolase) have been studied extensively. It is known that the dioxygenase is induced by glucocorticoids, which increase transcription of DNA. Furthermore, glucagon (via cyclic adenosine monophosphate, cAMP) increases the synthesis of dioxygenase by enhancing the translation of mRNA. Hence in starvation, the combined effects of these hormones will promote the oxidation of tryptophan released from muscle protein.

During the catabolism of tryptophan, the amino group is retained in the first three intermediates formed. The amino group in the form of alanine is then hydrolytically cleaved from 3-hydroxykynurenine by kynureninase. This alanine molecule can then be transaminated to pyruvate, thus qualifying tryptophan as a glucogenic amino acid. The other product of kynureninase is 3-hydroxyanthranilate, which is degraded to α-ketoadipate. This is oxidized by a pathway that is similar to β-oxidation to form acetoacetyl CoA. Hence tryptophan is both a ketogenic and a glucogenic amino acid.

Glutamate. This readily enters Krebs cycle following oxidative deamination by glutamate dehydrogenase as α-ketoglutarate. However, for complete oxidation its metabolites must temporarily leave the cycle for conversion to pyruvate. This can then be oxidized to acetyl CoA, which enters Krebs cycle for energy metabolism, generating ATP.

Histidine. Histidine is metabolized to glutamate by a pathway that involves the elimination of a 1-carbon group. In this reaction, the formimino group (–CH=NH) is transferred from N-formiminoglutamate (FIGLU) to THF, yielding N^5-formimino-THF and glutamate.

Arginine. This amino acid is a constituent of proteins as well as being an intermediate in the urea cycle. Arginine is cleaved by arginase to liberate urea, and ornithine is formed. Ornithine is transaminated by ornithine aminotransferase to form glutamate γ-semialdehyde. The semialdehyde is then oxidized by glutamate γ-semialdehyde dehydrogenase to form glutamate.

Proline. The catabolism of proline to glutamate differs from its biosynthetic pathway. Proline is oxidized by the mitochondrial enzyme proline oxygenase, to form pyrroline 5-carboxylate. This is probably an FAD-dependent enzyme, located in the inner mitochondrial membrane, which can donate electrons directly to cytochrome c in the electron transport chain.

Chart 46.2 For complete oxidation, amino acids must be converted to acetyl CoA. If amino acids are to be used as a respiratory fuel **it is obligatory that their carbon skeletons are converted to acetyl CoA,** which must then enter Krebs cycle for oxidation, producing ATP as described in Chapter 6. **NB:** The simple entry of the carbon skeletons into Krebs cycle as 'dicarboxylic acids' (α-ketoglutarate, succinate, fumarate or oxaloacetate) does not ensure their complete oxidation for energy metabolism.

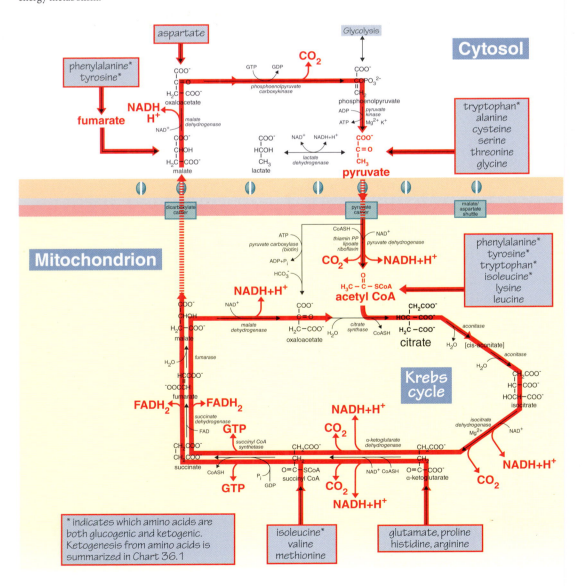

Metabolism at a Glance, Fourth Edition. J. G. Salway. © 2017 John Wiley & Sons Ltd. Published 2017 by John Wiley & Sons Ltd.

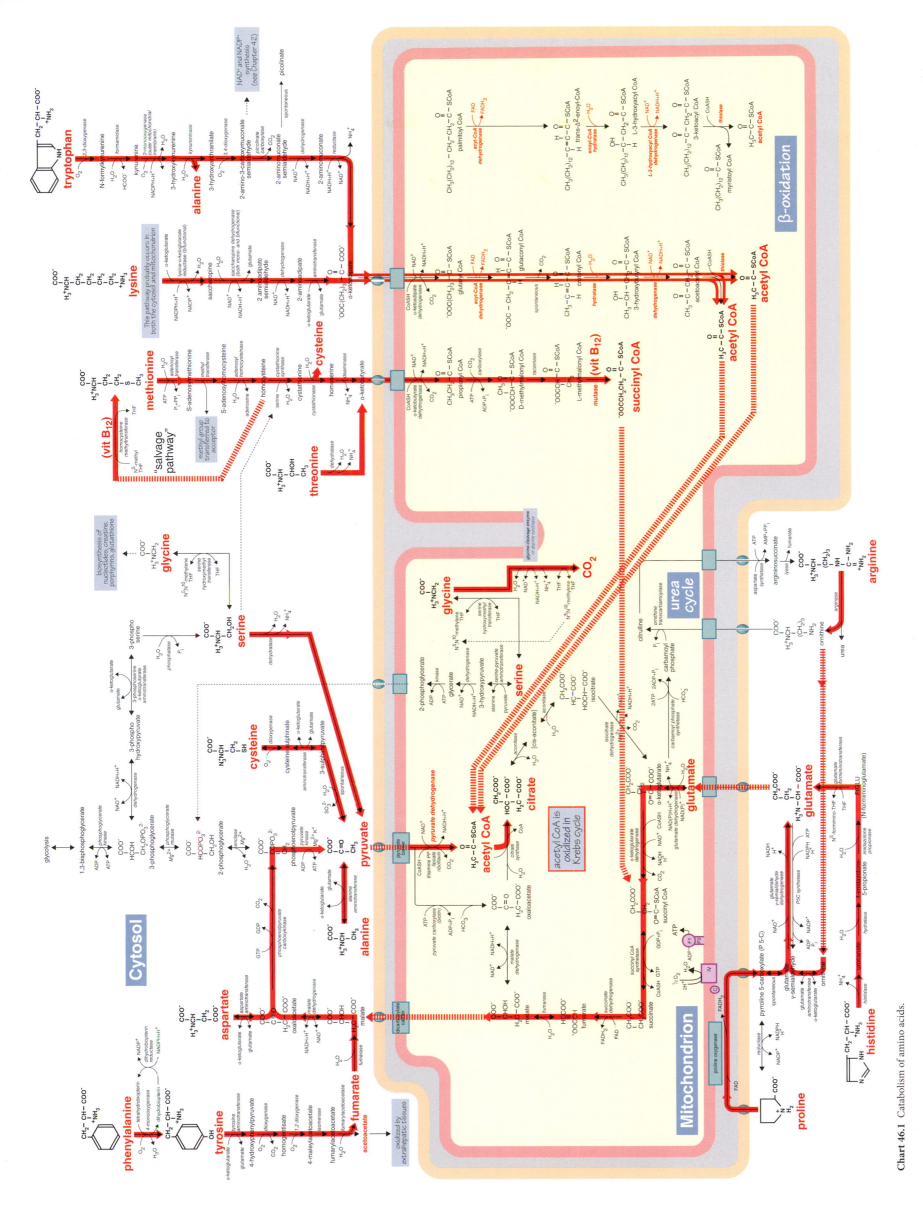

Chart 46.1 Catabolism of amino acids.

Metabolism of amino acids to glucose in starvation and during the period immediately after refeeding

47

In liver, the switch from gluconeogenic mode to glycolytic mode in the early fed-state is a slow process

During starvation, when the glycogen reserves have been exhausted, muscle proteins are degraded to amino acids and used by the liver for gluconeogenesis to maintain the supply of glucose, which is vital for the brain. The important role of alanine as a gluconeogenic precursor is described in Chapter 45.

Following refeeding after a period of starvation, the liver does not switch instantaneously from gluconeogenic to glycolytic mode even though it receives a large glucose load from the intestines. In the early fed state the effects of the gluconeogenic and lipolytic hormones linger, and β-oxidation of fatty acids continues. Consequently, large quantities of acetyl CoA are produced, which inhibit pyruvate dehydrogenase, thereby favouring gluconeogenesis in liver. Under these conditions, the amino acids derived from the gastrointestinal digestion of dietary protein can be used for gluconeogenesis, as shown in Chart 47.1 and described below.

Starvation

In starvation, hepatic gluconeogenesis is active under the hormonal influence of glucagon, cortisol and adrenocorticotropic hormone (ACTH) (see Chapter 18). Glycolysis in liver is inhibited because glucagon, through protein kinase A (cAMP-dependent protein kinase), causes the phosphorylation of hepatic pyruvate kinase, thereby causing inhibition. Moreover, the phosphorylation of hepatic pyruvate kinase is potentiated by its allosteric effector **alanine** (which is abundant in starvation), which therefore further enhances the inhibition of pyruvate kinase.

Role of acetyl CoA in promoting gluconeogenesis in starvation

During starvation, β-oxidation from fatty acids is very active in the liver, and large quantities of acetyl CoA are formed. The accumulated acetyl CoA inhibits pyruvate dehydrogenase and stimulates pyruvate carboxylase. This means that pyruvate (derived from alanine) does not enter Krebs cycle as acetyl CoA,

but is instead carboxylated by pyruvate carboxylase to oxaloacetate for metabolism to phosphoenolpyruvate and thence to glucose via gluconeogenesis.

Early fed state
Fate of the glucogenic amino acids

During refeeding after a period of starvation, the liver remains in the gluconeogenic mode for a few hours. Consequently, the glucogenic amino acids derived from dietary protein are metabolized to **2-phosphoglycerate**, which is their common precursor for gluconeogenesis (Chart 47.1 and Diagram 47.1).

NB: Evidence suggests that gluconeogenesis from serine originates in the mitochondrion. However, the mitochondrial carriers needed for the route shown, in particular the 2-phosphoglycerate carrier, have not been characterized.

In any event, 2-phosphoglycerate is metabolized to glucose 6-phosphate, which can be used to synthesize glycogen or glucose. The amino nitrogen derived from the amino acids is detoxified as urea.

Dietary glucose is converted by muscle to lactate prior to glycogen synthesis

It is emphasized that, in the early fed state, glucose cannot be used by the liver for glycolysis. Instead, high concentrations of glucose promote hepatic glycogen synthesis. Alternatively, in the presence of insulin, glucose enters the muscle cells where it undergoes glycolysis to lactate (Diagram 47.1). Remember that β-oxidation of fatty acids is active and produces an abundance of acetyl CoA, which inhibits muscle pyruvate dehydrogenase. This means that lactate is formed even though conditions are aerobic. The lactate is then transported to the liver, which can convert it to glycogen or glucose.

Diagram 47.1 Intermediary metabolism in the early fed state. β-Oxidation of fatty acids continues in the early fed state. The liver continues in ketogenic and gluconeogenic modes, using lactate (from muscle) and dietary amino acids as gluconeogenic substrates. Muscle uses fatty acids and ketone bodies as respiratory fuels. Also, glycolysis is active in muscle but, since pyruvate dehydrogenase is inactive, lactate is formed.

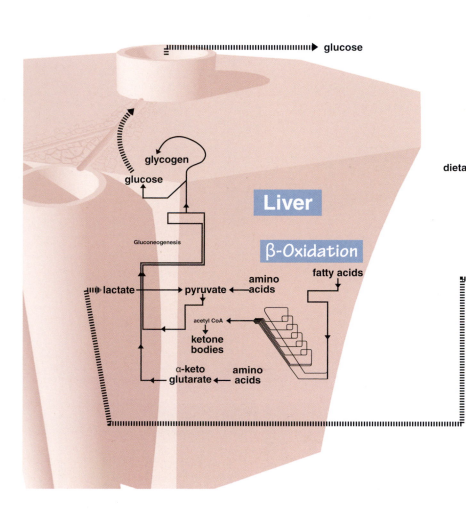

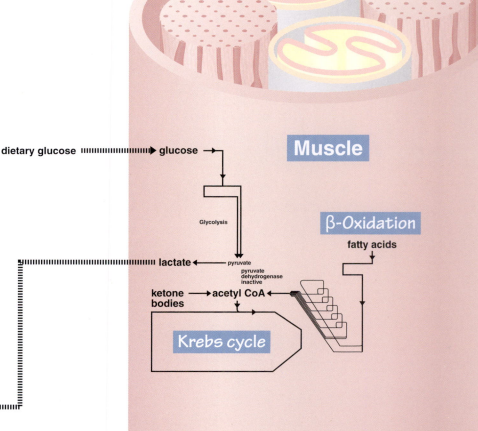

Metabolism at a Glance, Fourth Edition. J. G. Salway. © 2017 John Wiley & Sons Ltd. Published 2017 by John Wiley & Sons Ltd.

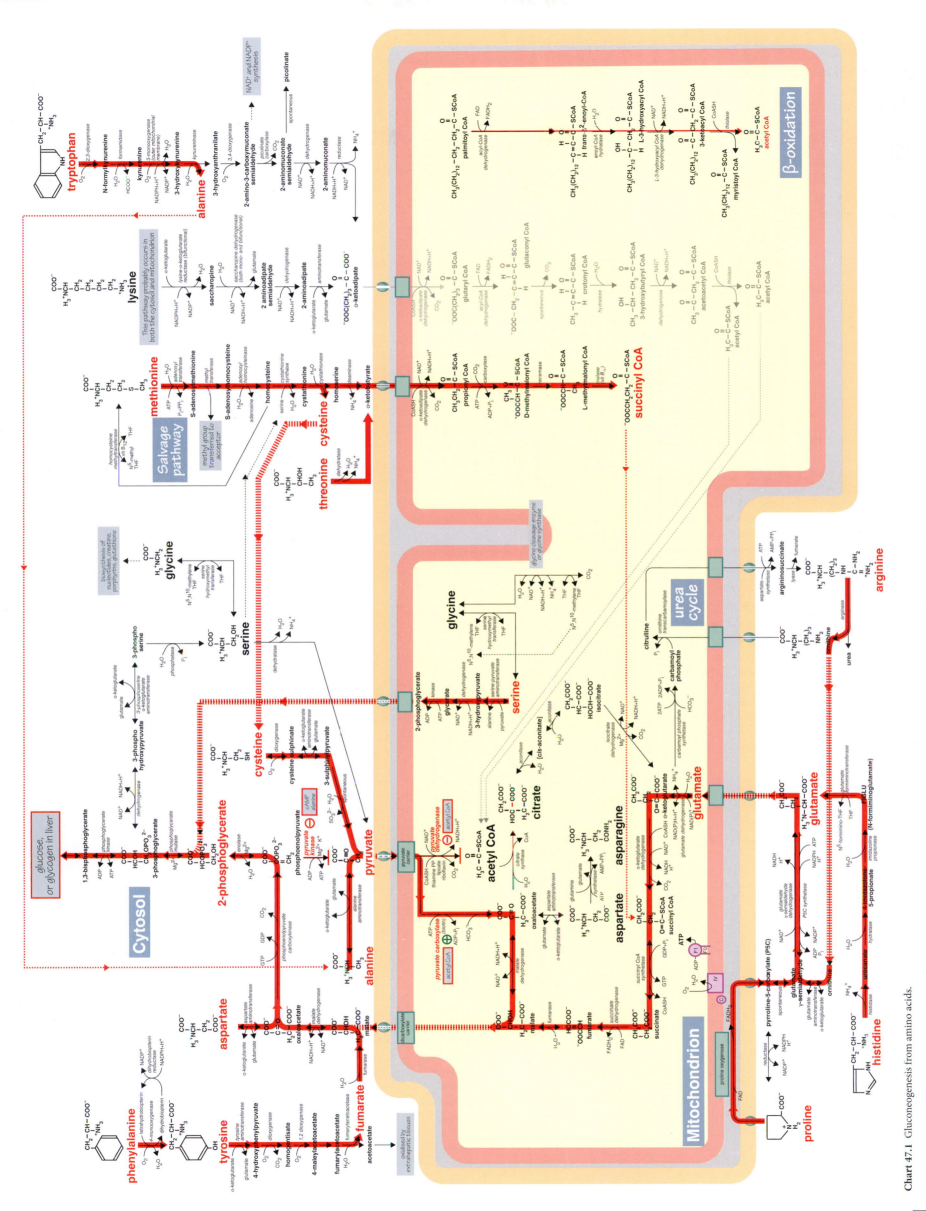

Chart 47.1 Gluconeogenesis from amino acids.

Disorders of amino acid metabolism

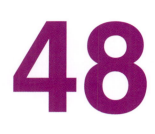

There is a very large body of literature on these rare inborn errors of amino acid metabolism, which has often contributed to our understanding of normal metabolic processes. A few examples are listed below and/or are indicated on Charts 48.1 and 48.2.

Phenylketonuria

This is an autosomal recessive disorder resulting from deficiency of **phenylalanine monooxygenase** (also known as phenylalanine hydroxylase, PAH) activity. Whereas the monooxygenase is usually directly involved, in 3% of cases the disorder is due to impaired synthesis of its coenzyme, **tetrahydrobiopterin**.

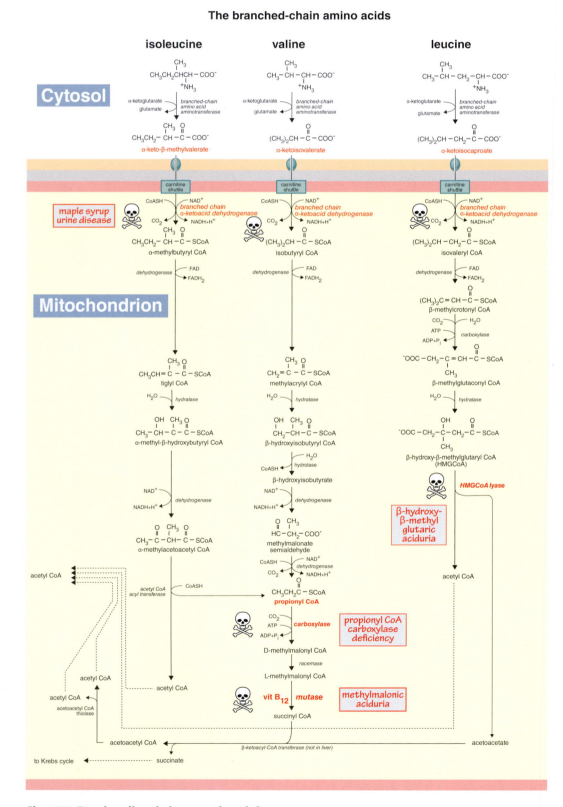

Chart 48.2 Disorders of branched amino acid metabolism.

Because phenylalanine cannot be metabolized to tyrosine, it accumulates and is transaminated to phenylpyruvate which is a 'phenylketone'. Phenylketonuria is described in Chapter 49.

Albinism

Tyrosine is metabolized by tyrosinase in melanocytes to form the pigment, melanin. Deficiency of **tyrosinase** results in albinism.

Alkaptonuria

This autosomal recessive condition is due to deficiency of **homogentisate 1,2-dioxygenase**. Homogentisate accumulates and is excreted in the urine where, under alkaline conditions, it can undergo oxidation and polymerization to form the black pigment alkapton.

Type I tyrosinaemia

Type I tyrosinaemia is an autosomal recessive disease due to a deficiency of **fumarylacetoacetase**. This causes accumulation of toxic intermediates, in particular fumarylacetoacetate, which causes DNA alkylation and tumour formation, and succinylacetone, which is an inhibitor of porphobilinogen synthase (see Chapter 57). Type I tyrosinaemia is described in Chapter 49.

Treatment of type I tyrosinaemia has been revolutionized using NTBC (2-(2-nitro-4-trifluoro-methylbenzoyl)-1,3-cyclohexanedione) to inhibit 4-hydroxy-phenylpyruvate dioxygenase. Also, restriction of dietary phenylalanine and tyrosine is necessary.

Non-ketotic hyperglycinaemia

This condition is due to deficiency of **glycine cleavage enzyme** and causes accumulation of glycine in body fluids including the nervous system, where it causes neurological symptoms. This is because glycine can function as a neurotransmitter and potentiates the N-methyl-D-aspartate (NMDA) receptor. Consequently, when glycine accumulates, neonates suffer feeding difficulties, myoclonic seizures, hypotonia and attacks of apnoea. In severe cases they may die or suffer severe neurological disease. In milder forms, patients survive with mental retardation without suffering the other features of the early onset form of the disease. Glycine is an inhibitory neurotransmitter in spinal cords. Finally, hyperglycinaemia can also occur during valproate therapy.

Histidinaemia

This is an autosomal recessive disorder in which deficiency of **histidase** causes an accumulation of histidine.

Maple syrup urine disease

In this autosomal recessive disorder, deficiency of the **branched-chain α-ketoacid dehydrogenase** complex causes accumulation of the branched-chain amino acids isoleucine, valine and leucine, and their corresponding α-ketoacids, α-methylbutyrate, isobutyrate and isovalerate. These compounds smell like maple syrup, hence the name of this condition. However, some clinicians liken the odour to fenugreek.

Methylmalonic aciduria

This condition is caused by deficiency of L-methylmalonyl CoA mutase or by vitamin B_{12} deficiency. Patients suffer lethargy, delayed psychomotor development, seizures and acute encephalopathy. Most die in infancy or childhood.

ß-Hydroxy-ß-methylglutaric aciduria

ß-Hydroxy-ß-methylglutaryl CoA lyase (3-hydroxy-3-methylglutaryl CoA lyase) deficiency is an autosomal recessive disorder of leucine catabolism and ketogenesis that is associated with hypoketotic hypoglycaemia, hyperammonaemia and metabolic acidosis (see Reye-like syndrome, Chapter 58).

Metabolism at a Glance, Fourth Edition. J. G. Salway. © 2017 John Wiley & Sons Ltd. Published 2017 by John Wiley & Sons Ltd.

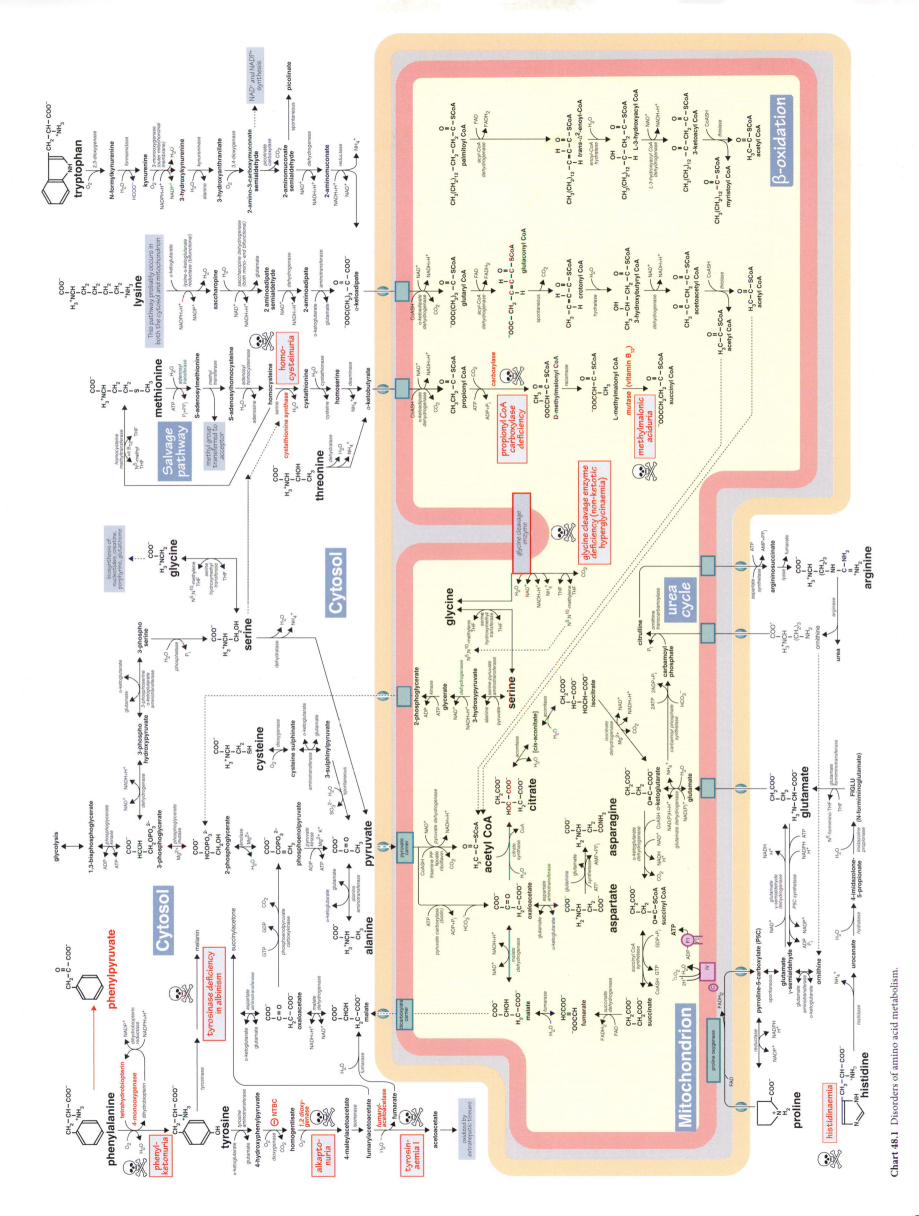

Chart 48.1 Disorders of amino acid metabolism.

Phenylalanine and tyrosine metabolism

49

Phenylalanine can be hydroxylated to: (i) tyrosine, which is the precursor of the pigment melanin; (ii) the thyroid hormones thyroxine (T_4) and tri-iodothyronine (T_3); and (iii) the catecholamines dopamine, noradrenaline and adrenaline. Any additional phenylalanine or tyrosine surplus to requirement for protein synthesis will be oxidized to acetoacetate and fumarate.

Inborn errors of phenylalanine metabolism
Phenylketonuria (PKU)
This autosomal recessive disorder, the most common inborn error of amino acid metabolism in the UK, is caused by deficiency of **phenylalanine monooxygenase** (also known as **phenylalanine hydroxylase, PAH**). Usually the monooxygenase is directly involved but in 3% of cases the disorder is due to impaired synthesis of its coenzyme, **tetrahydrobiopterin**. In both cases, because phenylalanine cannot be metabolized to tyrosine, it accumulates and is transaminated to the phenylketone, **phenylpyruvate**.

PKU patients not treated with a phenylalanine-free diet suffer neurological symptoms and have a low IQ. There are two hypotheses to explain this:
1 **The toxic metabolite hypothesis.** Phenylpyruvate and its metabolite phenyllactate can inhibit metabolic processes. However, they do so only at concentrations greater than those found in PKU patients.
2 **The transport hypothesis.** This proposes that high concentrations of phenylalanine competitively interfere with the transport into the brain of other large neutral amino acids including tryptophan (a precursor of serotonin, see Chapter 50), and tyrosine (a precursor of dopamine, Chart 49.1).

Inborn errors of tyrosine metabolism
Tyrosinaemia I (hepatorenal tyrosinaemia)
This is an autosomal recessive disorder of **fumarylacetoacetase**. Patients suffer severe liver disease and develop carcinoma caused by accumulation of the toxic, electrophilic metabolites, **fumarylacetoacetate** and **succinylacetone** (Chart 49.1). Succinylacetone can also cause porphyria-like attacks because it is a competitive inhibitor of porphobilinogen synthase (see Chapter 57). Because oxidation of tyrosine is inhibited, tyrosine is diverted towards the catecholamines which are produced in increased amounts and may cause hypertension. Patients also develop **hypermethioninaemia** and have a 'cabbage-like' odour.

Traditionally, type I tyrosinaemia was treated with low-tyrosine and low-tryptophan diets and liver transplantation. However, since 1991 a trial of the **4-hydroxyphenylpyruvate oxidase** inhibitor, **NTBC** (2-(2-nitro-4-trifluoromethylbenzoyl)-1,3-cyclohexanedione), plus dietary restriction of tryptophan and tyrosine, has been conducted with great success.

NTBC is a weed killer that, during toxicity trials (for its herbicidal use), caused hypertyrosinaemia in experimental animals. It was shown to inhibit 4-hydroxyphenylpyruvate oxidase. Then, following inspired and bold lateral thinking (and no doubt much trepidation at the thought of using a weed killer as a therapeutic drug), it was given to children with tyrosinaemia I, with remarkable results. NTBC stopped the production of fumarylacetoacetate and succinylacetone, thereby preventing the severe liver damage caused by these hepatotoxins. This clinical trial was successful and in 2002 the US Food and Drug Administration approved the use of NTBC.

Tyrosinaemia II (Richner–Hanhart syndrome; oculocutaneous tyrosinaemia)
This is an autosomal recessive disorder of **tyrosine aminotransferase** that affects the eyes, skin and central nervous system. The eye problems are due to accumulation of tyrosine in the cornea. Once diagnosed, this condition is successfully treated and the lesions are reversed with low dietary tyrosine and phenylalanine formulations.

Tyrosinaemia III
This is a very rare autosomal recessive disorder caused by deficiency of **4-hydroxyphenylpyruvate oxidase**. Tyrosine and phenolic metabolites accumulate and patients suffer neurological symptoms and mental retardation.

Hawkinsinuria
This is a rare autosomal dominant disorder caused by a partial defect of **4-hydroxyphenylpyruvate oxidase** activity. This partial defect prevents the **epoxide** intermediates produced during the reaction from rearranging to form homogentisate and instead they react with **glutathione** to form **hawkinsin** (which is an amino acid named after the Hawkins family in which the disorder was discovered). Infants present with metabolic acidosis, a body odour 'like a swimming pool' and excrete hawkinsin. They also excrete 5-oxoproline (pyroglutamic acid), presumably secondary to glutathione depletion (see Chapter 15). In later life, they excrete **4-hydroxycyclohexylacetic acid (4-HCAA)**.

Other inborn errors of tyrosine metabolism
Albinism and alkaptonuria are described in Chapter 48.

Parkinson's disease
This disease, which usually develops from age 60 onwards, is caused by destruction of the brain region, known as the substantia nigra, that produces the neurotransmitter **dopamine**. The symptoms of Parkinson's disease include tremor, muscular rigidity and akinesia. The use of the dopamine precursor L-DOPA (levodopa) was a landmark in the treatment of Parkinson's disease, and was subsequently refined by combining it with a peripheral (i.e. extracerebral) **L-DOPA decarboxylase** inhibitor (e.g. carbidopa or benserazide). Other therapeutic drugs used are dopamine agonists and the catechol-O-methyltransferase (**COMT**) inhibitors entacapone and tolcapone, which prevent the catabolism of L-DOPA to form 3-O-methyldopa (**3-OMD**).

Phaeochromocytoma
This rare condition is usually caused by a tumour of the adrenal medulla, which produces excessive amounts of the catecholamines **adrenaline** (epinephrine) and **noradrenaline** (norepinephrine), and their catabolic products **metadrenaline** (metepinephrine), **normetadrenaline** (normetepinephrine) and vanillylmandelic acid (**VMA**; also known as hydroxymethoxymandelic acid (HMMA)). However, 10% of cases occur in the sympathetic nerve chain and overproduce noradrenaline. If the tumour releases a surge of catecholamines, patients suffer a hypertensive attack associated with severe headache, sweating, palpitations, anxiety, glucosuria and, if adrenaline predominates, tachycardia. The tumour can be surgically removed but handling of the tumour during the operation can cause a surge of catecholamines, precipitating a hypertensive crisis. Patients are therefore prepared preoperatively with adrenergic blockers. There are reports that treatment with **α-methyl-p-tyrosine**, which inhibits **tyrosine 3-monooxygenase**, has been used to deplete the tumour of catecholamines prior to the operation.

Neuroblastoma
This rare tumour usually presents in children less than 5 years old and 70% have metastatic disease at diagnosis. During the last decade, mass screening trials of children were conducted, the outcome of which remains controversial. Urine was dried onto filter paper and used for assays of **homovanillic acid (HVA)** and **VMA**, which are excreted in increased amounts in neuroblastoma.

Dopamine and mental illness
The 'dopamine hypothesis' for schizophrenia postulates increased brain dopaminergic activity. Although several research approaches suggest an association of psychosis with altered dopaminergic transmission, the evidence is not conclusive. The *COMT* gene is receiving special attention as a candidate risk factor for schizophrenia.

Metabolism at a Glance, Fourth Edition. J. G. Salway. © 2017 John Wiley & Sons Ltd. Published 2017 by John Wiley & Sons Ltd.

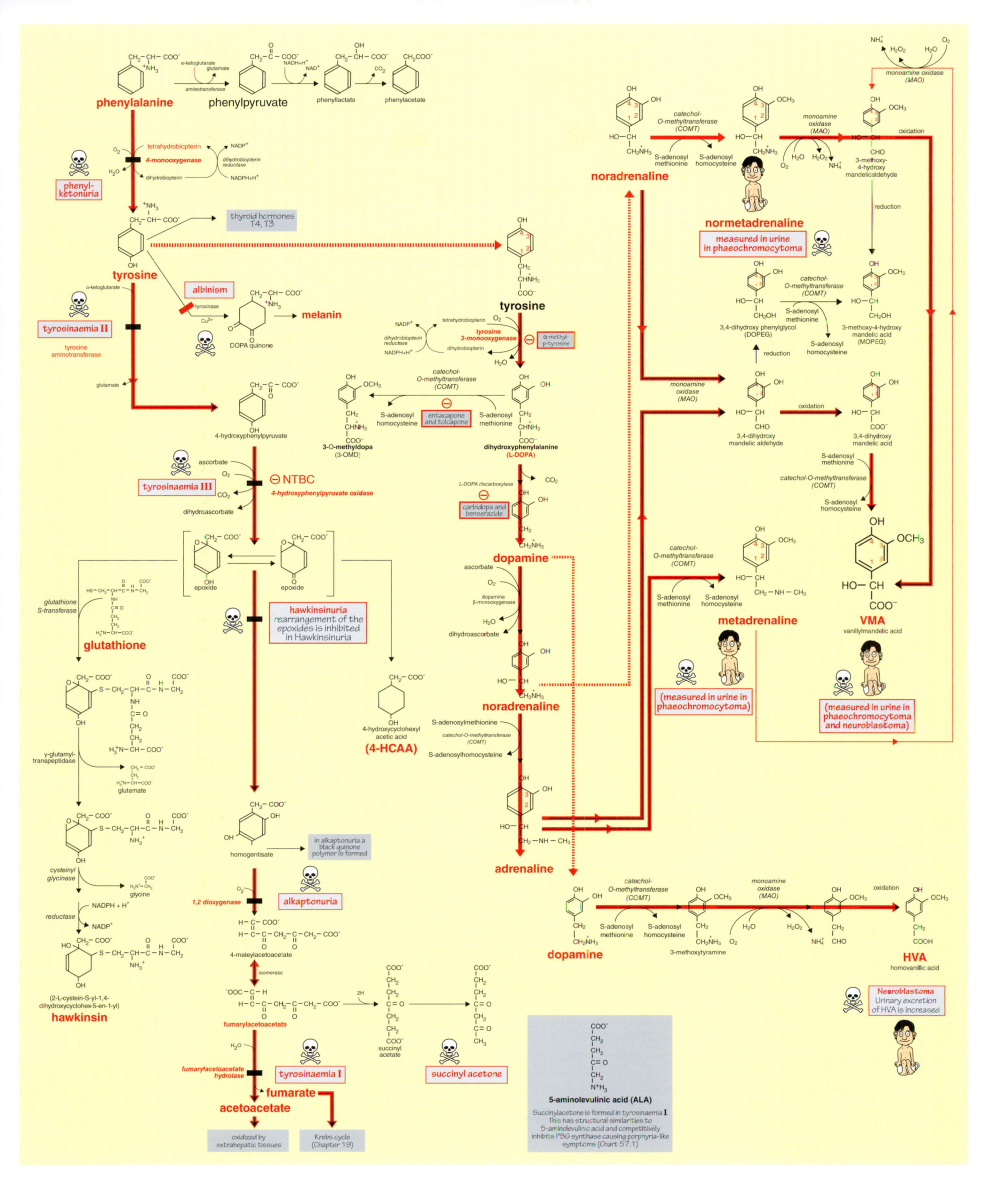

Chart 49.1 Phenylalanine and tyrosine metabolism.

Tryptophan metabolism: the biosynthesis of NAD⁺, serotonin and melatonin

50

Chart 50.1 (opposite) Tryptophan metabolism.

Hartnup disease, niacin deficiency and pellagra

Tryptophan is an essential amino acid whose importance is demonstrated in **Hartnup disease**. This is an autosomal recessive disorder in which renal loss and intestinal malabsorption of tryptophan and other neutral amino acids occurs. Patients with Hartnup disease suffer neurological symptoms and skin lesions resembling severe sunburn, which are similar to pellagra. Pellagra is classically seen in dietary **niacin** deficiency, niacin being the collective term for the NAD⁺ precursors **nicotinic acid** and **nicotinamide**. However, tryptophan metabolism via the **kynurenine pathway** also produces precursors of NAD⁺.

Kynurenine pathway

The regulatory enzymes for the kynurenine pathway are **tryptophan 2,3-dioxygenase (TDO)** and the less specific **indoleamine 2,3-dioxygenase (IDO)** (Chart 50.1).

Production of NAD⁺ and NADP⁺

The kynurenine pathway is the main pathway for tryptophan metabolism and it provides precursors that supplement dietary niacin (i.e. nicotinic acid and nicotinamide) for the biosynthesis of **NAD⁺** and **NADP⁺**. It is generally accepted that 60 mg of tryptophan is equivalent to 1 mg of niacin. Because kynureninase needs **vitamin B₆**, deficiency of the latter can cause secondary pellagra. In a malnourished population with marginally sufficient dietary tryptophan, women of childbearing age are twice as vulnerable as men to suffer pellagra. This is because oestrogens inhibit several enzymes of the kynurenine pathway that produce the precursors of NAD⁺. Conversely, when tryptophan is abundant, any surplus to requirement is metabolized via α-ketoadipate to acetyl CoA for oxidation in Krebs cycle and ATP production by oxidative phosphorylation.

Kynurenine and its metabolites prevent maternal rejection of the fetus

Upstream products of the kynurenine pathway may have several important functions, for example, in immunology and regulation of cell proliferation, and the pathway is attracting attention as a target for the development of new drugs. Work in mice suggests that placental trophoblasts express IDO, which is involved in feto-maternal tolerance. The production of kynurenine, picolinate and quinolinate prevent maternal T cells from activating a lethal anti-fetal response, and they may also have antimicrobial functions.

Indoleamine pathway for the formation of serotonin (5-hydroxytryptamine) and melatonin

A pathway of major neuroendocrinological importance is the **indoleamine pathway**, which makes the neurotransmitter **serotonin** and the hormone **melatonin** in the pineal gland and retina (Chart 50.1). Because impaired serotonin metabolism has been associated with the 'affective disorders' (disorders of mood), this pathway has been a target for the treatment of depression. Indeed, tryptophan and 5-hydroxytryptophan have historically been used to treat depression. Also, melatonin has been associated with **seasonal affective disorder** (SAD) but this remains unproven. This depression is thought to be caused by the long, dark nights of winter. Many sufferers benefit from light treatment by exposure to 2500 lux for 2 hours each morning.

Depression as a neurochemical disease

Although one in four people experience mental disease, it is a sad fact that sufferers are frequently stigmatized, even in the 21st century, because of the debilitating effect it has on their personalities. All too frequently depression is unfairly considered to be self-indulgent weakness due to lack of resolve and determination. This is despite the fact that a psychiatric condition such as **endogenous depression** is a disease with a substantial biochemical component. *Perhaps it is time to refer to these disorders as 'neurochemical diseases' to prevent the stigmatizing effect that 'mental illness' can have on people.*

Of course, not all depression is **primarily** of neurochemical origin. For example, bad news such as failing exams or bereavement will quite naturally cause a period of '**reactive**' depression secondary to the tragic event.

However, there are people with a happy, contented lifestyle who for no apparent reason slip into a period of inconsolable depression. It is these people who are probably suffering from an '**endogenous**' biochemical failure to make sufficient brain serotonin and consequently their brain function is depressed. Clearly, lack of space here permits only a simplistic view of reactive and endogenous depression since it is likely there is an interaction between the two. However, there is an urgent need for an enlightened public attitude to these 'taboo' diseases.

The **indoleamine-amine hypothesis for affective disease** proposes that brain concentrations of neuroactive amines, e.g. serotonin, are associated with mood disorders. In depression, there is insufficient serotonin present for neurotransmission so brain function is depressed. Successful treatment of depression with serotonin reuptake inhibitors such as Prozac, which increase synaptic concentrations of serotonin, supports this hypothesis. Conversely, it is hypothesized that excessive concentrations of serotonin cause mania.

Serotonin metabolism

The regulatory enzyme for serotonin biosynthesis is **tryptophan hydroxylase**. Note that tryptophan hydroxylase has to compete for tryptophan with its rivals TDO and IDO. It is possible that if the hydroxylase is insufficiently active, brain concentrations of serotonin would be depleted and cause depression.

Catabolism of serotonin occurs when it is deaminated by monoamine oxidase and then oxidized to **5-hydroxyindoleacetic acid (5-HIAA)**. 5-HIAA is excreted in excessive amounts in patients with carcinoid syndrome.

Melatonin metabolism

Melatonin is made from its precursor **serotonin** in the pineal gland normally during periods of darkness. Melatonin is almost totally absent in daylight. The regulatory enzyme is **arylalkylamine *N*-acetyltransferase (AANAT)**. AANAT is **up-regulated** by noradrenergic stimulation that normally occurs during the **dark phase** of the day. It is **down-regulated** by light, which stimulates photoreceptors in the retina and initiates signals that are transmitted through a neural circuit including the **suprachiasmatic nuclei** (SCN, also called the '**biological clock**') and then onwards towards the pineal gland. **NB:** During continuous darkness melatonin varies up and down, driven by the SCN, i.e. a light/dark cycle is not needed to produce a rhythm.

Melatonin biosynthesis: AANAT is up-regulated in the dark by noradrenaline

Noradrenergic stimulation of primarily β- but also α-adrenergic receptors on pinealocytes and retinal photoreceptors activates **protein kinase A (PKA)** which phosphorylates and activates AANAT (Chart 50.1). Phosphorylated AANAT is now protected from degradation by binding to its 'bodyguard' **14-3-3 protein** (named after the laboratory number of the fraction from which it was isolated by its discoverers).

Melatonin biosynthesis: AANAT is down-regulated by light

Light, via the SCN, adjusts the time duration of sympathetic input to the pineal which inhibits synthesis of melatonin in the pineal gland. Light causes a rapid decrease in both the activity of AANAT and the amount of AANAT protein, which has a $t_{1/2}$ of 3 minutes. When noradrenergic stimulation ceases, PKA activity also decreases, and protein phosphatase dephosphorylates AANAT which loses its protective 14-3-3 protein and is exposed to and destroyed by **proteosomal proteolysis**.

Catabolism of melatonin

Melatonin is hydrophobic and must be conjugated with hydrophilic groups before it can be excreted in the urine. It is metabolized by **CYP 1A2** to **6-hydroxymelatonin**, which can be conjugated in two ways. The principal excretory product is **6-sulphatoxymelatonin** with the sulphate donated by **3′-phosphoadenosine-5′-phosphosulphate (PAPS)**. Alternatively, it forms **6-hydroxymelatonin glucuronide**.

Metabolism at a Glance, Fourth Edition. J. G. Salway. © 2017 John Wiley & Sons Ltd. Published 2017 by John Wiley & Sons Ltd.

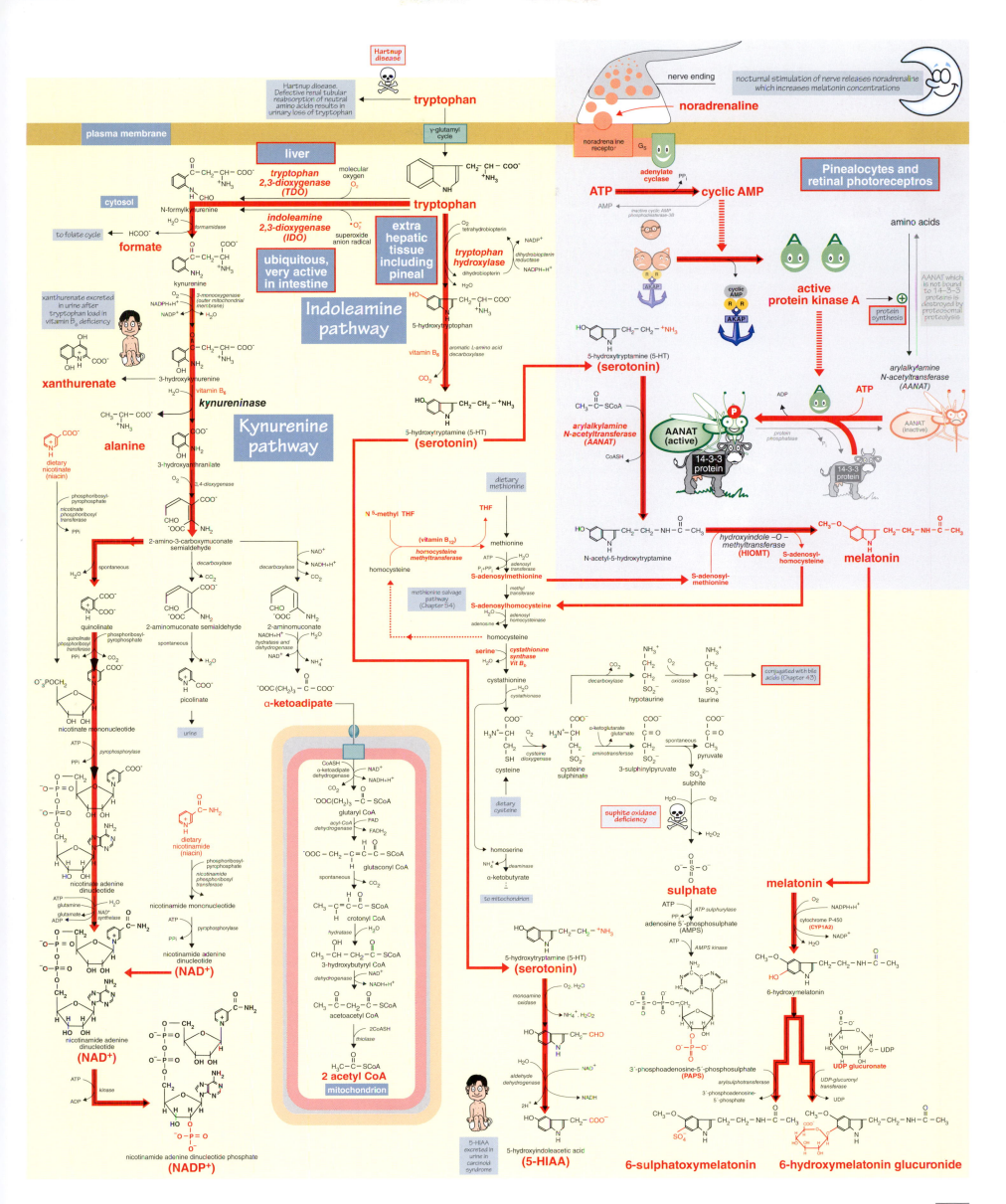

Ornithine cycle for the production of urea: the 'urea cycle'

51

A study of another metabolic cycle elucidated by Krebs, the Krebs–Henseleit ornithine cycle – popularly (but inaccurately) known as the 'urea cycle' – offers an overview of amino acid metabolism. In the fed state, any amino acids surplus to requirement for protein synthesis can be metabolized to non-nitrogenous substances such as glucose, glycogen or fatty acids, or they can be oxidized to generate ATP. On the other hand, during fasting or starvation, catabolic wasting of muscle occurs thereby yielding amino acids that are used for gluconeogenesis to maintain normoglycaemia. Because the ammonia derived from these amino acids is extremely toxic, it is converted to non-toxic **urea** for urinary excretion. Any ammonia that evades detoxification as urea can alternatively be incorporated into **glutamine** by glutamine synthetase, which has been described by Häussinger as serving as a scavenger for stray ammonium ions.

Origins of the nitrogen used for urea synthesis

In the fed state, amino acids are formed from dietary proteins by proteolytic digestion in the gastrointestinal tract. The amino acids are then absorbed into the bloodstream and may be used intact for protein synthesis. Alternatively, surplus amino acids can be metabolized to glucose, be used for fatty acid synthesis, or be catabolized to generate ATP. The amino groups are removed by transamination and deamination prior to urea synthesis in the periportal hepatocytes. The residual carbon skeletons are metabolized to the gluconeogenic precursors: pyruvate, succinyl CoA, fumarate, α-ketoglutarate and oxaloacetate or, alternatively, to the ketone bodies or their precursors (see Chapters 47 and 36, respectively).

In starvation, the circulating amino acids are derived mainly from proteolysis of muscle protein. Transamination of the amino acids, particularly the branched-chain amino acids isoleucine, valine and leucine (Chart 51.1), occurs in the muscle in partnership with pyruvate, so that the amino acid pool in the venous blood draining from the muscle is enriched with alanine (see Chapter 45). This alanine is transported to the liver, entering via the hepatic artery, where transamination with α-ketoglutarate (α-KG) occurs to form glutamate.

Chart 51.1: nitrogen, in the form of ammonium ions or glutamate, is used for urea synthesis

As shown in Chart 51.1, amino acids, whether of dietary or endogenous (muscle) origin, enter the pathway for urea synthesis by the **transdeamination route** or the **transamination route**.

Transdeamination route

This route consists of an initial transamination in the cytosol, followed by deamination in the mitochondrion. Initially **α-ketoglutarate** accepts an amino group from the donor amino acid to form **glutamate** in a cytosolic reaction catalysed by an **aminotransferase**. The glutamate is then transported by the glutamate carrier into the mitochondrion where it is oxidatively deaminated by **glutamate dehydrogenase** to form α-ketoglutarate and **ammonium ions**. The ammonium is incorporated into **carbamoyl phosphate**, which in turn reacts with **ornithine** to enter the urea cycle as **citrulline**.

Transamination route

Alternatively, nitrogen from the amino acids can enter the urea cycle via the transamination route, which involves two transamination reactions. Again, **α-ketoglutarate** initially accepts the amino group from the donor amino acid and once again **glutamate** is formed as described above. However, a second transamination now follows, with **oxaloacetate** accepting the amino group from glutamate to form **aspartate** in a reaction catalysed by **aspartate aminotransferase (AST)**. This aspartate now carries the second amino group into the urea cycle by condensing with **citrulline** to form **argininosuccinate**. Argininosuccinate is then cleaved to form **fumarate** and **arginine**. Finally, arginine is hydrolysed to **ornithine** and **urea**, and ornithine is regenerated for another rotation of the cycle.

Regulation of the urea cycle

The condensation of ammonia with bicarbonate to form carbamoyl phosphate is catalysed by **carbamoyl phosphate synthetase (CPS)**, which is only active in the presence of its allosteric effector, **N-acetylglutamate (NAG)**. NAG is synthesized from acetyl CoA and glutamate by **N-acetylglutamate synthase**.

Disorders of the urea cycle

The most common urea cycle disorder is ornithine transcarbamoylase (OTC) deficiency, which is X-linked. Affected boys develop severe hyperammonaemia, which often leads to early death. However, in heterozygous

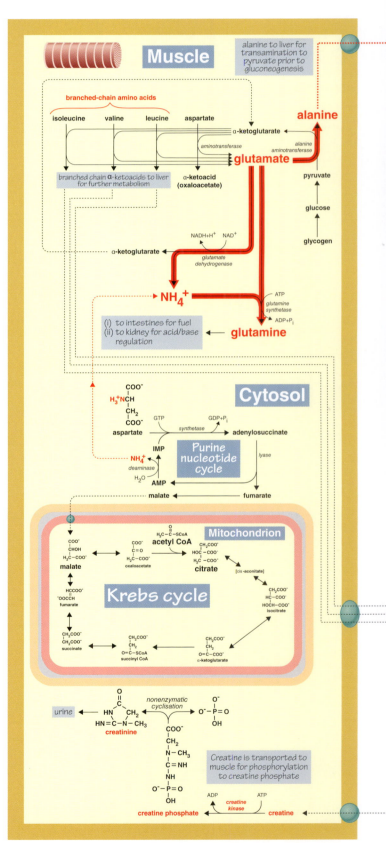

Chart 51.1 (this page and opposite) Nitrogen, in the form of ammonium ions or glutamate, is used for urea synthesis.

Metabolism at a Glance, Fourth Edition. J. G. Salway. © 2017 John Wiley & Sons Ltd. Published 2017 by John Wiley & Sons Ltd.

girls, the condition can vary from being undetectable to a severity equal to that in boys. In this condition, carbamoyl phosphate accumulates and passes into the cytosol where it reacts with aspartate to form carbamoyl aspartate. This is metabolized to form orotate by the reactions described for pyrimidine synthesis in Chapter 55. The detection of orotic acid (orotic aciduria) in urine is used to diagnose OTC deficiency.

OTC deficiency and gene therapy

There was considerable optimism that OTC deficiency would be a model candidate for liver-directed gene therapy. Unfortunately, a pilot study on 17 subjects with partial OTC deficiency using an adenoviral vector was very disappointing. There was very little gene transfer and when subject 18 suffered lethal complications, the trial was stopped.

Creatine and creatinine

The main function of the ornithine cycle is to produce urea. However, as shown in the chart, a small but significant quantity of arginine is diverted to form creatine. This is phosphorylated by creatine kinase to produce **creatine phosphate**, which is the phosphagen used to generate ATP during short bursts of intensive exercise. Approximately 2% of the body pool of creatine phosphate spontaneously cyclizes each day and is excreted in the urine as creatinine.

Purine nucleotide cycle

The purine nucleotide cycle described by Lowenstein, although present in many types of tissues, is particularly active in muscle. During vigorous exercise in rats, the blood concentration of ammonium ions can increase five-fold. This ammonium is thought to be derived from aspartate via the purine nucleotide cycle. This cycle is mentioned in Chapter 19.

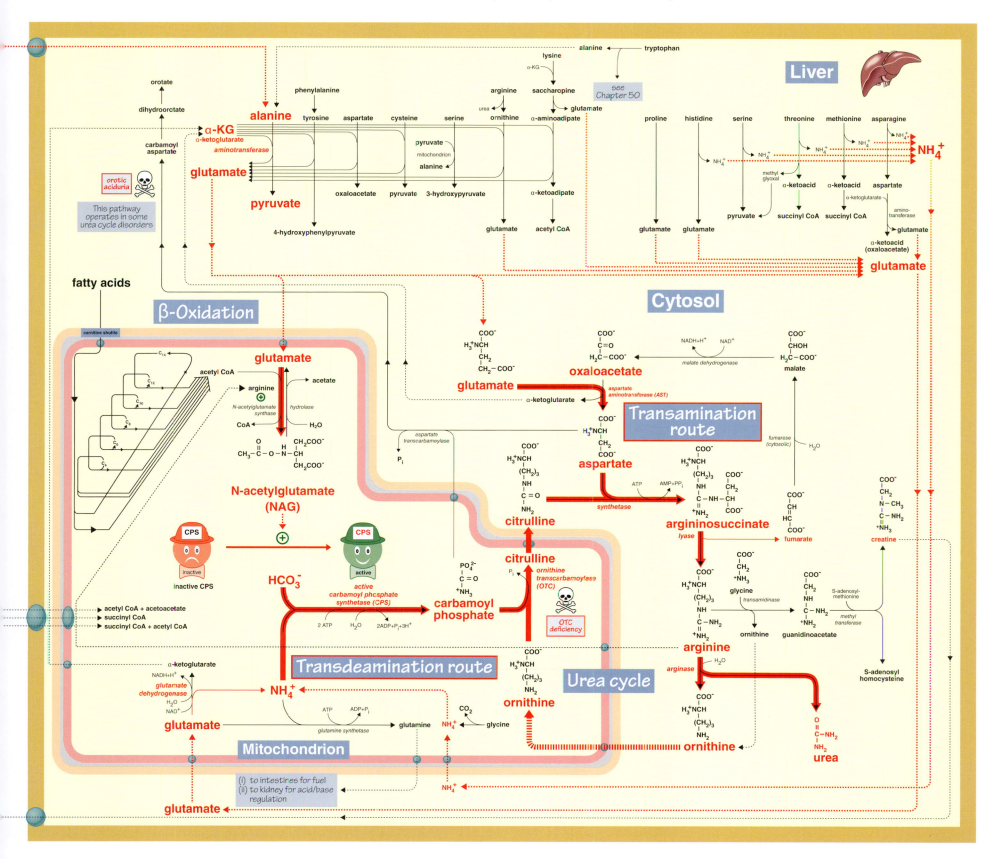

Metabolic channelling I: enzymes are organized to enable channelling of metabolic intermediates

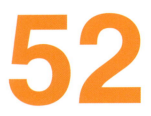

Metabolic intermediates are channelled from enzyme to enzyme

When I was a student it was rather assumed that the cell was 'a bag of enzymes' and that their substrates were randomly moving throughout the cytoplasm until a chance collision brought enzyme and substrate together, enabling the reaction to proceed. It was imagined that the product of this reaction would diffuse through the aqueous environment until a chance encounter with the next enzyme and substrate occurred to form the next product, and so on through to the end of the metabolic pathway. However, this simplistic idea is very inefficient and P. A. Srere introduced the hypothesis of **metabolic channelling**. This concept proposes that the products of an enzyme reaction are passed directly from the enzyme to the next enzyme in the metabolic sequence. This was defined by Srere as follows:

> 'Metabolic channelling of an intermediate can be defined as the passage of a common intermediate between two enzymes. The intermediate is localised and is out of equilibrium with the bulk solution.'

Experimental evidence supporting 'metabolic channelling'
Co-precipitation of enzymes

One of several experimental approaches that provides compelling evidence in support of metabolic channelling is provided by the tendency of enzymes that are sequential in a metabolic pathway to associate and co-precipitate when studied under certain conditions. Although enzymes when studied in dilute solution *in vitro* are free to diffuse in search of their substrates, this is not the case *in vivo*. For example, the proportion of soluble protein in the mitochondrial matrix is approximately 500 mg/ml of water. This water is approximately 50% water of hydration leaving just 50% free. These conditions can be simulated *in vitro* by adding to an enzyme preparation a volume-excluder, such as polyethyleneglycol, that removes water causing the enzymes to crowd together. This results in enzymes that are next to each other in a metabolic sequence to associate and co-precipitate. For example, the mitochondrial enzyme **citrate synthase** has been shown to bind to and co-precipitate with **pyruvate carboxylase**, the **pyruvate carrier**, **pyruvate dehydrogenase** and the **tricarboxylate transporter**. As shown in Diagram 52.1, these enzymes and carrier proteins are sequential in the pathways for pyruvate metabolism in mitochondria. Moreover, the binding is specific; for example, **citrate synthase** binds to the **mitochondrial** isoform of **malate dehydrogenase** but not to the **cytosolic** isoform of this enzyme.

Isotope dilution studies

Further evidence for metabolic channelling is provided by radioisotope dilution studies. Diagram 52.2a represents a metabolic pathway in which a radiolabelled substrate A is metabolized via intermediates B and C to

product D. If the substrates and their enzymes are free to diffuse in solution (**i.e. if there is no channelling of the metabolites**), then at steady state the specific activity of B, C and D will be the same as A. If, as shown in Diagram 52.2b, a 200-fold excess of non-radioactive C is added, then **in the absence of channelling** the specific radioactivity of C and product D will be diluted 200-fold, i.e. to 0.5% of the original value.

However, as represented metaphorically in Diagram 52.2c, if the metabolites and their enzymes are prevented from freely diffusing in the surrounding solution (i.e. the intermediates are passed from enzyme to enzyme and **metabolite channelling is occurring**), then the addition of a 200-fold excess of non-radioactive C will not dilute the specific radioactivity of product D. Instead, D is formed from the channelled radioactive C rather than from the pool of non-radioactive C in the bulk solution.

Metabolic channelling in the urea cycle

Experiments using radioisotope dilution studies suggest that metabolic channelling occurs in the urea cycle, albeit incompletely (Diagram 52.3). An experiment used **α-toxin** to make pores in the plasma membrane of hepatocytes. The hepatocytes were incubated in a physiological medium with ^{14}C-labelled HCO_3^-, **aspartate** and **ammonium chloride** as carbon and nitrogen sources plus other essential compounds. The ^{14}C label appeared in **urea** as would be anticipated. When a 200-fold excess of **non-radioactive arginine** was added, there was no decrease in the specific radioactivity of the urea formed. This suggests that metabolic channelling

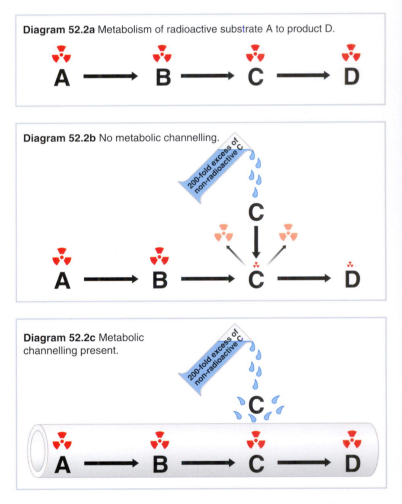

Diagram 52.2a Metabolism of radioactive substrate A to product D.

Diagram 52.2b No metabolic channelling.

Diagram 52.2c Metabolic channelling present.

Diagram 52.2 Experimental approach to demonstrate metabolic channelling by radioisotope dilution. (a) This represents a pathway from substrate A, which is metabolized via intermediates B and C to product D. If A is radioactive, then the specific radioactivity of intermediates B and C and product D will all be the same. (b) If a 200-fold excess of non-radioactive C is added, then provided substrate channelling does not occur, radioactive C will equilibrate with non-radioactive C and the specific radioactivity of product D will be diluted 200-fold. (c) If the experiment in (b) is repeated but metabolic channelling does occur, then the 200-fold excess of non-radioactive C will not equilibrate with radioactive C and the specific radioactivity of D will be the same as A.

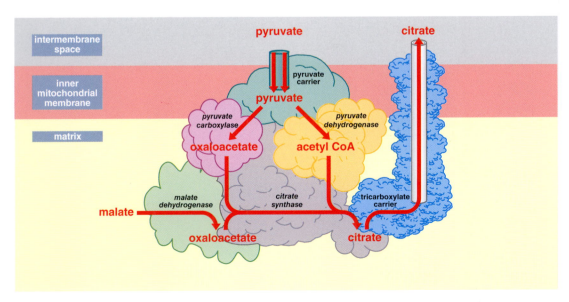

Diagram 52.1 Enzymes associating with citrate synthase. A schematic representation of how the enzymes and carrier proteins involved in the reactions adjacent to citrate synthase might be organized to allow metabolic channelling.

Metabolism at a Glance, Fourth Edition. J. G. Salway. © 2017 John Wiley & Sons Ltd. Published 2017 by John Wiley & Sons Ltd.

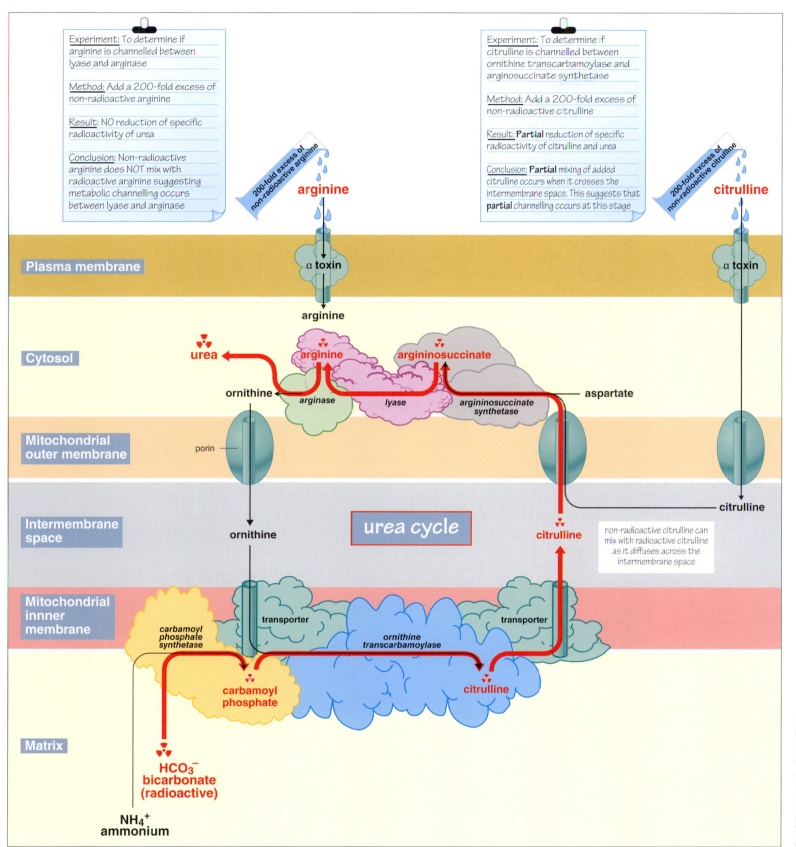

Diagram 52.3 Partial metabolic channelling in the urea cycle. Channelling is interrupted when ornithine and citrulline diffuse across the intermembrane space. During this stage of the journey, the molecules are free to equilibrate with other molecules in the intermembrane space and so metabolic channelling does not occur.

occurs between the **lyase** and **arginase** enzymes. However, when a 200-fold excess of **non-radioactive citrulline** was added, the specific radioactivity of the urea formed was reduced. This is because **citrulline** is formed by enzymes on the mitochondrial inner membrane and must diffuse across the intermembrane space to **argininosuccinate synthetase**, which is located on the outer side of the outer mitochondrial membrane. While ^{14}C citrulline is diffusing across the intermembrane space metabolic channelling

is not occurring and the radiolabelled citrulline is diluted with the added non-radioactive citrulline.

Reference

Cohen N.S., Cheung C.W., Raijman L. (1996) The urea cycle. In: *Channelling in Intermediary Metabolism* (L. Agius & H.S.A. Sherratt, eds), pp. 183–99. Portland Press, London and Miami.

Metabolic channelling II: fatty acid synthase

53

The *de novo* biosynthesis of **palmitate** from its precursor **acetyl CoA** involves the formation of 34 intermediate metabolites, which takes metabolic channelling to an extraordinary level of sophistication. It is represented in its familiar format in Chart 53.1 and as a cartoon in Diagram 53.4.

Fatty acid synthase complex

In animals, **fatty acid synthase** consists of two polypeptide chains. The two subunits are identical and are organized in a head-to-toe configuration (Diagrams 53.1 and 53.2). The component enzymes of the fatty acid synthase complex (Diagram 53.2) are:

1 **β-Ketoacyl ACP synthase (KS)** (also known as condensing enzyme or 3-oxoacyl synthase). The sulphydryl group of cysteine 161 has a vital function in the 'condensation reaction'. This is the process of chain elongation that occurs when malonyl acyl carrier protein (ACP) condenses with acyl ACP (or the initial acetyl ACP).
2 **β-Ketoacyl ACP reductase (KR)** (also known as 3-oxoacyl reductase).
3 **β-Hydroxyacyl ACP dehydratase (HD)** (also known as 3-hydroxyacyl hydratase).

4 **Enoyl ACP reductase (ER)** (also known simply as enoyl reductase).
5 **Thioesterase (TE)**. Once the fatty acyl chain is complete (palmitate is formed), it is thiolytically cleaved from ACP by thioesterase.
6 **Malonyl-acetyl CoA-ACP transacylase (MAT)** (also known as malonyl/acetyltransferase). This transfers the malonyl group of malonyl CoA to ACP, forming malonyl ACP. It also transfers the acetyl group of acetyl CoA to ACP, forming **acetyl ACP**. This acetyl group provides the ω and ω-1 carbon atoms of the fatty acid chain with **all** subsequent carbon atoms being provided by malonyl CoA.

In addition, there are two proteins:

1 **Acyl carrier protein (ACP)**. ACP is a relatively small protein of 54 kD. The prosthetic group **phosphopantetheine** (Diagram 53.3a) is attached to serine-2151 (Diagram 53.3b). This long prosthetic group carries the acyl groups sequentially from enzyme to enzyme as they grow, in the manner of a robotic arm on an assembly line which would rival a modern motor car factory.
2 **Core protein.** The core protein of each monomer is a component that stabilizes the structure of the dimer and is without enzymic activity.

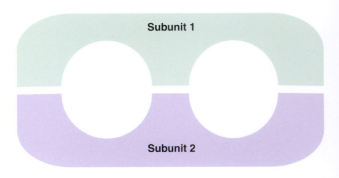

Diagram 53.1 In animals, fatty acid synthase is a dimer of two subunits that associate to form a complex with two holes.

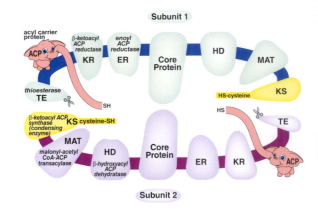

Diagram 53.2 **The protein components of each monomer are organized in a head-to-toe manner.** For example, in the diagram **thioesterase (TE) of subunit 1 is on the left**, while **TE of subunit 2 is on the right**. This arrangement allows cooperation between the subunits; that is that TE, ACP, KR and ER of subunit 1 collaborate with HD, MAT and KS of subunit 2 (and *vice versa* for the similar enzymes on the right of the diagram).

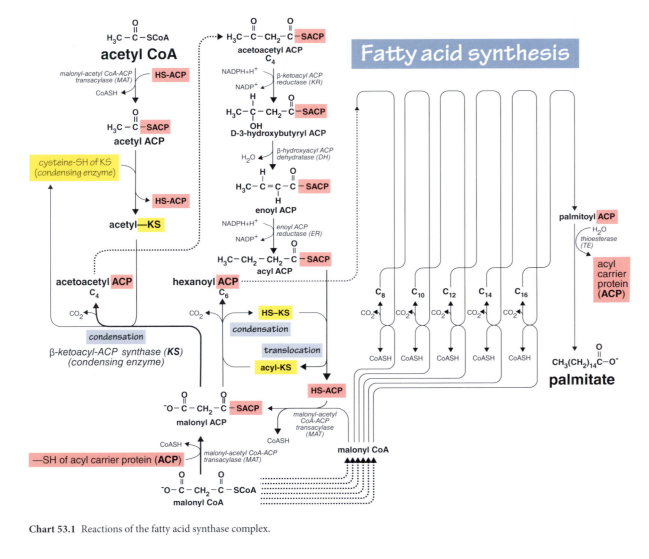

Chart 53.1 Reactions of the fatty acid synthase complex.

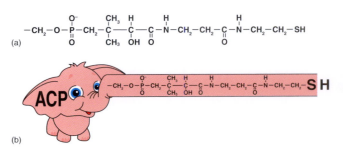

Diagram 53.3 (a) Phosphopantetheine. (b) Phosphopantetheine is attached to acyl carrier protein (ACP) to form a long prosthetic group.

Metabolism at a Glance, Fourth Edition. J. G. Salway. © 2017 John Wiley & Sons Ltd. Published 2017 by John Wiley & Sons Ltd.

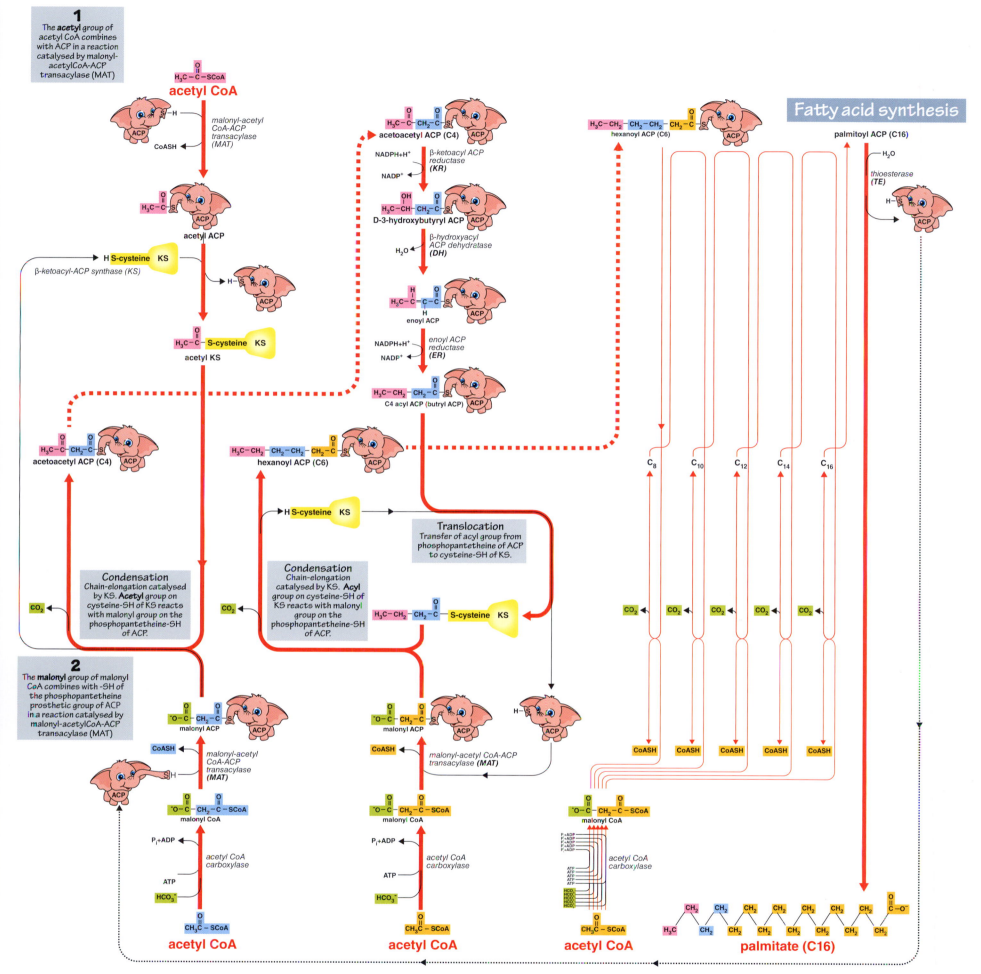

Diagram 53.4 Reactions of the fatty acid synthase complex (cartoon version).

Amino acid metabolism, folate metabolism and the '1-carbon pool' I: purine biosynthesis

54

Chart 54.1 (opposite) **Purine biosynthesis.** *For an explanation of low-dose methotrexate functioning as an antirheumatic drug, see Chapter 55.*

The '1-carbon pool'

This term describes the 1-carbon residues associated with *S-adenosylmethionine* (**SAM**) and **folate** that are available for metabolic reactions. *S*-adenosylmethionine (**SAM**). SAM, which is formed from methionine, is the major donor of methyl groups for biosynthetic reactions. It can, for example, methylate noradrenaline to form adrenaline, as shown in Chart 49.1. Other important reactions involving SAM include the methylation of phosphatidylethanolamine to phosphatidylcholine, and the formation of creatine.

Folate '1-carbon' units. The vitamin folate is reduced in two stages by dihydrofolate reductase to produce the active form, **tetrahydrofolate** (**THF**) (Chart 54.1). THF is a versatile carrier of 1-carbon units in the following oxidation states: formyl, methenyl, methylene and methyl. These THF compounds, which are interconvertible, together with SAM, comprise what is known as the '1-carbon pool'.

Amino acids and the '1-carbon pool'

Serine is converted to **glycine**, in a reaction catalysed by **serine hydroxymethyl transferase**, with the transfer of a methyl group to THF forming N^5,N^{10}-**methylene THF**. This reaction is particularly important in the thymidylate synthase reaction described in Chapter 55. Oxidation of glycine in mitochondria by the glycine cleavage enzyme also produces N^5,N^{10}-methylene THF (see Chapter 46).

Tryptophan is oxidized to *N*-formylkynurenine, which, in the presence of formamidase, yields kynurenine and the toxic product **formate**. THF accepts the formate, producing N^{10}-**formyl THF**.

Methionine, as mentioned above, is the precursor of SAM, which, following transfer of the methyl group to an acceptor, e.g. noradrenaline, forms homocysteine. Methionine can be regenerated from homocysteine by methylation using N^5-methyl THF in a salvage pathway. **NB:** This reaction, catalysed by homocysteine methyltransferase, requires **vitamin B$_{12}$**, and deficiency can lead to folate being caught in the 'methyl-folate' trap (see below).

Amino acid metabolism and purine synthesis

Glycine contributes the C-4, C-5 and N-7 atoms to the purine ring in a reaction catalysed by glycinamide ribonucleotide (GAR) synthetase (Chart 54.1).

Aspartate is an important donor of nitrogen atoms during purine biosynthesis, contributing the N-1 atom to the purine ring. Aspartate also donates the –NH$_2$ group in the adenylosuccinate synthetase reaction of the pathway that forms AMP from inosine monophosphate (IMP) (Chart 54.2).

Chart 54.2 Conversion of IMP to ATP, the purine nucleotide cycle. IMP reacts with aspartate in the presence of GTP to form adenylosuccinate, which is cleaved to form fumarate and AMP. The AMP can be phosphorylated to ADP, which undergoes oxidative phosphorylation to form ATP. The purine nucleotide cycle has an anaplerotic role in Krebs cycle.

Conversion of IMP to GTP. IMP is oxidized to xanthine monophosphate (XMP), which is aminated to form GMP, which is phosphorylated to form GDP. GDP is phosphorylated by ATP in a reaction catalysed by nucleoside diphosphate kinase. Alternatively, when Krebs cycle is active, GTP is formed from GDP by succinyl CoA synthetase (see Chapter 19).

Formation of dATP (deoxyadenosine triphosphate) and dGTP (deoxyguanosine triphosphate). The deoxy-ribonucleotides dATP and dGTP are formed by first reducing ADP and GDP to dADP and dGDP in the presence of ribonucleotide reductase. These are subsequently phosphorylated to form dATP and dGTP, which can be used for the synthesis of DNA.

Glutamine plays a very important role in nucleotide metabolism. It donates the nitrogen atoms that form N-9 and N-3 of the purine ring. It also participates in the amination of xanthine monophosphate (XMP) to form guanosine monophosphate (GMP) (Chart 54.2).

Biosynthesis of purines

Purine nucleotides can be synthesized *de novo*. They can also be reclaimed from existing nucleosides by the so-called 'salvage pathway' (see Chapter 55). The *de novo* pathway needs '1-carbon' units from the folate pool, and several amino acids as detailed below.

De novo pathway for purine biosynthesis

The pathway starts with **ribose 5-phosphate** formed by the pentose phosphate pathway (Chart 54.1). This is activated to form **phosphoribosyl pyrophosphate** (**PRPP**). A total of 11 reactions are needed to form **IMP** (or inosinic acid), which is the precursor of the adenine- and guanine-containing nucleotides. The important roles of glutamine and aspartate as amino donors are emphasized. A total of **3 glutamine** molecules and **1 aspartate** molecule are needed for the synthesis of GMP. Similarly, a total of **2 glutamine** and **2 aspartate** molecules are needed for AMP synthesis. A molecule of **glycine** is needed in each case.

The *de novo* pathway is controlled by feedback inhibition of PRPP amidotransferase by AMP and GMP. In **primary gout** this feedback control is impaired, causing increased production of purines resulting in the increased formation of their sparingly soluble excretory product, uric acid.

Vitamin B$_{12}$ and the 'methyl-folate trap'

Vitamin B$_{12}$, or more precisely its methyl cobalamin derivative, is an essential coenzyme for the transfer of methyl groups in the **methionine salvage pathway** (Chart 54.1). Accordingly, in B$_{12}$ deficiency, THF cannot be released and remains trapped as N^5-methyl THF. Eventually, all the body's folate becomes trapped in the N^5-methyl THF form, and so folate deficiency develops secondary to B$_{12}$ deficiency. Because blood cells turn over rapidly, they need nucleotides for nucleic acid synthesis and are vulnerable to folate deficiency, which causes megaloblastic anaemia. Another effect of folate/B$_{12}$ deficiency is increased plasma concentration of homocysteine, which is associated with cardiovascular disease.

The methyl-folate trap hypothesis explains the observation that, although the haematological symptoms of B$_{12}$ deficiency respond to folate treatment, the neurological degeneration progresses. Remember that the other enzyme for which B$_{12}$ is a coenzyme is methylmalonyl CoA mutase (see Chapters 45 and 46). Accumulation of methylmalonyl CoA may interfere with the biosynthesis of lipids needed for the myelin sheath.

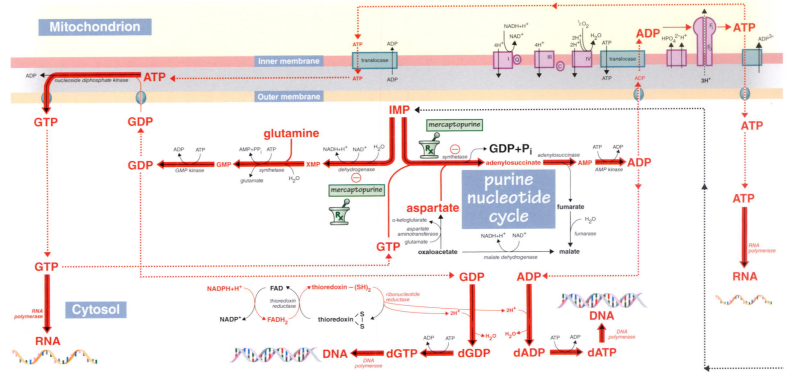

Metabolism at a Glance, Fourth Edition. J. G. Salway. © 2017 John Wiley & Sons Ltd. Published 2017 by John Wiley & Sons Ltd.

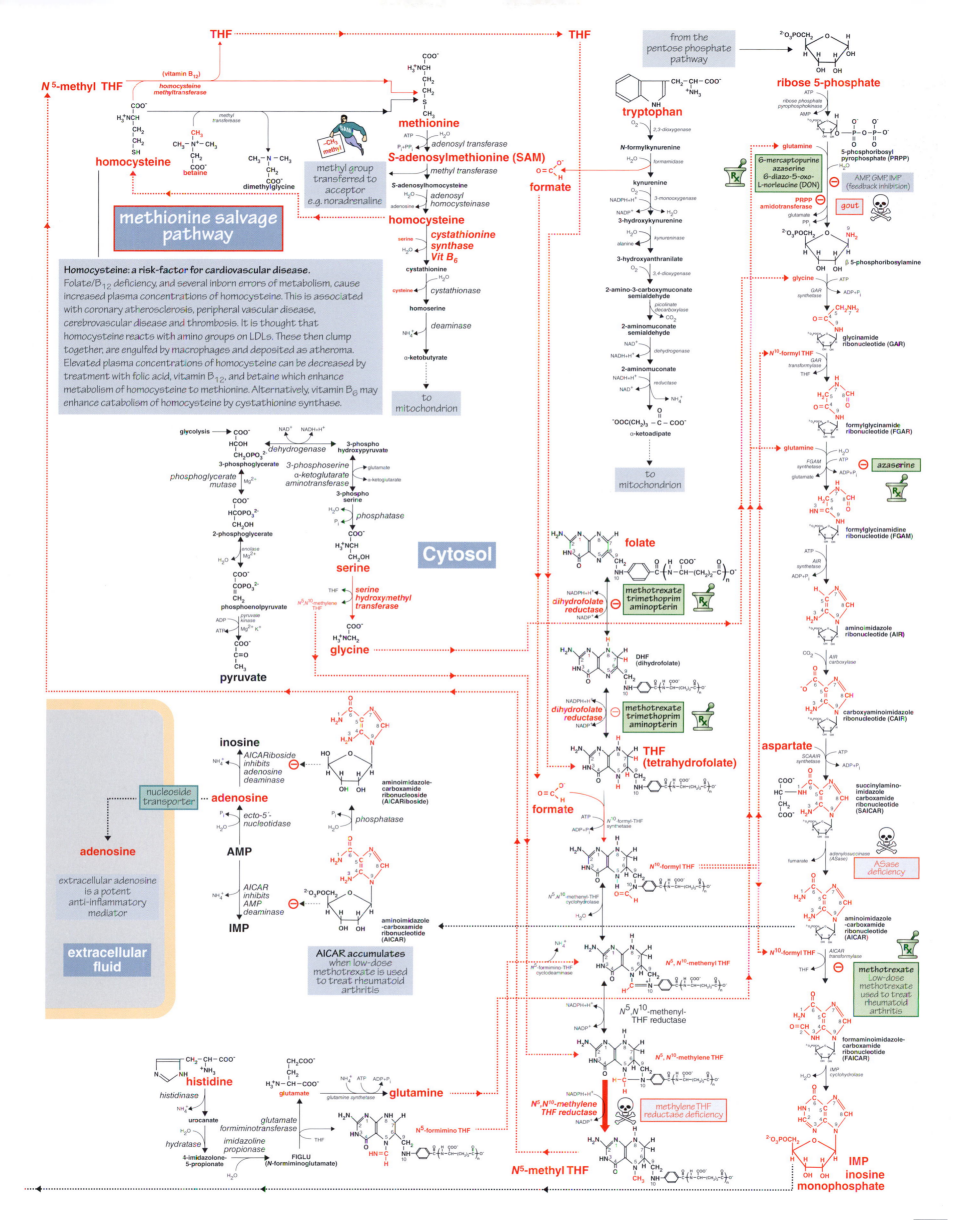

Amino acid metabolism, folate metabolism and the '1-carbon pool' II: pyrimidine biosynthesis

55

Chart 55.1 (opposite) Biosynthesis *de novo* of pyrimidines.

Amino acid metabolism and pyrimidine biosynthesis

The pyrimidine ring is derived from bicarbonate, glutamine and aspartate. The first reaction, catalysed by **carbamoyl phosphate synthetase II (CPS II)**, occurs in the cytosol and produces **carbamoyl phosphate** from bicarbonate, glutamine and two molecules of ATP. This is similar to the mitochondrial reaction involved in the urea cycle, which differs in that it forms carbamoyl phosphate from bicarbonate and NH_4^+ ions. Another difference is that CPS II does not require *N*-acetyl glutamate as an allosteric stimulator. The rest of the pyrimidine ring is donated by aspartate and, after ring closure and oxidation, **orotate** is formed. It is at this stage that **phosphoribosyl pyrophosphate (PRPP)** is added to yield **orotidine monophosphate (OMP)**, which, following decarboxylation, produces **uridine monophosphate (UMP)**, which is the common precursor of the pyrimidine-containing nucleotides (Chart 55.1).

Conversion of UMP to UTP and CTP

UMP is phosphorylated by a specific UMP kinase to form uridine diphosphate (UDP), which in turn is phosphorylated by the non-specific nucleoside diphosphate kinase to yield **uridine triphosphate** (**UTP**). When UTP is aminated, **cytidine triphosphate** (**CTP**) is formed.

Formation of deoxycytidine triphosphate (dCTP) and deoxythymidine triphosphate (dTTP)

dCTP is formed from cytidine diphosphate (CDP) by ribonucleotide reductase, by a mechanism analogous to the production of purine-containing deoxyribonucleotides (see Chapter 54).

The pathway for the formation of dTTP is quite distinct from that used to produce deoxyadenosine triphosphate (dATP), deoxyguanosine triphosphate (dGTP) and dCTP. The pathway starts with deoxycytidine diphosphate (dCDP), which is dephosphorylated and deaminated to yield deoxyuridine monophosphate (dUMP). This is methylated by N^5,N^{10}-methylene tetrahydrofolate (THF), which is oxidized to dihydrofolate (DHF) in the reaction catalysed by **thymidylate synthase**, and deoxythymidine monophosphate (dTMP) is formed. The dTMP is now phosphorylated by dTMP kinase and nucleoside diphosphate kinase to produce dTTP.

Let us return to DHF, which is formed by the **thymidylate synthase** reaction. This is reduced by **dihydrofolate reductase**, which regenerates **THF**. The cycle is completed when this THF participates in the **serine hydroxymethyltransferase** reaction, producing glycine and N^5,N^{10}-methylene THF; the latter is now available once more for thymidylate synthase.

Cancer chemotherapy

Because rapidly dividing cancer cells have a great demand for DNA synthesis, much attention has been directed at the pathways for nucleotide synthesis as a target for chemotherapeutic intervention. These drugs are classified by pharmacologists as 'antimetabolites' and fall into the following categories: glutamine antagonists, folate antagonists, antipyrimidines and antipurines.

Glutamine antagonists

The importance of glutamine for the biosynthesis of purines and pyrimidines has been emphasized already (see Chapter 54). Azaserine and diazo-oxo-norleucine (DON) irreversibly inhibit the enzymes involved in the glutamine-utilizing reactions (see Chart 54.1), reducing the DNA available to cancer cells.

Folate antagonist

Methotrexate, which is a close structural analogue of folate (Diagram 55.1), inhibits **DHF reductase**. This prevents the reduction of DHF to THF, as shown in Chart 55.1. Consequently, in the absence of THF, serine hydroxymethyltransferase is unable to generate the N^5,N^{10}-methylene THF needed by thymidylate synthase for dTMP production.

The clinical benefit to patients treated with high doses of methotrexate is enhanced by the use of folinic acid, N^5-formyl THF (also known as **leucovorin**), which 'rescues' normal cells from the toxic effects of methotrexate.

Methotrexate and rheumatoid arthritis. Intermittent weekly low-doses of methotrexate (5–25 mg/week; cf. 5000 mg weekly for treatment of malignancy) is an important therapy for rheumatoid arthritis. The mechanism is thought to be as shown on Chart 54.1. Methotrexate inhibits aminoimidazole-carboxamide ribonucleoside (AICAR) transformylase causing accumulation of **AICAR** and its dephosphorylated metabolite, **AICARiboside**. AICAR inhibits AMP deaminase and AICARiboside inhibits adenosine deaminase causing **adenosine** to accumulate. Extracellular adenosine is a potent anti-inflammatory mediator.

Antipyrimidines and antipurines

1 **Antipyrimidines, e.g. flurouracil.** Fluorouracil inhibits thymidylate synthase and thus prevents the conversion of dUMP to dTMP.
2 **Antipurines, e.g. mercaptopurine.** Mercaptopurine inhibits purine biosynthesis at several stages. It inhibits PRPP amidotransferase (see Chart 54.1), IMP dehydrogenase and adenylosuccinate synthetase (see Chart 54.2).

Salvage pathways for the recycling of purines and pyrimidines

When nucleic acids and nucleotides are degraded, the free purine and pyrimidine bases are formed. These can be recycled by 'salvage pathways' (Diagram 55.2), which require much less ATP compared with the energy-intensive *de novo* pathways shown in Charts 54.1 and 55.1. The salvage pathways for purines require specific **phosphoribosyl transferases (PRTs)** that transfer **PRPP** in reactions analogous to that of **orotate PRT** (Chart 55.1).

Lesch–Nyhan syndrome

This is an extremely rare disorder caused by almost total deficiency of **hypoxanthine-guanine PRT**. In this condition, which is characterized by severe self-mutilation, the salvage pathway is inactive. Consequently, the free purines hypoxanthine and guanine are instead oxidized by xanthine oxidase to uric acid which is sparingly soluble and causes gout.

Antiviral drug azidothymidine (AZT)

AZT is an analogue of thymidine that can be phosphorylated to form the nucleotide triphosphate, azidothymidine triphosphate (AZTTP). AZTTP inhibits the viral DNA polymerase, which is an RNA-dependent polymerase. The host cell's DNA-dependent polymerase is relatively insensitive to inhibition by AZTTP.

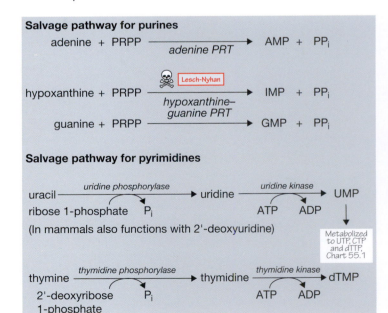

Diagram 55.2 Salvage pathways for purines and pyrimidines.

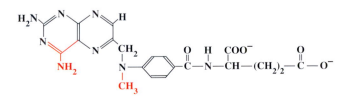

Diagram 55.1 Methotrexate.

Metabolism at a Glance, Fourth Edition. J. G. Salway. © 2017 John Wiley & Sons Ltd. Published 2017 by John Wiley & Sons Ltd.

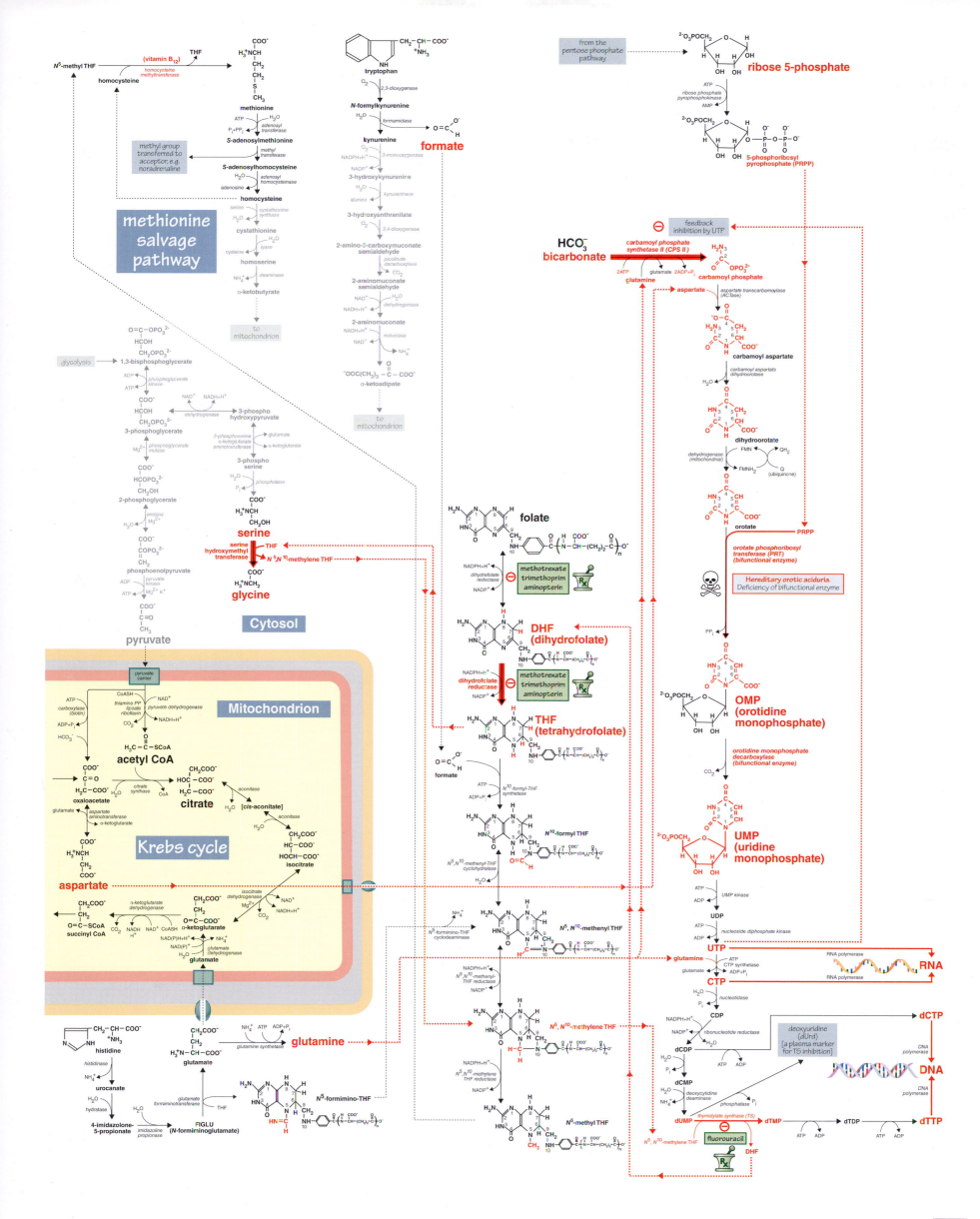

Krebs uric acid cycle for the disposal of nitrogenous waste

56

Krebs and his trinity of cycles

The distinguished biochemist from Oxford University, Sir Hans Krebs (1900–1981), discovered three biochemical cycles which have been described elsewhere in this book. Earlier we met the **Krebs citric acid cycle** or **TCA cycle**, referred to in this book simply as **Krebs cycle** (see Chapter 19), and a truncated version of this, the **glyoxylate cycle** (see Chapter 20). Also, we have seen how mammals dispose of their toxic nitrogenous waste from amino acid catabolism by using the **ornithine** or **urea cycle** (see Chapter 51) to form urea for urinary excretion. Hans Leo Kornberg wrote in 2000, 'Everyone who has taken biology at school has heard of the Krebs cycle, but few realize that Krebs also discovered **two** other cycles.' It is remarkable that even Kornberg, ironically co-discoverer of the glyoxylate cycle, had overlooked a fourth Krebs cycle which was published in 1978.

A fourth Krebs cycle in uricotelic animals

There is a fourth Krebs cycle which has been almost totally overlooked by text books and biochemists. This is the **uric acid cycle**, which operates in birds and probably in other uricotelic animals (e.g. land reptiles) and insects. The term uricotelism is used to describe animals that dispose of their nitrogenous waste from protein metabolism as uric acid. Similarly, the terms ureotelism and ammonotelism apply to the excretion of nitrogen as urea and ammonia respectively. **NB:** It should be emphasized that whereas mammals dispose of nitrogenous waste from **protein catabolism as urea** (see Chapter 51, they dispose of **purine waste as uric acid or allantoin** (Diagram 56.1).

Origin of the nitrogen used for uric acid synthesis

Nitrogen from the catabolism of amino acids is incorporated into **glutamate** or converted to **ammonium ions** by a process analogous to that used for the urea cycle (Chart 56.1). Ammonium ions are very toxic and react with glutamate to form **glutamine**. Uric acid contains four nitrogen atoms: two of these are derived from glutamine, one from glutamate and one from glycine. The uric acid cycle is a cyclic adaptation of the process used for mammalian purine catabolism shown in Chapter 54. **Inosine monophosphate (IMP)** is formed, which reacts with pyrophosphate to form **hypoxanthine** and **5-phosphoribosyl pyrophosphate (PRPP)**. This reaction is catalysed by **hypoxanthine phosphoribosyl transferase** (EC 2.4.2.8), otherwise known as IMP pyrophosphorylase. The phosphoribosyl transferases (PRTs) have

been referred to in Chapter 55 in connection with the salvage pathway for recycling purines and pyrimidines. Pyrophosphate is regenerated by the **PRPP amidotransferase** reaction. **NB:** The substrate that is recycled is PRPP, so strictly speaking this should be called the '**PRPP cycle for the production of uric acid**'.

Energy considerations

Formation of uric acid by the cycle requires hydrolysis of 6-phosphoanhydride bonds (see Chapter 2. The reactions are: glutamine synthetase (2 bonds); FGAM synthetase (1 bond); AIR synthetase (1 bond); SAICAR synthetase (1 bond); and GAR synthetase (1 bond). Thus for the excretion of four nitrogen atoms as uric acid, six phosphoanhydride bonds are hydrolysed, which is equivalent to 1.5 per nitrogen atom. This compares favourably with excretion of urea by mammals where two phosphoanhydride bonds are used for each nitrogen atom synthesized.

What about glycine? When considering the energy for the biosynthesis of uric acid it is easy to overlook that a molecule of glycine is incorporated. If this glycine was oxidized as fuel it would generate ATP as follows. Chart 46.2 shows that glycine can be metabolized to pyruvate and oxidized in Krebs citric acid cycle. The following NADH + H⁺-dependent reactions – pyruvate dehydrogenase, isocitrate dehydrogenase, α-ketoglutarate dehydrogenase and malate dehydrogenase – generate a total of 4 NADH + H⁺ which, assuming a P/O ratio of 2.5 (see Chapter 6), yield **10 ATP**. Succinyl CoA synthetase produces **1 GTP** (equivalent to ATP) and succinate dehydrogenase produces 1 FADH₂ yielding **1.5 ATP**. Thus a glycine molecule has the potential to produce 12.5 molecules of ATP.)

Ammonotelic, uricotelic and ureotelic animals

Although all animals have the challenge of disposing toxic ammonia from protein catabolism, there are three main nitrogenous waste products: ammonium ions, uric acid and urea. For animals such as bony fish and larval amphibians, which inhabit an aquatic environment with an unlimited supply of water, ammonia is the principal excretory product. Approximately 400 ml of water is needed to excrete 1 g of ammonia. However, terrestrial animals such as insects, terrestrial reptiles and birds, can tolerate a dry environment and excrete uric acid requiring only approximately 8 ml of water per gram of nitrogen – whereas urea needs 40 ml of water.

Diagram 56.1 Metabolism of uric acid to ammonium ions. This sequence of enzymatic reactions is mainly (but not entirely) contained within the intestinal flora of the species. For example, uricase is present in the liver of mammals with the notable exception of the primates. Therefore, this diagram should be used with judicious caution as the excretion of nitrogenous waste is complicated by many anomalies in response to environmental adaptation. It is a fascinating topic for the study of evolutionary biochemistry.

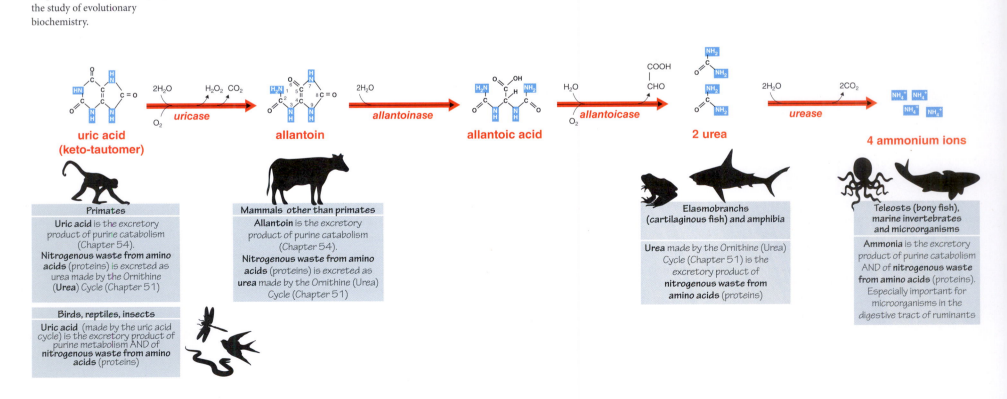

Metabolism at a Glance, Fourth Edition. J. G. Salway. © 2017 John Wiley & Sons Ltd. Published 2017 by John Wiley & Sons Ltd.

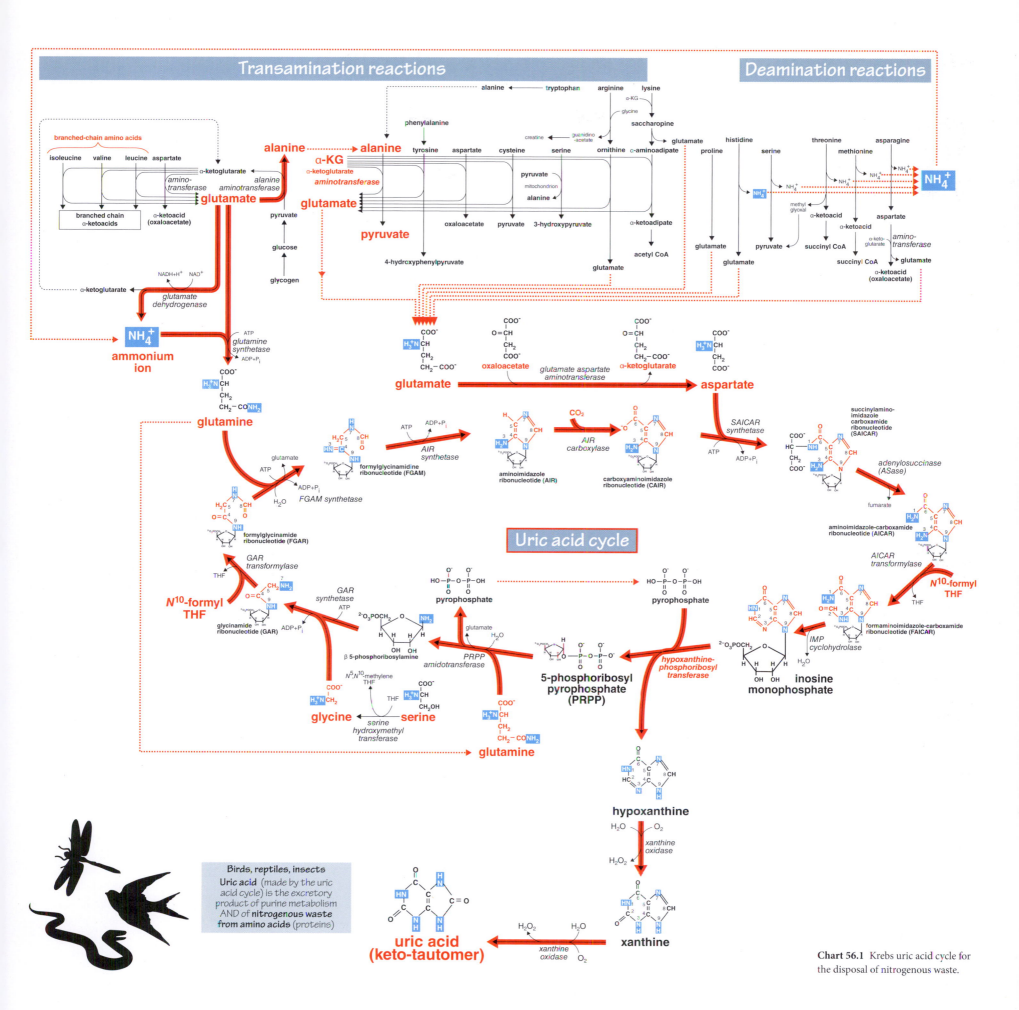

Chart 56.1 Krebs uric acid cycle for the disposal of nitrogenous waste.

Although other biochemists established the intermediates involved in purine metabolism as a **linear process**, it was Mapes and Krebs who organized the **pathway as a cycle**. The Krebs uric acid cycle described here is in their publication cryptically entitled: 'Rate-limiting factors in urate synthesis and gluconeogenesis in avian liver'.

References

Kornberg H. (2000) Krebs and his trinity of cycles. *Nature Rev Cell Biol*, **1**, 225–8.

Mapes J.P., Krebs H.A. (1978) Rate-limiting factors in urate synthesis and gluconeogenesis in avian liver. *Biochem J*, **172**, 193–203.

Porphyrin metabolism, haem and the bile pigments

57

Haem biosynthesis

The porphyrin-iron complex, haem, is a component of the cytochromes (e.g. those of the respiratory chain and cytochrome P450, or CYP, family), several enzymes, myoglobin and haemoglobin. Haem is therefore formed in most cells but especially in erythropoietic bone marrow and liver. The latter are particularly affected in the porphyrin disorders, which can be classified as 'erythroid' and 'hepatic' porphyrias, respectively.

As shown in Chart 57.1, **succinyl CoA** and **glycine** condense to form **5-aminolevulinic acid (ALA)** in a reaction catalysed by **ALA synthase**, which is the regulatory enzyme for haem biosynthesis. Two molecules of ALA combine to form the monopyrrole **porphobilinogen (PBG)**. Four molecules of the latter react to form the tetrapyrrole **hydroxymethylbilane**, which cyclizes in a reaction catalysed by uroporphyrinogen III cosynthase to form **uroporphyrinogen III**. Note that hydroxymethylbilane can also cyclize non-enzymically to form an isomer, **uroporphyrinogen I**, differing in the positions of the propionic and acetic acid substituents in the D ring.

Disorders of porphyrin metabolism: 'the porphyrias'

There is a principle common to many of the porphyrias. The porphyrin pathway is regulated by feedback inhibition of ALA synthase by haem. If an enzyme in this pathway is deficient, the consequent tendency for the haem concentration to fall is compensated by de-repression of ALA synthase, thus favouring haem biosynthesis. This causes moderately increased concentrations of the metabolites upstream of the enzyme deficiency and maintains haem formation without affecting the subject; i.e. the disorder is 'clinically silent'. A crisis occurs if the patient takes drugs (such as barbiturates, sex steroids or ethanol), which can dramatically increase the activity of ALA synthase. This results in a massive surge of intermediates, which accumulate proximally to the deficient enzyme causing distressing symptoms.

Neurological or photosensitizing effects of metabolites in porphyria

Deficiency of PBG deaminase results in a chronic, but clinically silent, accumulation of PBG and ALA. An acute crisis is precipitated by the ingestion of ethanol or drugs, which can cause up to a 50-fold increase in ALA synthase activity. The consequent dramatic increase in these porphyrin precursors is associated with the onset of **neuropsychiatric** features of the acute crisis, which may be caused by a neurotoxic effect of ALA. Nowadays, it is thought that an acute porphyria was responsible for the bizarre behaviour of King George III towards the end of his reign (1760–1820), which led to the Regency Period following the appointment of his son George as Prince Regent in 1811.

If the enzyme deficiency is after PBG deaminase, then **photosensitivity** is a major feature. This is because porphyrinogens accumulate and are oxidized non-enzymically to their corresponding porphryins. The latter are activated by light and generate singlet oxygen, which is very cytotoxic and causes the dermatological features of porphyria.

Porphyrin metabolism and the treatment of skin cancer by photodynamic therapy (PDT)

In PDT for cancer, a photosensitizing drug (or a precursor molecule that can be metabolized into a photosensitizer) is administered topically or systemically to a patient with a tumour. The cancer site is then irradiated with light of a suitable wavelength, determined by the photosensitizer absorption spectrum. In combination with molecular oxygen, this induces the formation of reactive 'singlet oxygen', which causes local destruction of tissue, but only at the precise area where the light is applied.

The approach is now widely used in the treatment of non-melanoma skin cancers by topical application of ALA, the first dedicated metabolic precursor of protoporphyrin IX and haem. ALA then enters the tumour haem biosynthetic pathway but, because of the artificially high loading on this pathway, relatively large concentrations of protoporphyrin IX build up transiently in tumours, where ferrochelatase activity is relatively low compared with healthy tissue. Since protoporphyrin IX is a powerful photosensitizer, tumour destruction occurs rapidly when light is applied. This is a relatively selective process, not only because of the targeting of the light, but also because of the greater accumulation of protoporphyrin IX in tumours compared with normal tissue.

Since protoporphyrin IX is strongly fluorescent, this approach is also being widely used to diagnose certain cancers (e.g. in the bladder), which 'light up' under UV light.

Catabolism of haem to bilirubin

Following the death, damage or turnover of cells, the various haem proteins (cytochromes, enzymes, haemoglobin and myoglobin) are degraded to release haem. The cyclic tetrapyrrole ring of haem is split at the α-methene bridge by **haem oxygenase** in a reaction that liberates iron, forms the green linear tetrapyrrole called **biliverdin** and, curiously, emits carbon monoxide. Next, the methene bridge between the C and D rings is reduced to a methane bridge and the major orange/brown bile pigment **bilirubin** is formed. Bilirubin is **hydrophobic** and binds to albumin for transport in the blood to the liver (obviously, this stage is not necessary for bilirubin derived from haem *in situ* in liver). At the hepatocyte surface bilirubin changes its means of transport for a protein called ligandin, which carries it to the endoplasmic reticulum. Here, it conjugates with two molecules of uridine diphosphate (UDP) glucuronide forming bilirubin diglucuronide, which is **hydrophilic**. Bilirubin diglucuronide is secreted in the bile and is further metabolized by the intestinal flora to urobilinogen, urobilin and stercobilin.

Treatment of neonatal jaundice with Sn (tin) mesoporphyrin

Although mild, transient neonatal jaundice is common and is not usually cause for concern. Severe neonatal jaundice caused, for example, by immune haemolysis or glucose 6-phosphate dehydrogenase deficiency (see Chapter 15) can be life-threatening, as explained below.

In Chart 57.1 we see how haem is metabolized to bilirubin, which is a **hydrophobic**, fat-soluble molecule. Bilirubin normally combines with UDP glucuronate to form a **hydrophilic** conjugate prior to excretion in the bile. However, in infants, especially premature infants, the conjugating enzyme **UDP glucuronyl transferase** can be insufficiently developed and so the unconjugated, fat-soluble form of bilirubin accumulates causing neonatal jaundice. In extreme hyperbilirubinaemia, the fat-soluble bilirubin is toxic to the brain causing kernicterus (brain jaundice). Fortunately, hyperbilirubinaemia can often be treated by light therapy, which destroys the bilirubin. However, if this is not successful then exchange transfusion is needed. **Sn-mesoporphyrin** can help avoid this treatment and has been used to treat babies of Jehovah's Witness parents who oppose exchange transfusion on religious grounds.

Sn-mesoporphyrin is a tin-containing metalloporphyrin derived from Sn-protoporphyrin by reducing the vinyl groups at C-2 and C-4 to ethyl groups. It is a potent competitive inhibitor of haem oxygenase, thereby restricting formation of bilirubin, and it has been used to treat neonatal jaundice. A single dose of Sn-mesoporphyrin has been shown to prevent development of severe hyperbilirubinaemia in neonates with glucose 6-phosphate dehydrogenase deficiency.

Metabolism at a Glance, Fourth Edition. J. G. Salway. © 2017 John Wiley & Sons Ltd. Published 2017 by John Wiley & Sons Ltd.

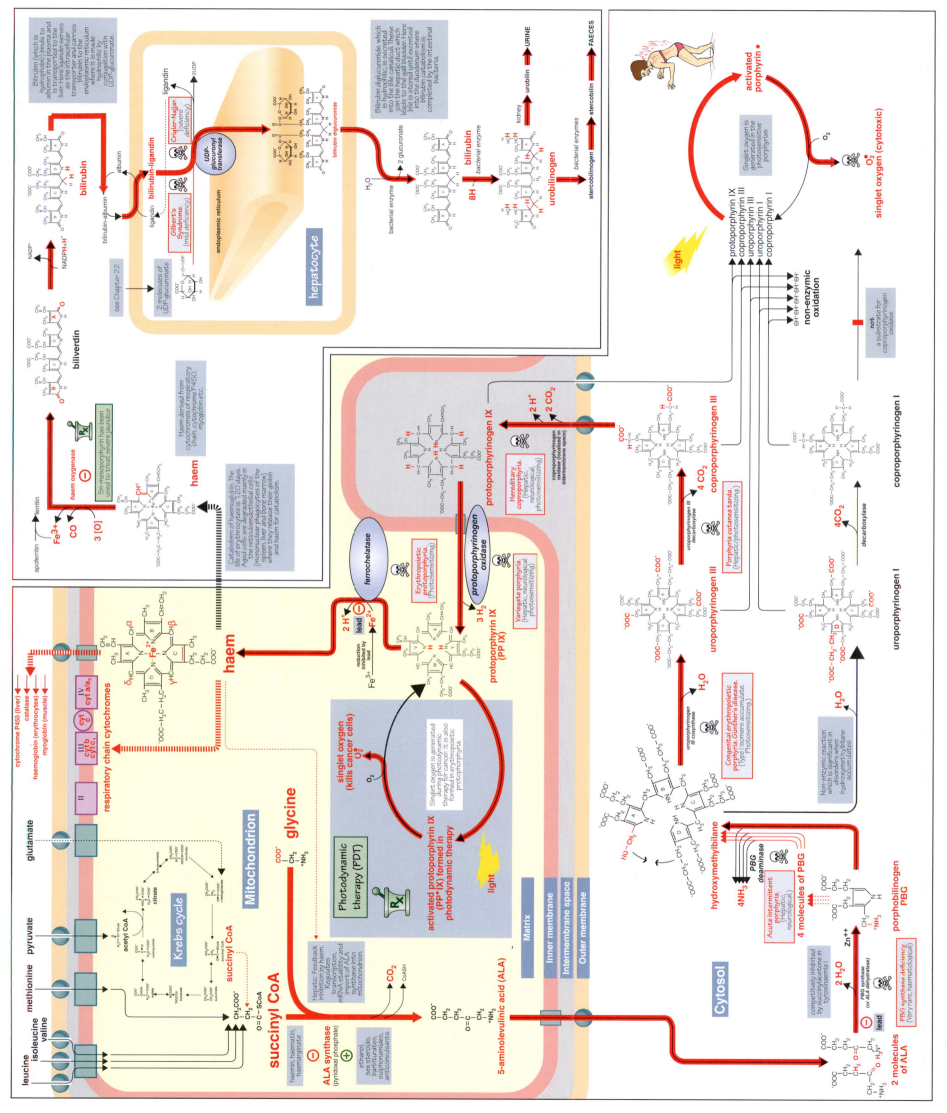

Chart 57.1 Biosynthesis of haem and its catabolism to the bile pigments.

Metabolic pathways in fasting liver and their disorder in Reye's syndrome

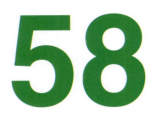

58

Metabolic mutual dependence

In a splendid example of '*United we stand, divided we fall*' the pathways for **gluconeogenesis**, **β-oxidation**, the **urea cycle**, **ketogenesis** and the **respiratory chain** are mutually dependent (Chart 58.1). The demand for ATP in liver during fasting arises from: (i) the need for ATP by **gluconeogenesis**, to maintain the blood glucose concentration; and (ii) the need for ATP by the **urea cycle**, which disposes of nitrogen from amino acids. To generate ATP in the **respiratory chain**, $FADH_2$ and NADH are supplied by **β-oxidation**, which produces acetyl CoA that is deployed for **ketogenesis**. If all the pathways are functioning optimally, all is well. However, if **even one** of these pathways is not operating adequately, this failure might compromise the functioning of **all** the other pathways. Their mutual dependency is summarized in Table 58.1.

Reye's syndrome

In 1963, R. D. Reye (pronounced 'rye') described a syndrome characterized by **microvesicular accumulation of fat** in the liver, **cerebral oedema**, **swollen mitochondria**, **hyperammonaemia** and **hypoglycaemia**. Subsequently, it has also been shown to be associated with **increased blood concentrations of free fatty acids** and **amino acids**, such as glutamine, alanine and lysine. The disease occurs in children suffering from a viral infection **treated with aspirin**. In what has been declared a 'public health triumph', by withholding aspirin from children the disease is now very rare. Furthermore, early diagnosis and treatment has dramatically reduced mortality (originally 50%) and neurological damage. It has been shown that metabolites of aspirin, namely salicylate and hydroxyhippurate, inhibit long-chain hydroxyacyl CoA dehydrogenase of the trifunctional enzyme (see Chapter 35), thereby inhibiting **β-oxidation**. When this happens in fasting liver, **all the other** pathways dependent on **β-oxidation** (Chart 58.1) are restricted, as shown in Chart 58.2 and Table 58.1.

Reye-like syndrome

About 30 inborn errors of metabolism have been shown to mimic classic aspirin-induced Reye's syndrome. Although at first glance they may seem many and varied, nearly all of them can be classified into groups causing impaired functioning of either **β-oxidation**, **gluconeogenesis**, **ketogenesis**, the **urea cycle** or the **respiratory chain** (Chart 58.2). Failure of just **one** of these pathways leads to restriction of them **all** with microvesicular fat accumulation in liver, hypoglycaemia and hyperammonaemia as in classic Reye's syndrome.

Chart 58.1 (below) **Mutual dependency of the metabolic pathways operating in liver in the fasting state.** In liver during fasting, gluconeogenesis, ketogenesis, β-oxidation, the respiratory chain and the urea cycle operate as outlined on the chart. Their mutual dependency is based on their need for a supply of cofactors such as ATP, NAD⁺, FAD, etc.

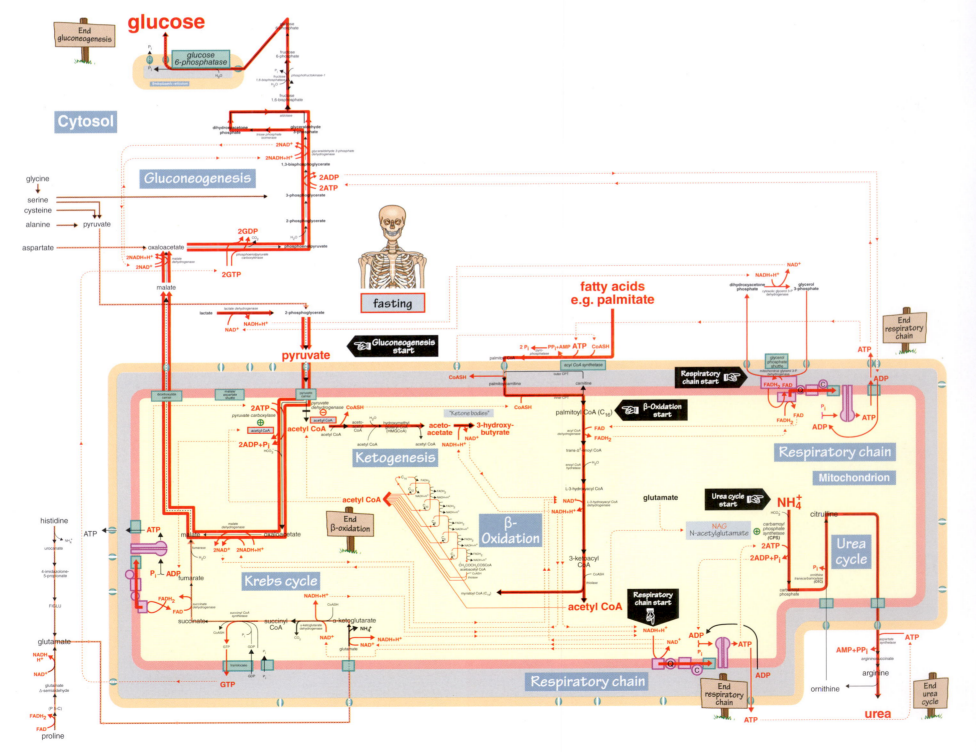

Metabolism at a Glance, Fourth Edition. J. G. Salway. © 2017 John Wiley & Sons Ltd. Published 2017 by John Wiley & Sons Ltd.

Table 58.1 Mutual interdependence of the metabolic pathways operating in liver during fasting.

Pathway	Substrates or cofactors needed for the pathway to operate during starvation	Function of the pathway	Consequences of pathway malfunction (*Signs characteristic of Reye's syndrome)
Gluconeogenesis (Chapter 18)	• Carbon source such as the glycogenic amino acids • ATP from the respiratory chain and GTP from Krebs • Acetyl CoA from β-oxidation activates pyruvate carboxylase	• Produces glucose during fasting which prevents hypoglycaemia	• **Hypoglycaemia***, which if severe can cause brain damage
β-Oxidation (Chapters 9 and 35)	• ATP for the acyl CoA synthetase reaction is supplied by the respiratory chain • FAD and NAD⁺ from the respiratory chain and NAD⁺ from ketogenesis • CoASH is supplied by ketogenesis	• Produces acetyl CoA mainly for ketogenesis • Acetyl CoA is also used to make N-acetyl-glutamate (NAG), an allosteric stimulator of the urea cycle, which produces urea • $FADH_2$ and NADH are oxidized in the respiratory chain to form ATP	• **Fatty acids and triacylglycerol (microvesicular fat) accumulate in liver*** because they cannot be oxidized • **Ketogenesis is impaired, hypoketonaemia*** • Impaired production of NAG restricts function of the urea cycle causing neurotoxic **hyperammonaemia*** • $FADH_2$ and NADH are not available for ATP production by the respiratory chain
Ketogenesis (Chapter 36)	• Acetyl CoA provided by β-oxidation forms the ketone bodies, i.e. acetoacetate and 3-hydroxybutyrate • NADH is supplied by β-oxidation	• Ketone bodies are used by the brain during starvation thus sparing glucose	• The supply of ketone bodies is decreased so the brain must use glucose as a fuel. But if gluconeogenesis is also impaired, glucose supply is restricted, hence **hypoglycaemia***
Urea cycle (Chapter 51)	• ATP supplied by the respiratory chain • NAG an allosteric stimulator of CPS	• Detoxifies ammonia, which is a waste product of amino acid metabolism	• **Hyperammonaemia***, which can cause brain damage
Respiratory chain (Chapter 3)	• $FADH_2$ and NADH supplied by β-oxidation • ADP and Pi supplied by the hydrolysis of ATP in gluconeogenesis and the urea cycle	• Produces ATP • Produces FAD and NAD⁺ which are needed for β-oxidation	• Because ATP is needed for gluconeogenesis, the urea cycle and β-oxidation, these pathways will be inhibited if ATP production is impaired

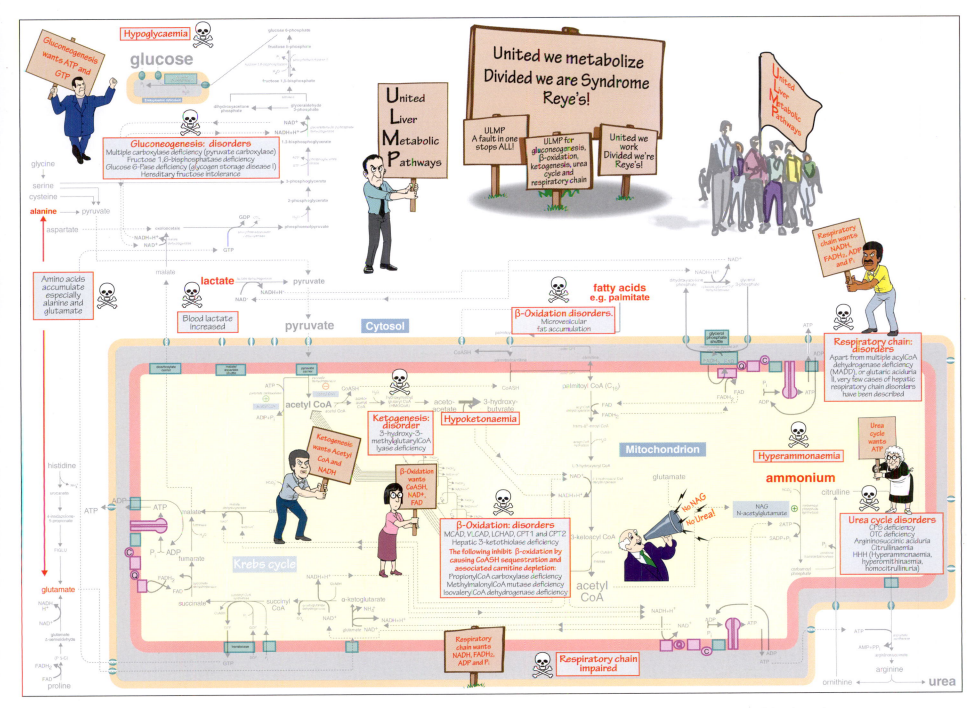

Chart 58.2 Failure of metabolic pathways seen in Reye's syndrome. Impaired functioning of any individual pathway shown in Chart 58.1 can impair the activity of any or all the other pathways.

Diabetes I: metabolic changes in diabetes

59

Hyperglycaemia and ketoacidosis in diabetes

In severely uncontrolled diabetes, many metabolic pathways are directed towards the breakdown of body protein and fat which are used to synthesize **glucose** and the **ketone bodies**. This is a consequence of failure of the balance between anabolism and catabolism, which is the basis of metabolic homeostasis in healthy adults. In diabetes, the anabolic state is impaired because insulin, an anabolic hormone, is not available to maintain this balance. Consequently, catabolism predominates inducing the following alterations in lipid, protein and carbohydrate metabolism.

Metabolism of triacylglycerol in diabetes

In adipose tissue, insulin prevents triacylglycerol catabolism by inhibiting lipolysis (see Chapter 30). In uncontrolled diabetes, therefore, increased lipolysis results in a 300% enhancement of fatty acid and glycerol mobilization.

1 **Fatty acid metabolism in diabetes.** In white adipose tissue in the healthy fed state, fatty acids formed by lipolysis undergo a cyclic process in which they are re-esterified with glycerol 3-phosphate to re-form triacylglycerol (see Chapter 31). In diabetes, this cycle is interrupted due to lack of glycerol 3-phosphate, which is unavailable because it is formed from glucose, which in turn needs insulin to enter the fat cell. Furthermore, cortisol is increased in diabetes and this will inhibit PEPCK, preventing glyceroneogenesis, which provides glycerol 3-phosphate for re-esterification (see Chapter 32). Consequently, since re-esterification of the fatty acids is decreased, they are instead released into the blood. Normally, fatty acids would be oxidized as a respiratory fuel by most tissues, especially red skeletal muscle. In diabetes, however, surplus fatty acids are transported to the liver where they enter the β-oxidation spiral to form acetyl CoA. In the healthy state, this condenses with oxaloacetate producing citrate for oxidation in Krebs cycle. In the diabetic state, oxaloacetate is removed from the mitochondrion for gluconeogenesis and is in short supply. Consequently, acetyl CoA molecules combine with each other to form the '**ketone bodies**': **acetoacetate** and **D-3-hydroxybutyrate** (see Chapter 36). Moreover, in the cytosol, acetyl CoA may be diverted in the direction of cholesterol synthesis, which is often increased in diabetes. In severely uncontrolled type 1 diabetes, metabolic regulation is deranged (Chart 59.1 and see also Chapter 61) and may

be associated with a massive production of acetoacetic acid and D-3-hydroxybutyric acid. In serious cases this overwhelms the pH buffering capacity of the blood causing diabetic ketoacidosis.

2 **Glycerol metabolism.** The glycerol released from adipose tissue is phosphorylated in liver to glycerol 3-phosphate. This is metabolized to glucose, which is released into the blood, contributing to the hyperglycaemia.

Metabolism of protein and amino acids in diabetes

Insulin enhances the uptake of amino acids into muscle from the blood thus favouring protein synthesis. In diabetes, the process is reversed and muscle protein breaks down to form amino acids. Some of these, particularly alanine and glutamine, may be released from muscle and used by the liver for gluconeogenesis (see Chapter 45).

Metabolism of glucose and glycogen in diabetes

Insulin recruits to the plasma membrane the GLUT4 glucose transporters needed for glucose to enter muscle cells and adipocytes. Consequently, in diabetes, glucose accumulates in the extracellular fluids causing hyperglycaemia, while paradoxically the muscle and fat cells are starved of glucose: a situation described as '*starvation in the midst of plenty*'.

Insulin stimulates glycogen synthesis and increases glucokinase activity. Consequently, in the absence of insulin, glycogen synthesis ceases and **glycogenolysis** occurs with glucose being exported from liver into the blood, once again compounding the hyperglycaemic state.

Glucagonocentric diabetes

Hitherto, lack of insulin or reduced insulin action has been blamed for causing diabetes. However, recently it has been proposed that the insulin counter-regulatory partner, **glucagon**, is a major contributor to the pathophysiology of diabetes. In liver, glucagon increases glycogenolysis, gluconeogenesis and ketogenesis (see Chapter 61). This suggest that treatment of diabetes should also be directed at suppressing glucagon secretion or action.

Reference

Unger R.H., Cherrington A.D. (2012) Glucagonocentric restructuring of diabetes: a pathophysiologic and therapeutic makeover. *J Clin Invest*, **122**(1), 4–12.

Diagram 59.1 Metabolic relationship of adipose tissue, muscle and liver in diabetes mellitus.

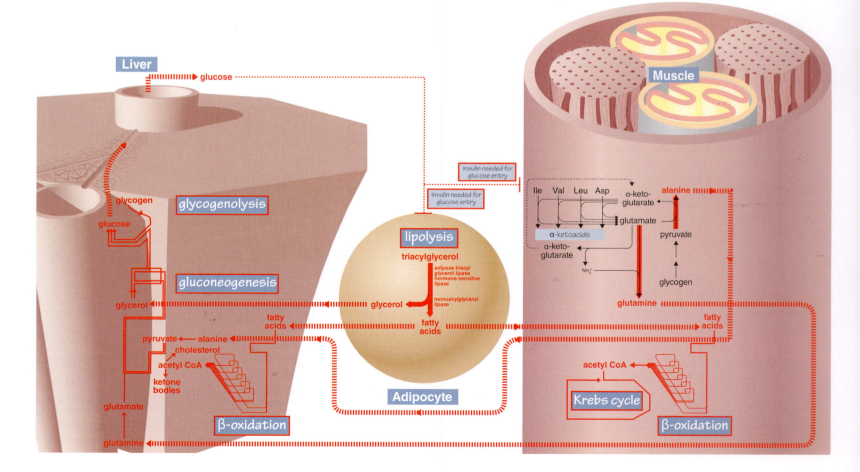

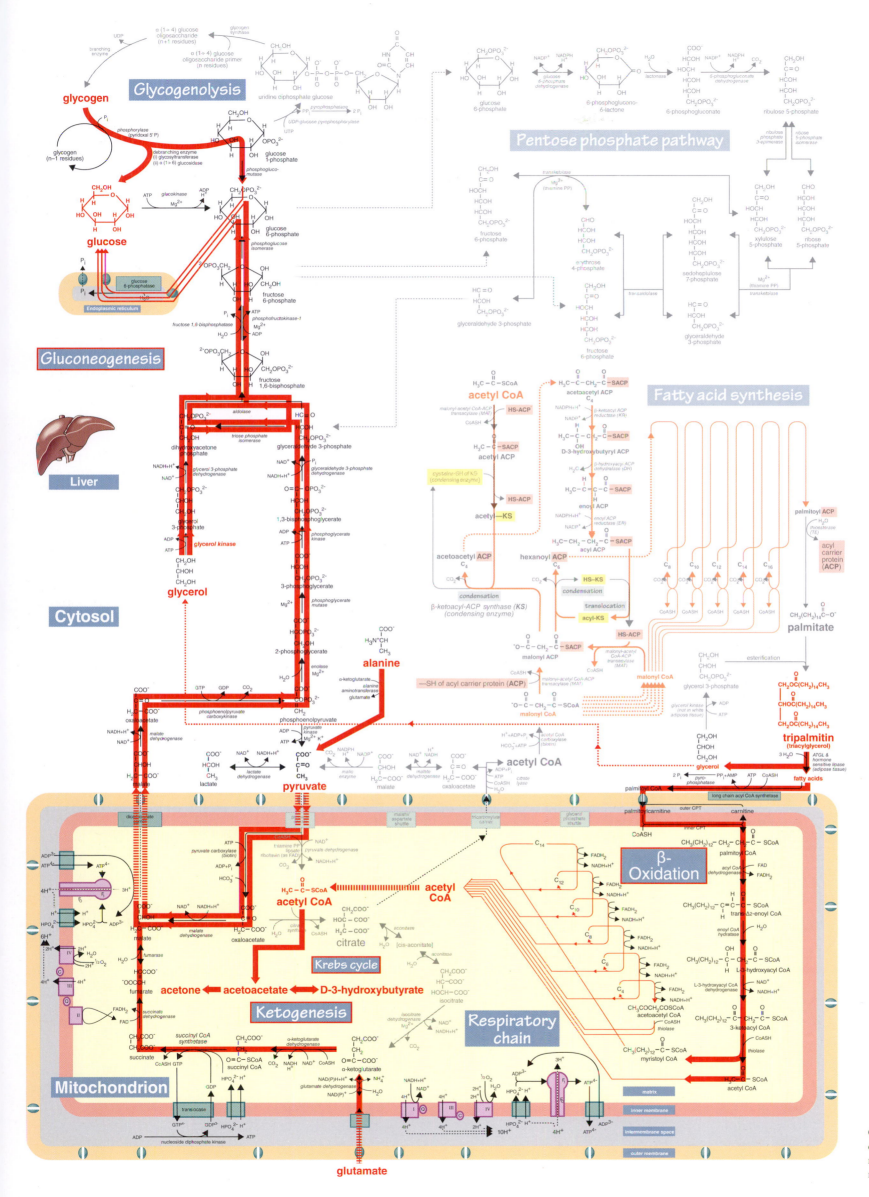

Chart 59.1 An overview of intermediary metabolism in diabetes mellitus.

Diabetes II: types I and II diabetes, MODY and pancreatic β-cell metabolism

60

Chart 60.1 (opposite) Glucose metabolism in pancreatic β-cells causes secretion of insulin.

Type 1 diabetes mellitus (T1DM)

T1DM (previously known as insulin-dependent diabetes mellitus (IDDM), and historically as juvenile-onset diabetes), is the result of β-cell death, for example following viral/autoimmune attack. Consequently, **T1DM is characterized by failure of pancreatic β-cells to produce and secrete insulin**. It is treated by insulin replacement therapy.

Type 2 diabetes mellitus (T2DM)

Patients with T2DM (previously known as non-insulin-dependent diabetes mellitus (NIDDM), and historically as maturity-onset diabetes (MOD)), **usually suffer from a combination of defective insulin secretion plus resistance to the action of insulin**. Within the population of patients with T2DM, there are probably scores of individual biochemical causes with differing degrees of pathological severity. However, it is postulated that the biochemical cause common to all variants of T2DM is that the insulin produced is relatively ineffective. This could be for several reasons, which are the subject of research focused on pancreatic β-cells, skeletal muscle, adipose tissue and liver. For example, following a carbohydrate meal, secretion of insulin from β-cells may be inadequate (insufficient or too slow); or (very rarely) the insulin released is structurally abnormal and thus only partially functional. Alternatively, the defects could be in the tissues targeted by insulin, especially skeletal muscle, adipose tissue and liver. It is possible that the insulin receptor is defective, or that transduction and/or amplification of the insulin signal to intracellular metabolic processes is impaired. Finally, it is possible that regulation, by gene expression or phosphorylation, of an enzyme crucial to glucose homeostasis underlies an abnormal response to the insulin signal. In all the above cases, the consequence could be hyperglycaemia and the diabetic state.

Maturity-onset diabetes of the young (MODY)

MODY is a rare and clinically diverse form of T2DM with autosomal dominant inheritance, and onset at usually less than 25 years of age. It is characterized by **impaired glucose-stimulated insulin secretion from the β-cell** resulting in hyperglycaemia usually in the absence of insulin resistance. Whereas T2DM is a complex genetic disorder, **MODY is due to a single gene defect**. There are several genetic causes for MODY, but the most common aetiologies are mutations in the *HNF1A* and *HNF4A* genes. These encode transcription factors for β-cell development and function called **hepatocyte nuclear factor 1α** and **hepatocyte nuclear factor 4α** respectively. Patients with these subtypes of diabetes respond better to sulphonylurea tablets than insulin injections. **Heterozygous** *inactivating* **mutations** in the glucokinase (*GCK*) gene cause a glucose-sensing defect resulting in mild, fasting *hyper*glycaemia which does not need treatment. However, **homozygous** individuals with **two** *inactivating* copies of the *GCK* gene have a severe form of diabetes, called **neonatal diabetes**. Conversely, those with **heterozygous** *activating* mutations of the *GCK* gene suffer *hypo*glycaemia (**persistent hyperinsulinaemic hypoglycaemia of infancy (PHHI)**).

Neonatal diabetes

Diabetes presenting in the first 6 months of life is termed **neonatal diabetes**. The most common genetic causes are **heterozygous** *activating* **mutations** in the pancreatic **β-cell K-ATP channel genes *KCNJ11* and *ABCC8***. These encode the channel components **Kir6.2** (the inwardly rectifying potassium channel subunit) and **SUR1** (the sulphonylurea receptor subunit 1) (Chart 60.1). **NB:** Patients with this type of diabetes are treated with **oral sulphonylureas** rather than insulin injections. Conversely, **inactive mutations** in both of these genes cause **hypoglycaemia (PHHI)**. Mutations in *SLC2A2* encoding the **β-cell glucose transporter 2 (GLUT2)** are a rare cause of neonatal diabetes. This is in addition to their role in **Fanconi–Bickel syndrome** (glycogen storage disease type XI) characterized by **post-prandial** *hyper*glycaemia, **fasting** *hypo*glycaemia and hepatorenal glycogen accumulation due to dysfunctional GLUT2 in liver and kidney (see Chapters 11 and 18).

Biochemical aetiology of type 2 diabetes (T2DM)

Glucose homeostasis depends on coordination between the following: (i) the **pancreatic β-cell** for insulin synthesis, storage and secretion; (ii) **skeletal muscle** for glucose utilization and, in starvation, provision of amino acids for gluconeogenesis; (iii) **adipose tissue** for triacylglycerol storage/mobilization; and (iv) **liver** for gluconeogenesis, glycogen storage/mobilization, and synthesis of triacylglycerol. An abnormality of any of these can cause hyperglycaemia and lead to type 2 diabetes.

T2DM has been described as the '*geneticists' nightmare*'. This is consistent with the multitude of possible biochemical mechanisms for the development of T2DM and the key roles both genetics and environment play in governing who develops this disorder. In the 21st century, there has been unprecedented progress in dissecting out the various regions of the genome that alter T2DM risk. From the 100 regions of the genome identified to date, it is clear that β-cell dysfunction is at the heart of diabetes pathogenesis. Another striking feature is that many of the genes that are involved in monogenic forms of diabetes harbour genetic variants that are common in the population and influence the risk of developing T2DM. Examples include *KCNJ11/ABCC8*, *GCK* and *HNF1A*.

Metabolic fuel hypothesis for insulin secretion

Oxidative metabolism of glucose by β-cells involves glycolysis, Krebs cycle and the respiratory chain. This increases the intracellular concentration **ratio of ATP to ADP** which provides the metabolic signal for insulin secretion (Chart 60.1). This in turn causes the **ATP-sensitive K⁺ channel** in the β-cell plasma membrane to close, resulting in membrane depolarization which activates the **voltage-dependent Ca²⁺ channels** causing calcium influx. The consequential increased concentration of intracellular Ca²⁺ is thought to activate **calmodulin-dependent protein kinase-2** (CaMPK-2), which phosphorylates a protein (or proteins) causing secretion of insulin. **Synaptotagmin** might also act as a Ca²⁺ sensor for the regulation of exocytosis.

Other notable compounds that, when metabolized, stimulate insulin secretion are **leucine** and, under experimental conditions, **mannose**, **glyceraldehyde** and **α-ketoisocaproate**.

Another metabolic mechanism for insulin secretion has been proposed. It has been suggested that, when glucose is abundant, it is metabolized to **malonyl CoA** (see Chapter 35), which inhibits transport of acyl molecules by the carnitine shuttle into the mitochondrion for β-oxidation. Instead, the consequent elevation of cytosolic fatty acyl esters, either directly or indirectly (i.e. as lysophosphatidate, phosphatidate or diacylglycerol (DAG)), stimulate secretion of insulin by an unknown mechanism.

Potentiation of glucose-stimulated insulin secretion

Whereas insulin secretion is primarily stimulated by metabolic fuels, such as glucose, this effect can be potentiated by several endocrine and pharmacological agonists that stimulate plasma membrane receptors. For example, **acetylcholine** acts on muscarinic receptors, thus activating phospholipase C, producing **diacylglycerol**, which activates **protein kinase C** (Chart 60.1). Also, several hormones that use **cyclic AMP** as an intracellular signal are potentiators of glucose-stimulated insulin secretion, for example, **GIP** (glucose-dependent insulinotrophic polypeptide) and **GLP-1** (glucagon-like peptide-1). They activate **protein kinase A**, which is thought to phosphorylate the same or similar substrates acted on by calmodulin-dependent protein kinase-2 and the other kinases mentioned previously.

Metabolism at a Glance, Fourth Edition. J. G. Salway. © 2017 John Wiley & Sons Ltd. Published 2017 by John Wiley & Sons Ltd.

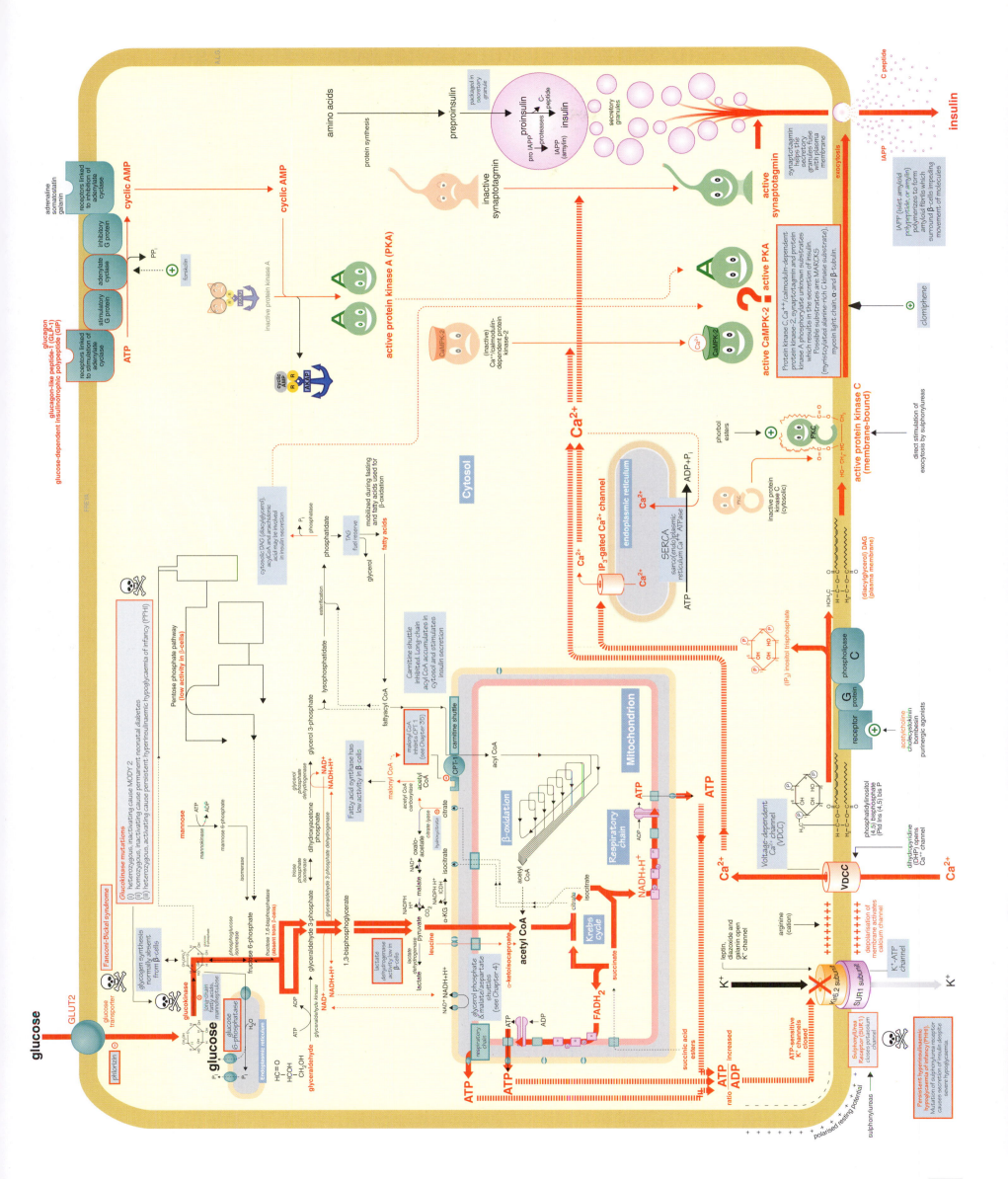

Diabetes III: type 2 diabetes and dysfunctional liver metabolism

61

Insulin promotes the metabolism of glucose to glycogen and triacylglycerol

Insulin **stimulates** transcription of certain genes involved in hepatic lipogenesis, including genes encoding glucokinase, glyceraldehyde 3-phosphate dehydrogenase, pyruvate kinase, malic enzyme, acetyl CoA carboxylase and fatty acid synthase. Conversely, insulin **inhibits** transcription of the gluconeogenic genes encoding phosphoenolpyruvate carboxykinase (PEPCK), fructose 1,6-bisphosphatase and glucose 6-phosphatase. Consequently, in diabetes, gluconeogenesis is stimulated resulting in hyperglycaemia.

Increased hepatic glucose output by liver: glycogenolysis and gluconeogenesis

Hepatic glycogenolysis contributes to hyperglycaemia in diabetes. NB: In liver, unlike muscle, no evidence has been found for regulation of the regulatory subunits of protein phosphatase-1 by phosphorylation/dephosphorylation. Instead, as shown in Chart 61.1, **phosphorylase a** binds to an inhibitory binding site on the regulatory subunit and blocks phosphatase activity.

Gluconeogenesis and diabetes. As shown in Chart 61.1, in type 2 diabetes mellitus (T2DM) the liver is presented with an abundance of gluconeogenic substrates, notably **lactate** from skeletal muscle and red blood cells (see Chapter 7), **alanine** from muscle (see Chapter 45) and **glycerol** from adipose tissue (see Chapter 30). The ATP for gluconeogenesis is provided by β-oxidation of fatty acids, the latter being in abundant supply because of the inappropriately high rate of lipolysis in adipocytes as mentioned above. Consequently, an abundance of acetyl CoA is produced, which both inhibits pyruvate dehydrogenase while stimulating pyruvate carboxylase, a regulatory enzyme for gluconeogenesis. The next flux-regulating step involves PEPCK, which is regulated at the level of DNA transcription. Cyclic AMP mediates the production of PEPCK, whereas insulin inhibits its production. In T2DM where there is diminished repression by insulin, PEPCK will be produced, favouring gluconeogenesis.

Glucagoncentric diabetes

Insulin and glucagon collaborate in glucose homeostasis. In the **fed state**, insulin is secreted and causes surplus dietary glucose to be stored as glycogen or triacylglycerol. Conversely, during **fasting or starvation**, glucagon promotes glycogenolysis and gluconeogenesis. Glucagon is stored and released from the α-**cells of the pancreas** on which there are insulin receptors. When insulin binds to these receptors, the secretion of glucagon is inhibited. Consequently, in diabetes when insulin availability is diminished, the α-cells secrete glucagon which promotes gluconeogenesis causing hyperglycaemia.

Hyperlipidaemia

As mentioned in Chapters 29 and 30, in the healthy fed state when **insulin is present**, surplus dietary glucose is metabolized to triacylglycerol, which is stored in white adipose tissue. Conversely, when **insulin levels are very low** during fasting, or inactive in diabetes, fatty acids will be mobilized from adipose tissue and delivered to liver. Here they will be esterified to triacylglycerol and secreted as very-low-density lipoproteins (VLDLs) causing the hyperlipidaemia frequently seen in T2DM. Fatty acids are also metabolized by β-oxidation to form acetyl CoA, which is used for ketogenesis.

Hypothesis for the pathogenesis of T2DM

Diagram 61.1 illustrates current opinion on the interplay between genetic and lifestyle influences that interact initially to cause mild hyperglycaemia. However, as the years pass, a vicious cycle of ever-increasing hyperglycaemia insidiously contributes to glucose toxicity, eventually manifesting as clinical T2DM.

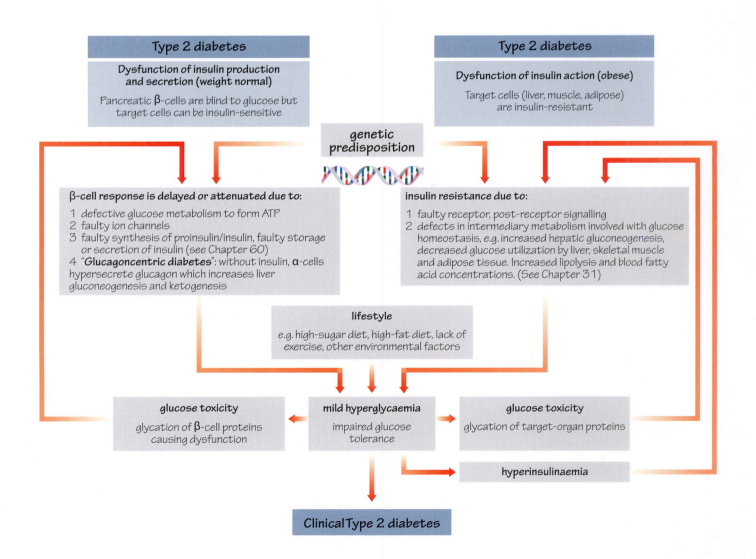

Diagram 61.1 Interplay between genetic and lifestyle influences: a hypothesis for the early stages in the pathogenesis of T2DM.

Metabolism at a Glance, Fourth Edition. J. G. Salway. © 2017 John Wiley & Sons Ltd. Published 2017 by John Wiley & Sons Ltd.

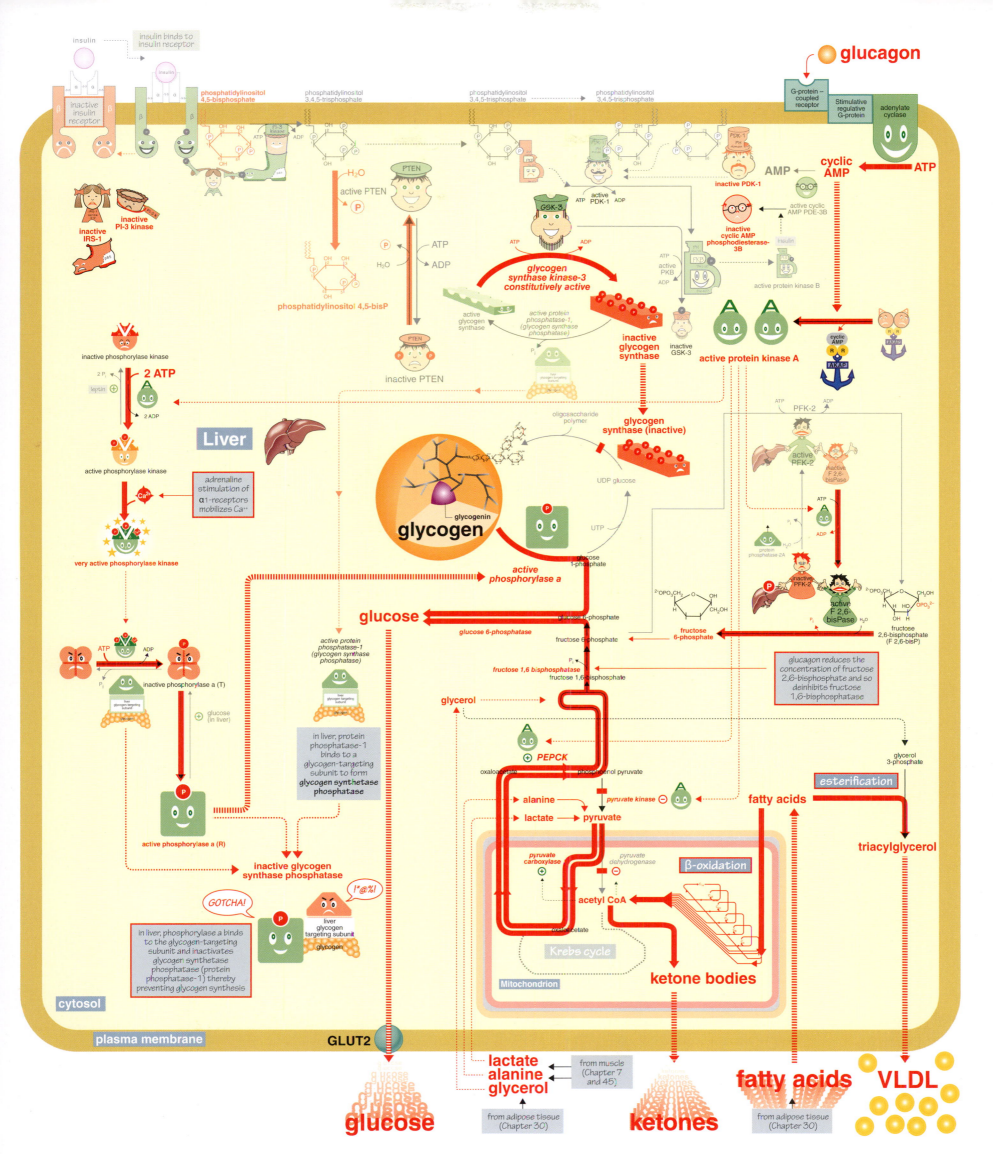

Chart 61.1 Metabolic pathways and possible sites of insulin resistance in liver in T2DM. When insulin action fails, cyclic AMP phosphodiesterase-3B is inactive and so cyclic AMP accumulates. This enables the effects of the counter-regulatory hormone glucagon to dominate and the pathways highlighted in red operate.

Index

Page numbers in **bold** denote tables.

AANAT *see* arylalkylamine *N*-acetyltransferase
ABCC8, β-cell KATP channel gene mutation 120
ABCD1 transporter and X-ALD 78
ABCD3 transporter 78
acetaldehyde, metabolism 48
acetoacetate 66, 118
   in ketogenesis 72, 73, 74, 75, 90, 91
acetoacetyl CoA, biosynthesis 72, 73
acetoacetyl CoA thiolase, catalysis 72, 73, 74, 75
acetone 72, 73
acetylcholine, insulin secretion stimulation 120, 121
acetyl CoA
   biosynthesis 40, 43, 54, 72, 92
   gluconeogenesis in fasting 94
   in ketogenesis 72
   oxidation 40
   pyruvate dehydrogenase inhibition 36, 38, 39, 56, 94
   roles 50, 66
acetyl CoA carboxylase 52, 56
   activation 54
N-acetylglutamate (NAG), biosynthesis 102
N-acetylglutamate synthase, catalysis 102
acetyl transferase 38
ackee fruit 71
ACP (acyl carrier protein) 54, 106
acyl carrier protein (ACP), roles, in fatty acid biosynthesis 54, 106
acyl CoA dehydrogenases 70, 71, 76, 77
   localization 70
acyl CoA esters, transport 60
acyl CoA oxidase, catalysis 78, 79
acyltransferase 56
adenosine
   accumulation following AICAR 110
   biosynthesis 34
adenosine diphosphate (ADP), phosphorylation 4
adenosine monophosphate (AMP)
   biosynthesis 18
   fatty acid oxidation 18, **19**, 70, 71
   phosphorylation 4
   see also cyclic AMP
adenosine monophosphate deaminase, deficiency 38
adenosine triphosphate (ATP) 2, 4, 10
   aerobic, production 34, 35
   anaerobic, production, 34
   biosynthesis 4–7, 12–13
   in glucose metabolism 14
   D-3-hydroxybutyrate oxidation 74
   β-oxidation 18, **19**
   phosphoanhydride bonds 4
   phosphofructokinase-1 inhibition 30
   structure 4
   as substrate 4
S-adenosylmethionine (SAM) 92
   biosynthesis 92, 93
   as methyl donor 108
adenylate cyclase, activation 26
adenylate kinase, catalysis 34
adenylosuccinase (ASase) 108, 109, 113
   deficiency 39
adipic acid (hexanedioic acid) 70
adipocytes
   fatty acids 62, 63
   fructose transport 46
   glucose transport 32, 64, 118
   glycerol kinase expression 62
   insulin receptors 32
   lipolysis 122
   lipoprotein lipase 59
   triacylglycerol biosynthesis 52
adipose triacylglycerol lipase (ATGL) 60
   regulation of 60
adipose tissue
   brown 7, 64
   fatty acid mobilization 34, 60–3
   free fatty acids 40
   glyceroneogenesis 64
   hormone-sensitive lipase 18, 60, 61
   lipogenesis 30
   lipolysis 60–3
   pentose phosphate pathway in 30
   pyruvate dehydrogenase phosphatase in 38
   thermogenesis 64
   triacylglycerol biosynthesis 52
   triacylglycerol storage 18
   white 5, 59, 60, 61, 62
ADP *see* adenosine diphosphate (ADP)

adrenal leucodystrophy protein (ALDP) 79
   see also ABCD1 transporter and X-ALD
adrenaline 98
   biosynthesis 99, 108
   fight or flight response 20, 22, 26
   glycogenolysis stimulation 22, 24, 25, 26, 27
   glycolysis stimulation 14, 32, 34
   lipolysis stimulation 60, 61
   phaeochromocytoma 98
adrenoleukodystrophy, X-linked, aetiology of 78–9
aerobic ATP synthesis 10–13, 18, 19, 34, 35
affective disorders
   aetiology 100
   amine hypothesis 100
AICAR and rheumatoid arthritis 110
AICARiboside and rheumatoid arthritis 110
A-kinase anchoring protein 26
Akt *see* protein kinase B (PKB)
ALA *see* 5-aminolevulinic acid (ALA)
alanine
   biosynthesis in diabetes 90, 122, 123
      from muscle 90
   catabolism 92
   as gluconeogenic precursor 36
   glucose alanine cycle 90, 91
   pyruvate kinase inhibition 32
alanine cycle (glucose alanine cycle) 90, 91
albinism, aetiology 96
alcohol, metabolism 48–9
alcohol dehydrogenase, roles, in ethanol metabolism 15, 48, 49
alcoholic fermentation 15
alcoholism, treatment 48
ALD (adrenoleukodystrophy) 78–9
aldehyde dehydrogenase, deficiency 48
aldolase, deficiency 16,
aldolase A 25, 31, 45, 46, 47
aldolase B 46, 47
aldose reductase
   catalysis 44, 45
   in diabetes mellitus 44, 45
   inhibitors 44
aldosterone, biosynthesis 86, 87
ALDP *see* adrenal leucodystrophy protein (ALDP)
alkaptonuria, aetiology 96, 97
allantoin 112
amine hypothesis 100
aminoacetone pathway for threonine metabolism 92
   see also chart, back cover
amino acids
   branched-chain 90
   catabolism 90–3
   in diabetes 118
   glucogenic 94–5
   in ketogenesis 72, 90
   ketogenic 90
   metabolism disorders 96–7
   non-essential, biosynthesis 88–9
   in purine and pyrimidine biosynthesis 108, 109, 110–11
   in urea biosynthesis 50, 51, 92, 93
   see also individual amino acids
aminoimidazole-carboxamide ribonucleoside *see* AICAR and rheumatoid arthritis
5-aminolevulinic acid (ALA) 99
   biosynthesis 114, 115
   structural resemblance to succinyl acetone 99
5-aminolevulinic acid synthase, catalysis 114
aminopterin 109, 111
aminotransferase, transamination 102
ammonia
   biosynthesis 66
   incorporation into glutamine 102
ammonium chloride 104
ammonium ions 102, 112
ammonotelism 112
AMP *see* adenosine monophosphate (AMP)
AMP-dependent protein kinase 60
amytal, electron transport inhibition 7
anaerobic ATP synthesis 34
anaerobic glycolysis 14–15, 22
anaplerotic reactions 34, 38, 43
anastrozole, aromatase inhibitor and breast cancer 87
androstane 84
androstenedione, biosynthesis 87
Antabuse, in alcoholism treatment 48
antidiabetic drugs, glitazones 64
antimetabolites 110

antimycin A 7
antipurines, mechanisms 110
antipyrimidines, mechanisms 110
arachidic acid 78
arachidonic acid, as eicosanoid hormone precursor 68, 78
arachidonoyl CoA, biosynthesis 68
arginase 103, 105
arginine 88
   biosynthesis 102, **104**
   catabolism 92
argininosuccinate, biosynthesis in urea cycle 102, 105
argininosuccinate synthetase 105
argininosuccinic aciduria 117
aromatase inhibitors 87
arylalkylamine *N*-acetyltransferase (AANAT) 100
ASase (adenylosuccinase) deficiency 39, 109, 113
ascorbate, biosynthesis 44
asparagine, biosynthesis 88
aspartate
   biosynthesis 88, 102
   malate/aspartate shuttle 9
   and purine biosynthesis 108
   and purine nucleotide cycle 39
aspartate aminotransferase (AST), malate/aspartate shuttle 9
   and urea cycle 102, 103
aspirin, and Reye's syndrome 116, 117
AST *see* aspartate aminotransferase (AST)
atorvastatin 85
ATP *see* adenosine triphosphate (ATP)
ATP/ADP translocase 4
   inhibition 7
ATP synthetase 7
ATP synthetase complex 6
atractyloside 7
atrial natriuretic factor 60
axons 74
azaserine, inhibitory activity 110
azide, electron transport inhibition 7
azidothymidine (AZT), phosphorylation 110
azidothymidine triphosphate (AZTTP), inhibitory activity 110
AZT (azidothymidine), phosphorylation 110
AZTTP (azidothymidine triphosphate), inhibitory activity 110

Bai and Paik shunt 84
barbiturates
   potentiation of ALA synthase 114
   interaction with ethanol 48
BCAAs *see* branched-chain amino acids (BCAAs)
BCKADH (α-ketoacid dehydrogenase) 90
behenic acid 78
betaine, and homocysteine metabolism 109
bicarbonate ion, ^{14}C-labelled and metabolic channelling 104, 105
bifunctional enzyme PFK-2/F2,6 bisPase 32, 33
bile acids/salts 84, 86–7
   biosynthesis 86
bilirubin
   biosynthesis 114
   glucuronate conjugates 44
biliverdin, biosynthesis 114
biological clock 100
biotin, as cofactor 52
bipolar disease, amine hypothesis 100
1,3-bisphosphoglycerate, reduction 45
2,3-bisphosphoglycerate (2,3-BPG) 16–17
   adaptation to high altitude 16
   importance in medicine 16
bisphosphoglycerate mutase, deficiency 16
2,3-bisphosphoglycerate phosphatase (2,3-BPG phosphatase) 16, 17
   deficiency 16
2,3-bisphosphoglycerate shunt 16
Bloch pathway 84
blood glucose
   during fasting (gluconeogenesis) 90
   in type 2 diabetes (glyceroneogenesis) 64
blood transfusions, and 2,3-BPG 16
bombesin, insulin secretion stimulation 121
bongkrekic acid 7
2,3-BPG *see* 2,3-bisphosphoglycerate (2,3-BPG)
brain
   fuel requirements 10, 20, 36, 40
   kernicterus 44
branched-chain amino acids (BCAAs), catabolism 90, 96
branched-chain α-ketoacid dehydrogenase (BCKADH), activity 96
branched-chain fatty acids 80
branching enzyme, catalysis 3, 119

brown adipose tissue 64
  thermogenesis 64

calcium channels, voltage-dependent 120
calmodulin-dependent protein kinase-2, activation 120
cancer
  chemotherapy 110
  photodynamic therapy 114
capric acid 78
caproic acid 78
caprylic acid 78
carbamoyl aspartate, biosynthesis 103
carbamoyl phosphate 93, 95, 97, 102, 105
  accumulation 103
  biosynthesis (CPS) 102
  biosynthesis (CPS II) 111
carbamoyl phosphate synthetase (CPS) 102, 103, 105
carbamoyl phosphate synthetase II (CPS II), catalysis 110
carbohydrate response element binding protein see ChREBP
carbon monoxide, electron transport inhibition 7
carbonylcyanide-p-trifluoromethoxyphenylhydrazone (FCCP), protein
    transport inhibition 7
carcinoid syndrome 100
carcinoma of the liver in tyrosinaemia 98
cardiac muscle
  glycolysis 33
  phosphofructokinase-2/fructose 2,6-bisphosphatase 32
cardiomyocytes, insulin sensitivity 32
cardiovascular disease
  and cholesterol 84
  and homocysteine 108
caries see dental decay
carnitine/acylcarnitine translocase, in carnitine shuttle 70, 71
carnitine deficiency 70
carnitine-palmitoyl transferases (CPTs) 70
carnitine shuttle 70–1, 76
casein kinases, glycogen synthase phosphorylation 28
catalase
  ethanol oxidation 48
  fatty acid oxidation 78
cataracts, diabetic, polyol osmotic theory 44
catecholamines and lipolysis 60
  biosynthesis 98
  see also adrenaline
catechol-O-methyltransferase (COMT) 99
CDPX2 syndrome 85
cells
  concepts of 2
  energy conservation 4
  muscle 10, 28, 32, 35, 46, 94
  nerve 74
  see also adipocytes; hepatocytes; red blood cells
β-cells
  metabolism 121
  response 122
cerebral oedema 116
cerotic acid 78
  accumulation 79
cerotoyl CoA 78
cervonic acid see DHA (docosahexaenoic acid)
CGI-58 60
Chanarin–Dorfman syndrome 60
charge separation 6
chemiosmotic theory 6
chenodeoxycholate biosynthesis 86
CHILD syndrome 85
chlorpropamide, aldehyde dehydrogenase inhibition 48
chlorpropamide alcohol flushing 48
cholane 84
cholate, biosynthesis 86
cholecystokinin, insulin secretion stimulation 121
cholestane 84
5,7,9(11)-cholestatrien-3β-ol 84
19-nor-5,7,9,(10)-cholestatrien-3β-ol 84
cholesterol 84–5
  biosynthesis 84, 85
  and cancer 84
  metabolism disorders 84
cholesterol desmolase 86
ChREBP 56
chylomicrons 52, 59
citrate 20
  fatty acid synthesis 54
  glycolysis inhibition 32
citrate lyase, catalysis 50, 54, 56, 66
citrate synthase
  catalysis 72
  metabolic channelling 104
citric acid cycle see Krebs citric acid cycle
citrullinaemia and Reye's syndrome 117
citrulline
  biosynthesis 102
  diffusion (metabolic channelling) 105

clupanodonic acid 78
cofactors 10
  biotin 52
  pyruvate dehydrogenase reaction 10
  vitamins as 10
comparative gene identification 58 (CGI-58) 60
complexes I–IV 6
  proton transport 7
COMT (catechol-O-methyltransferase) 99
congenital adrenal hyperplasia 87
congenital erythropoietic porphyria 115
coproporphyria, hereditary, aetiology 115
coproporphyrinogens, biosynthesis 115
core protein of fatty acid synthase 106
Cori cycle
  muscle/liver 14
  red blood cells/liver 14
Cori's disease, aetiology 22
cortisol
  biosynthesis 86, 87
  effect on PEPCK 64
  starvation and HSL 60
cot death see sudden infant death syndrome (SIDS)
C peptide 121
CPS see carbamoyl phosphate synthetase (CPS)
CPS II (carbamoyl phosphate synthetase II) 110
CPTs (carnitine-palmitoyl transferases) 70
creatine, biosynthesis 102, 103
creatine phosphate, biosynthesis 103
Crigler–Najjar syndrome, aetiology 44
crotonic acid 78
CTP (cytidine triphosphate) 110
cyanide, electron transport inhibition 7
cyclic AMP 25, 120
  binding to receptor 26
  biosynthesis 25, 26, 32
  removal 28
cyclic AMP-dependent protein kinase see protein kinase A (PKA)
cyclic AMP phosphodiesterase-3, activation 61
cyclic AMP phosphodiesterase-3B (PDE-3B) 28
  activation 27, 29
CYP family
  melatonin catabolism 100
  ω-oxidation of fatty acids 82
  see also cytochrome P450
cystathionine β-synthase, catalysis 88
cysteine
  biosynthesis 88
  catabolism 92
  γ-glutamyl cycle 30
  uses 88
cysteinylglycine 30
cytidine triphosphate (CTP) 110
cytochrome b (cyt b), in Q cycle 7
cytochrome b_5, localization 68
cytochrome b_5 reductase, localization 68
cytochrome c (cyt c), electron transport 6
cytochrome P450
  adult Refsum's disease 82
  catalysis 79, 82
  deficiency in cholesterol biosynthesis (Antley–Bixler disease) 85
  need for NADPH + H^+ 30
  role in ethanol metabolism 48
  X-ALD 79
cytosol 2
  PEPCK overexpression in mouse muscle 43–4

dATP (deoxyadenosine triphosphate) 108
DCCD (dicyclohexylcarbodiimide) 7
dCTP (deoxycytidine triphosphate) 110
debranching enzyme, deficiency 22
decanoic acid 78
cis-Δ^4-decenoate, and MCAD deficiency 70, 71
cis-Δ^4-decenoyl CoA, oxidation 76
dehydratase and fatty acid elongation 68
7-dehydrocholesterol, biosynthesis 84
8-dehydrocholesterol, biosynthesis 84
7-dehydrocholesterol reductase 84
14-demethyllanosterol 84
dental decay
  absence in hereditary fructose intolerance 47
  xylitol chewing gum in prevention 44
dental enamel, remineralization 44
deoxyadenosine triphosphate (dATP), biosynthesis 108
deoxycytidine triphosphate (dCTP), biosynthesis 110
deoxyguanosine triphosphate (dGTP), biosynthesis 108
deoxythymidine monophosphate (dTMP), biosynthesis 110
deoxythymidine triphosphate (dTTP), biosynthesis 110
deoxyuridine (dUrd) as plasma marker for thymidylate synthase
    inhibition 111
deoxyuridine monophosphate (dUMP), biosynthesis 110
dephosphorylation, protein phosphatases 28
depression 100

Δ^4-desaturation of fatty acids 68, 69
14-desmethyllanosterol 84
desmolase, catalysis 86, 87
desmosterol, biosynthesis 85
desmosterolosis, aetiology 84
dexamethasone, effect on PEPCK 64
dGTP (deoxyguanosine triphosphate), biosynthesis 108
DHA (docosahexaenoic acid) 78
DHF (dihydrofolate) 110
DHT (dihydrotestosterone) 86, 87
diabetes mellitus
  aetiology 10
  antidiabetic drugs
    glitazones and glyceroneogenesis 56
    glucokinase activators as candidate drugs 64
  cataracts 44
  glucagonocentric diabetes 118, 122
  ketone body detection 72
  maturity-onset of young (MODY) 120
  metabolic processes in 118–19
  neonatal 120
  and sorbitol 44
  see also type 1 diabetes; type 2 diabetes
diacylglycerol (DAG) 58
diazoxide, insulin secretion inhibition 121
diazo-oxo-norleucin (DON), inhibitory activity 110
dicarboxylate carrier 2
dicarboxylic acids
  biosynthesis on MCAD deficiency 70, 71
  fatty 80
  Krebs cycle, arguably 'the dicarboxylic acid cycle' 38, 92
dicarboxylic fatty acids oxidation 78
dicyclohexylcarbodiimide (DCCD), proton transport inhibition 7
$\Delta^{3,5}$-$\Delta^{2,4}$-dienoyl CoA isomerase 78
2,4-dienoyl CoA reductase, catalysis 76, 77, 78, 79
dihomo-γ-linolenic acid, as eicosanoid hormone precursor 68
dihomo-γ-linolenoyl CoA, desaturation 68
dihydrofolate (DHF) 110
dihydrofolate reductase, catalysis 110
24,25-dihydrolanosterol 84
dihydrolipoyl dehydrogenase 38
dihydropyridine (DHP), calcium channel opening 121
dihydrotestosterone (DHT) 86
  biosynthesis 87
dihydroxyacetone phosphate
  biosynthesis 9, 12, 15, 36, 46
  reduction 8, 11, 64
4,4-dimethylcholesta-8(9),24-dien-3β-ol 84
4,8-dimethylnonanoyl CoA 80
2,4-dinitrophenol (DNP) 7
2,3-diphosphoglycerate (2,3-DPG) see 2,3-bisphosphoglycerate (2,3-BPG)
disulfiram, in alcoholism treatment 48
DNA, purine biosynthesis 108
DNP (2,4-dinitrophenol) 7
docasanoic acid 78
all cis-$\Delta^{4,7,10,13,16,19}$-docosahexaenoic acid (DHA) 78
cis-^{7,10,13,16,19}-docosapentaenoic acid 78
cis-Δ^{13}-docosenoic acid 78
dodecanoic acid 78
dolichol, precursors 84
DON (diazo-oxo-norleucin) 110
L-DOPA decarboxylase 98
L-DOPA (levodopa) 98
dopamine 98, 99
  and mental illness 98
2,3-DPG see 2,3-bisphosphoglycerate (2,3-BPG)
drug metabolites, glucuronide conjugates 45
dTMP (deoxythymidine monophosphate), biosynthesis 110
dTTP (deoxythymidine triphosphate), biosynthesis 110
dUMP (deoxyuridine monophosphate), biosynthesis 110

early fed state 94
eicosanoic acid 78
eicosanoid hormones, precursors 68
eicosapentaenoic acid (EPA) 68–9, 78
  in fish oils 68
all cis-$\Delta^{5,8,11,14}$-eicosatetraenoic acid see arachidonic acid
cis-Δ^{11}-eicosenoic acid 78
electron-transfer flavoprotein (ETF), in β-oxidation 70
electron transport
  inhibition 7
  processes 6
endogenous depression 100
endoplasmic reticulum 2
  and ethanol ingestion 48
  fatty acid elongation 68
  glucose 6-phosphatase 36
  glucose 6-phosphate translocator 22
energy conservation in cells 4
energy metabolism
  via glucose metabolism 20–1
  via triacylglycerol metabolism 18–19, **19**
energy storage, as fat 52, 56

enolase inhibition 14
enoyl ACP reductase 106
enoyl CoA hydratase, catalysis 78
Δ^2-enoyl CoA hydratases, localization 70
3,2-enoyl CoA isomerase, catalysis 76, 77, 79
trans-Δ^2-enoyl CoA isomerase, catalysis 76
enoyl CoA reductase, catalysis 68
entacapone 98
enzymes
    in cells 2
    co-precipitation and substrate channelling 104
EPA see eicosapentaenoic acid (EPA)
epimerase reaction 44
epinephrine see adrenaline
epoxides, in hawkinsuria 99
erucic acid 78
erythropoietic porphyria, aetiology 115
essential fatty acids, therapeutic benefits 68–9
essential fructosuria, aetiology 47
essential pentosuria, aetiology 44
esterification
    and fatty acid biosynthesis 54
    of fatty acids 58–9
estrane 84
ETF (electron-transfer flavoprotein) 70
ETF:ubiquinone oxidoreductase (ETF:QO), roles, in carnitine shuttle 70
ethanol
    biochemical effects 48
    drug interactions 48
    fasting hypoglycaemia 48
    metabolism 48–9
evening primrose oil, therapeutic benefits 68–9
exemestane, aromatase inhibitor and breast cancer 87
exercise
    biochemistry of 34–5
    cytosolic PEPCK overexpression 43–4
    effects on muscle protein 90
    hitting the wall 34, 43
exocytosis, regulatory mechanisms 120

FABP (fatty acid-binding protein) 60
FAD (flavine adenine dinucleotide) 4
FADH$_2$ (flavine adenine dinucleotide (reduced)) 10
Fanconi–Bickel syndrome 120
    aetiology 56, 57
farnesyl isoprenoid groups, precursors 84
farnesyl pyrophosphate (FPP) 85
fasting see starvation
fat
    biosynthesis see lipogenesis
    as energy store 52, 56
    microvesicular accumulation in Reye's syndrome 116
    metabolism see lipolysis
    sugar biosynthesis 40
fat cells see adipocytes
fatty acid-binding protein (FABP) 60
fatty acids 38
    activation in β-oxidation 18
    in adenosine triphosphate biosynthesis 18–19
    biosynthesis 40, 41, 50, 52, 53, 59, 66, 106, 107
        precursors 50, 54–5, 58–9, 66
    desaturation 68–9
    essential 68–9
    esterification, to triacylglycerols 54, 58–9, 66
    fuel reserve as triacylglycerol 34
    and glucose biosynthesis, problems in mammals 40–1
    metabolism, in diabetes mellitus 118
    mobilization 60–1, 62–3, 72
    nomenclature 76, 77, 78
    β-oxidation 70–1, 80
        in diabetes 118
    re-esterification 63
fatty acid synthase complex, metabolic channelling 106–7
fatty acyl CoA desaturases, activity 68
fatty aldehyde dehydrogenase 80
fatty dicarboxylic acids 80
favism 30
F 1,6-bisPase see fructose 1,6-bisphosphatase
F 2,6-bisPase see fructose 2,6-bisphosphatase
FCCP (carbonylcyanide-p-trifluoromethoxyphenylhydrazone), proton transport leakage 7
ferrochelatase, activity 114, 115
fetal haemoglobin, affinity for 2,3-bisphosphoglycerate 16
fetus, rejection 100
F$_o$/F$_1$ particles, roles 6, 7
fight or flight response 20, 22, 26
FIGLU (N-formiminoglutamate) 92
fish oils, therapeutic benefits 68–9
flavine adenine dinucleotide (FAD) 70
    as hydrogen carrier 4, 5, 10
    reduction 4, 37
flavine adenine dinucleotide (reduced) (FADH$_2$) 10
    biosynthesis 4, 8

phosphorylation 4
    P/O ratio 7
fluorouracil, inhibitory activity 110
folate, metabolism 108–9, 110, 111
folate antagonists, mechanisms 110
folinic acid, methotrexate toxicity 'rescue' 110
formate 108
N-formiminoglutamate (FIGLU) 92
N-formylkynurenine, biosynthesis 101
FPP (farnesyl pyrophosphate) 85
free fatty acids
    biosynthesis 60
    blood concentrations 116
    Reye's syndrome 116
    see also fatty acids
fructokinase
    catalysis 46
    deficiency 47
fructose
    intravenous, dangers of 46
    metabolism 46–7
fructose 1,6-bisphosphatase (F 1,6-bisPase) 36, 56, 122
    deficiency 47
    inhibition 36
    regulatory mechanisms 36
fructose 1,6-bisphosphate 32
    cleavage 12
    pyruvate kinase activation 32, 56
fructose 1,6-bisphosphate aldolase
    deficiency 47
    inhibition 47
fructose 2,6-bisphosphate
    biosynthesis 32
    fructose 1,6-biphosphatase inhibition 36
    roles 56
fructose 2,6-bisphosphatase, bifunctional enzyme 32
    in diabetes 123
fructose intolerance, hereditary 47, 117
fructose 1-phosphate, biosynthesis 46, 47
fructose 1-phosphate aldolase
    catalysis 46, 47
    deficiency 47
fructose 6-phosphate
    availability 32
    biosynthesis 31, 46, 56
    fate of 30
    glucokinase regulation 47
    'paradox' 47
fructose transporter (GLUT5) 10, 46, 47
fructosuria, essential 47
fumarate, biosynthesis (purine nucleotide cycle) 38, 102
fumarylacetoacetase
    deficiency 96, 98
    recessive disorders 96, 98
fumarylacetoacetate, accumulation 96, 98

galactitol, metabolism 44
galactokinase, deficiency 44
galactosaemia, aetiology 44
galactose 44
    inborn errors of metabolism 44
galactose 1-phosphate uridyltransferase (Gal-1-PUT), deficiency 44
galanin, insulin secretion inhibition 121
Gal-1-PUT (galactose 1-phosphate uridyltransferase), deficiency 44
GAR (glycinamide ribonucleotide), catalysis 108
GDP (guanosine diphosphate) 4
gene expression, insulin-regulated 120
gene therapy, OTC deficiency 103
George III, porphyria 114
geranyl isoprenoid group, precursors 84
geranyl pyrophosphate (GPP) 85
Gilbert's syndrome, aetiology 115
GIP (glucose-dependent insulinotrophic polypeptide) 120
GKRP (glucokinase regulatory protein) 32, 47
GLA (γ-linoleic acid) 68–9
GLP-1 (glucagon-like peptide-1) 120
glucagon
    in glycogenolysis 22, 23, 24, 26, 27
    in glycolysis 32, 33, 37, 47
    hormone-sensitive lipase activation 36
    lipolysis stimulation 60
glucagon-like peptide-1 (GLP-1), insulin secretion stimulation 120
glucagonocentric diabetes 118, 122
glucocorticoid steroids, biosynthesis 86
glucogenic amino acids 94–5
glucokinase
    catalysis 2, 3, 32
    localization 32
    metabolic roles 12, 13, 15, 23, 31, 32, 56
    translocation 47
    in diabetes 121, 122
    regulation 32, 47
glucokinase regulatory protein (GKRP)

mechanisms 32
    as nuclear anchor 47
gluconeogenesis 36, 37
    acetyl CoA in 94
    via amino acid metabolism 94–5
    in diabetes 122
    from fatty acids, problems in mammals 40–1
    inborn errors and Reye-like syndrome 116
    inhibition after ethanol consumption 48
    in liver 94
    precursors 36, 40–1, 90, 94
    regulatory mechanisms 36–7
    in Reye's syndrome 116, 117
gluconeogenesis–glycolysis switch 94
glucose
    accumulation 118
    brain requirements 10, 20, 36, 40
    homeostasis, requirements 36, 40, 47, 56, 90
    insulin-stimulated uptake 52
    metabolism see glycolysis
    nerve cell delivery 74
    phosphorylation 32
    roles, in liver phosphorylase inhibition 28
    synthesis see gluconeogenesis
    toxicity 122
    in type 2 diabetes 120
glucose alanine cycle 90, 91
glucose biosynthesis see gluconeogenesis
glucose-dependent insulinotrophic polypeptide (GIP), insulin secretion stimulation 120
glucose/fatty acid cycle 38
glucose 6-phosphatase 22, 122
    deficiency 22, 36
    localization 2, 36
glucose 1-phosphate
    biosynthesis 22, 24
    reactions, with uridine triphosphate 22
glucose 6-phosphate 26
    accumulation 25
    biosynthesis 12, 22, 24, 30
    glycolysis 24, 32
glucose 6-phosphate dehydrogenase 30, 56, 66
    deficiency 30
glucose transport
    insulin in 122
    in TAG synthesis 52–3, 54
glucose transporters (GLUTs) 32, 34, 46
    GLUT1 10
        in red blood cells 32
        in skeletal muscle 10, 35
    GLUT2 10, 23, 36, 37, 47
        abnormal 56, 57, 120, 123
        in liver 32, 56
    GLUT3 10
        in nerve 74
    GLUT4
        activation 52
        in adipose tissue 32
        in cardiomyocytes 32
        in skeletal muscle 10, 24, 25, 32, 35
        translocation 32, 52
    GLUT5 (fructose transporter) 10, 46, 47
        roles 10, 46, 47
        in skeletal muscle 10, 46
α$_1$→6-glucosidase (AGL), catalysis 22
glucuronate 44
    metabolism 45
    as vitamin C precursor 44
glucuronate/xylulose pathway, mechanisms 44
glucuronide conjugates 45
glutamate
    accumulation, in Reye's syndrome 117
    biosynthesis 66, 88, 90, 92, 102
    catabolism 92
    fatty acid synthesis 66
    γ-glutamyl cycle 30
    roles 88
glutamate dehydrogenase, in urea biosynthesis 102
glutamine
    acid/base regulation in kidney 88
    biosynthesis 88, 112
        of GMP 108
        in muscle 90
        of purines 108
    formation in diabetes 118
    as fuel for intestines 90
    roles 88
glutamine antagonists, mechanisms 110
glutamine synthetase, scavenger for ammonium ions 112
γ-glutamyl amino acid 30
γ-glutamyl cycle 30
γ-glutamylcyclotransferase 30
γ-glutamylcysteinylglycine see glutathione

γ-glutamyl transpeptidase (γ-GT) 30
glutarate, excretion 70
glutaric acidurias 70
glutaryl CoA dehydrogenase, deficiency 70
glutathione
 biosynthesis 30, 31
 depletion (Hawkinsinurea) 98
 oxidized 31
 reduced 30
 roles 30
 structure 30
glutathione peroxidase 31
glutathione reductase 30
GLUTs see glucose transporters
glyceraldehyde
 biosynthesis 46
 insulin secretion stimulation 120
glyceraldehyde 3-phosphate
 biosynthesis 12, 46, 56, 58, 59, 66
 oxidation 12
glyceraldehyde 3-phosphate dehydrogenase, catalysis 8
glycerol
 biosynthesis 49–51
 metabolism, in diabetes mellitus 118
 roles, as gluconeogenic precursor 36, 37, 40
glycerol kinase
 catalysis 36, 40, 58, 63, 64, 66, 67
 expression in white adipose tissue, debate 62
glycerol 3-phosphate
 biosynthesis see glyceroneogenesis
 fatty acid re-esterification 59, 63
 sources of 58, 59, 62, 63, 64, 65
glycerol 3-phosphate dehydrogenase 8, 12, 14
glycerol phosphate shuttle, mechanisms 8, 13
glyceroneogenesis 43, 59, 62, 63, 64–5, 66
glyceryl trierucate, Lorenzo's oil 79
glyceryl trioleate, Lorenzo's oil 79
glycinamide ribonucleotide (GAR), catalysis 108
glycine 30, 108
 accumulation, and non-ketotic hyperglycinaemia 96
 biosynthesis 88
 catabolism 92
 roles 88, 109, 111, 112, 115
glycine cleavage enzyme, deficiency 96
glycine cleavage system 92
glycine synthase, catalysis 88, 89
glycogen
 biosynthesis see glycogenesis
 exhaustion 34
 as fuel reserve 20, 34
 hepatorenal accumulation 56
 structure 20
glycogenesis 20–1, 22
 and 'fight or flight' response 20
 in liver 22, 23
 mechanisms 25
 regulatory mechanisms 25, 28–9
 in skeletal muscle 22, 23, 24, 25, 46
 and type 2 diabetes 122
 see also insulin-stimulated glycogen synthesis
glycogenin 20
glycogen metabolism 22–7
 anaerobic 14
 in diabetes mellitus 122
 in liver 22, 23
 in muscle 24–5
 metabolic demands 22
 regulatory mechanisms 26–7
 see also glycogenesis; glycogenolysis
glycogenolysis 14, 20
 in liver 22, 23
 mechanisms 22, 23, 24, 25
 in skeletal muscle 24
glycogen phosphorylase
 inhibition 47
 properties and regulation 26, 27
glycogen storage 22
glycogen storage diseases
 liver 22, 23
 muscle 25
 see also Fanconi–Bickel syndrome
glycogen synthase
 activation 28
 catalysis 22, 23
 inactivation 25, 26, 28
 properties 28
 regulatory mechanisms 28
glycogen synthase kinase-3 (GSK-3) 123
 functions 28
 glycogen synthase phosphorylation 28
glycolysis 2, 3, 5
 anaerobic 14–15, 22, 34
 enzymes in 10, 11, 32–3

inhibition 20, 22, 44
 in liver 22
 mechanisms 10–13
 and pentose phosphate pathway 30, 31, 54–7
 and Rapoport–Luebering shunt 16, 17
 regulatory mechanisms 32–3
 in skeletal muscle 34, 35
 unregulated after i.v. fructose 46
glycolytic enzymes, deficiency in red blood cells 16, 17
glycosyl transferase, catalysis 22
glyoxylate, biosynthesis 41
glyoxylate cycle 41, 112
glyoxysomes, roles, in germination 41
GMP (guanosine monophosphate) 108
gonane 84
gondoic acid 78
gout
 aetiology 22, 108, 109
 and hyperlactataemia 48
 low-fructose diet 30
GPP (geranyl pyrophosphate) 85
GSH see glutathione
GSK-3 (glycogen synthase kinase-3) 28
GSSG (oxidized glutathione) 31
γ-GT (γ-glutamyl transpeptidase) 30
GTP (guanosine triphosphate) 4, 13, 42, 43, 67
guanosine diphosphate (GDP) 4
guanosine monophosphate (GMP) 108
guanosine triphosphate (GTP) 4, 13, 42, 43, 67
L-gulonate, metabolism to vitamin C 44, 45
Günther's disease, aetiology 115

haem
 biosynthesis 114
 catabolism 114
haemoglobin, fetal 16
haem oxygenase, catalysis 114
Hartnup disease 100
hawkinsin, biosynthesis 98, 99
hawkinsinuria
 aetiology 98
 and 5-oxoprolinuria 30
HCAA (4-hydroxycyclohexylacetic acid) 98
hepatocyte nuclear factor 1α (HNF1A) mutations 120
hepatocyte nuclear factor 4α (HNF4A) mutations 120
hepatocytes 102
 glucokinase 32, 56
 glucose transport 56
 metabolic channelling studies 104
hepatorenal tyrosinaemia (tyrosinaemia, type I) 96, 98
hereditary fructose intolerance, aetiology 47, 117
hereditary orotic aciduria 103, 111
Hers' disease, aetiology 22
hexacosanoic acid see cerotic acid
hexadecanoic acid see palmitic acid
cis-Δ⁹-hexadecenoic acid 78
hexanedioic acid, biosynthesis in MCAD deficiency 71
hexanoic acid 78
hexanoyl carnitine, biosynthesis 71
hexanoylglycine, biosynthesis 70
hexokinase
 catalysis 32, 33
 deficiency 16, 17
hexose monophosphate shunt see pentose phosphate pathway
5-HIAA (5-hydroxyindoleacetic acid) 100
histidase, deficiency 96
histidinaemia, aetiology 96
histidine, catabolism 92
HMG CoA see 3-hydroxy-3-methylglutaryl CoA (HMG CoA) entries
HMMA (4-hydroxy-3-methoxymandelate) 98
HNF see hepatocyte nuclear factor entries
homocysteine, and cardiovascular disease 108
homocysteine methyltransferase, methionine salvage pathway 89, 92, 93, 95, 97, 101, 108, 109, 111
homogentisate 1,2-dioxygenase deficiency (alkaptonuria) 96
homovanillic acid (HVA) 98, 99
hormone-sensitive lipase (HSL)
 catalysis 18, 60, 61, 72
 regulatory mechanisms 60, 61
 roles, in ketone body biosynthesis 36, 72
HSL see hormone-sensitive lipase (HSL)
HVA (homovanillic acid) 98, 99
hydrogen carriers 4
hydrophilicity (bilirubin conjugates) 114
hydrophobicity (bilirubin) 114
β-hydroxyacyl ACP dehydratase (fatty acid synthase complex) 106
L-3-hydroxyacyl CoA dehydrogenase
 bifunctional enzyme 78
 catalysis 19, 41, 70, 78
 role, in β-oxidation 70, 71
3-hydroxyacyl CoA epimerase, issues 76–7
3-hydroxyanthranilate, biosynthesis 92
D-3-hydroxybutyrate

biosynthesis 72, 118
 oxidation 74
D-3-hydroxybutyrate dehydrogenase, catalysis 74
4-hydroxycyclohexylacetic acid (HCAA) 98
5-hydroxyindoleacetic acid (5-HIAA) 100
7-α-hydroxylase (cholesterol 7-α-hydroxylase), regulatory mechanisms 86
6-hydroxymelatonin 100
6-hydroxymelatonin glucuronide, biosynthesis 100
hydroxymethylbilane, biosynthesis 114
β-hydroxy-β-methylglutaric aciduria (3-hydroxy 3-methylglutaric aciduria) 96
3-hydroxy-3-methylglutaric aciduria (HMG CoA lyase deficiency and leucine catabolism) 96
3-hydroxy-3-methylglutaryl CoA (HMG CoA), and leucine catabolism 91
3-hydroxy-3-methylglutaryl CoA (HMG CoA) lyase, and ketogenesis 72, 73
 deficiency 96
3-hydroxy-3-methylglutaryl CoA (HMG CoA) reductase, and cholesterol biosynthesis 84, 85
3-hydroxy-3-methylglutaryl CoA (HMG CoA) synthase
 cholesterol biosynthesis 84–5
 ketogenesis 72–3
4-hydroxy-3-methoxymandelate (HMMA) 98
4-hydroxyphenylpyruvate dioxygenase 95
4-hydroxyphenylpyruvate oxidase 98
 deficiency 98
16-hydroxyphytanic acid 82
2-hydroxyphytanoyl CoA 80, 81
2-hydroxyphytanoyl CoA lyase 80, 81
5-hydroxytryptamine see serotonin
hyperammonaemia, in Reye's syndrome 116
hyperbilirubinaemia 114
hypercholesterolaemia, treatment 84
hyperglycaemia
 aetiology 10, 56, 118
 and glyceroneogenesis 64
 post-prandial 120
 see also persistent hyperinsulinaemic hypoglycaemic of infancy (PHHI)
hyperglycinaemia, non-ketotic, aetiology 96
hyperinsulinaemia, aetiology 122
hyperlactataemia
 aetiology 14
 and ethanol 48
 and thiamine deficiency 14
hyperlipidaemia in diabetes, aetiology 122
hypermethioninaemia 98
hypertension
 11-hydroxylase deficiency 87
 17-hydroxylase deficiency 87
 phaeochromocytoma 98
hypoglycaemia 120
 aetiology 10, 20, 22, 47, 71
 and ethanol 48
 fasting 48, 56, 120
 prevention by proteolysis and gluconeogenesis 117
 and Reye's syndrome 96, 116
hypoglycin A, metabolism 71
hypoketonaemia and Reye's syndrome 117, 117
hypophosphataemia, and diabetic ketoacidosis 16
hypoxanthine 112
hypoxanthine–guanine phosphoribosyl transferase, deficiency 110
hypoxanthine phosphoribosyl transferase 112

IAPP (islet amyloid polypeptide) 121
ICDH (isocitrate dehydrogenase) 36, 38, 54
IDO (indoleamine 2,3-dioxygenase) 100
immune haemolysis, jaundice 114
IMP (inosine monophosphate) and uric acid cycle 112
inborn errors of metabolism
 amino acid disorders 96–9
 cholesterol biosynthesis disorders 84, 85
 essential pentosuria 44
 fatty acid oxidation disorders 70, 71, 78–83
 fructokinase deficiency 47
 fructose 1,6-bisphosphatase deficiency 47
 fructose 1-phosphate aldolase deficiency 47
 galactose 44
 glycogen storage disorders 16, 17
 glycolytic enzymes (red blood cells) 16, 17
 phenylketonuria 96, 98, 99
 porphyrias 114–15
 purine and pyrimidine disorders 108–11
 Reye's syndrome and Reye-like syndrome 116, 117
 tyrosinaemias 96, 98, 99
 urea cycle disorders 51, 52
indoleamine-amine hypothesis for affective (bipolar) disease 100
indoleamine 2,3-dioxygenase (IDO) 100
indoleamine pathway 100
inner membrane, composition 2
inosine monophosphate (IMP)
 Krebs uric acid cycle 112, 113
 as purine precursor 108
 purine salvage pathway 109
 stimulation of glycogen phosphorylase 34

insects, glucose metabolism 8, 13
insulin 10–11
  gene transcription inhibition 56
  gene transcription stimulation 56
  glucose uptake stimulation 32, 122
  IRS-1 inhibition 123
  lipolysis inhibition 52
  PEPCK inhibition 36, 67
  roles 120, 121
  signal transduction 29
insulin-dependent diabetes (IDDM) 120
insulin-dependent glucose transporter see GLUT4
insulinoma 10
insulin receptors
  in adipocytes 52
  defective 120
  functions 10, 29, 52
  in muscle cells 10
insulin resistance 38
  in liver 123
  in type 2 diabetes 120, 122
insulin secretion, metabolism 120
insulin-stimulated glycogen synthesis 28, 29
  mechanisms 28, 29
intermembrane space 2, 3, 4, 6, 7, 8, 13
IPP (isopentenyl pyrophosphate) 85
iron-sulphur complexes (ETF:QO and fatty acid oxidation) 70
IRS-1 (insulin receptor substrate-1) 123
islet amyloid polypeptide (IAPP), polymerization 121
isobutyrate (maple syrup urine disease) 35, 96
isocitrate dehydrogenase (ICDH), inhibition 36, 38, 52, 54
isocitrate lyase, in glyoxylate cycle 41
isoleucine
  exercise metabolism 34
  metabolism disorders 96
  oxidation 90, 91
  transamination 102
isopentenyladenosine, biosynthesis 85
isopentenyl pyrophosphate (IPP), biosynthesis 85
isotope dilution studies and metabolic channelling 104
isovalerate 96
isovaleryl CoA dehydrogenase 91, 96
  deficiency 117

Jamaican vomiting sickness (JVS) 71
jaundice, neonatal 114
juvenile-onset diabetes 120
JVS (Jamaican vomiting sickness) 71

Kandutsch and Russell pathway (cholesterol biosynthesis) 84
KCNJ11, β-cell KATP channel gene mutation 120
kernicterus, aetiology 114
α-ketoacid dehydrogenase, branched-chain (BCKADH), deficiency 90
ketoacidosis, diabetic 118
β-ketoacyl ACP reductase (fatty acid synthase complex) 106
β-ketoacyl ACP synthase (fatty acid synthase complex) 106
3-ketoacyl CoA transferase, catalysis 74
α-ketoadipate 92
ketogenesis
  mechanisms 72
  in Reye's syndrome 117
ketogenic amino acids 72, 90
α-ketoglutarate biosynthesis 48, 92, 102
α-ketoisocaproate, insulin secretion stimulation 120
ketone bodies
  biosynthesis 72–3, 118
  oxidation 74
  utilization 74–5
ketosis, regulatory mechanisms 72
ketothiolases
  deficiency 117
  localization 70
Kir6.2 (potassium inwardly rectifying channel 6.2) 120
knockout mice (HSL knockout in mouse) 60
Krebs citric acid cycle
  acetyl CoA oxidation 38, 39
  in ATP biosynthesis 13
  catalytic mechanisms 4
  in fatty acid oxidation 19
  in glucose metabolism 10, 11–13
  glyoxylate shunt 40, 41
  inhibition following ethanol consumption 48
  ketone body utilization 74
  in mitochondrion 2, 3
  regulatory mechanisms 38–9
Krebs–Henseleit ornithine cycle 102–3
Krebs–Kornberg glyoxylate cycle 41
Krebs uric acid cycle 112–13
kynureninase
  biosynthesis 100, 101
  catalysis 92, 93
kynurenine, biosynthesis 100, 101
kynurenine pathway 100

lactate dehydrogenase, catalysis 14
lactate (lactic acid)
  accumulation in liver 22
  alcohol (ethanol) induced production 48
  biosynthesis 14, 94
  Cori cycle 14
  excess see lactic acidosis
  in fatty acid biosynthesis 50
  glycogen storage disease I 22–3
  roles 22, 36, 122
lactic acidosis 14
lactonase, catalysis 30
lanosterol
  biosynthesis 84
  demethylation 84
lanosterol 14-α-demethylase 84
lathosterol, biosynthesis 84
lauric acid 78
LCAD (long-chain acyl CoA dehydrogenase) 70, 71
LCHAD (long-chain hydroxyacyl CoA dehydrogenase) 70
  deficiency 70
leptin 121, 123
Lesch–Nyhan syndrome 110
leucine 96
  catabolism 42, 96, 102
  insulin secretion stimulation 120
  glyceroneogenesis 65
  ketogenesis 72, 73, 90, 91
  metabolic disorders 96
  oxidation 90
leucovorin, methotrexate toxicity rescue 110
levodopa (L-DOPA) 98
ligandin, bilirubin transport 114
lignoceric acid 78
linoleic acid 78
  as eicosanoid hormone precursor 68
  β-oxidation 70, 76, 77
α-linolenic acid 78
γ-linolenic acid (GLA) 68–9, 78
lipase, hormone-sensitive 18, 60–5
lipogenesis 52–7, 66–7
  NADPH + H⁺ 30
  fatty acid synthase complex 106, 107
lipolysis 18, 19, 43
  in adipose tissue 60–3
  signalling defects in diabetes 118, 122
  regulation of 60, 61
  sport and exercise metabolism 34, 35
  fatty acid esterification and re-esterification 58, 59
liver
  Cori cycle 14, 15
  fatty acid esterification 58–9
  fatty acid transport inhibition 70
  fructose metabolism 46
  functions 56
  gluconeogenesis 36, 37
  gluconeogenesis and Cori cycle 14
  glutathione in 30
  glycogenesis in 20, 22, 28, 29
  glycogen metabolism 22, 26
  glycogen storage 20, 22
  glycogen storage diseases 22, 23
  glycolysis in 32, 56–7
  insulin resistance see insulin resistance
  ketone bodies in 70, 72, 74
  Krebs cycle inhibition after ethanol consumption 48
  metabolic pathways 2–3
  pentose phosphate pathway 31–7, 56–7
  PFK-2/F 2,6-bisPase bifunctional enzyme, isoenzymes 32
  phosphorylase inhibition 28
liver cells see hepatocytes
London Underground map 2
long-chain acyl CoA dehydrogenase (LCAD), localization 71
long-chain acyl CoA synthetase, catalysis 18, 71
long-chain hydroxyacyl CoA dehydrogenase (LCHAD), specificity 70
  deficiency 70, 117
Lorenzo's oil, studies 78–9
lovastatin 85
Lowenstein's cycle see purine nucleotide cycle
lyase (arginosuccinate lyase) 105
lysine, metabolism to fat 66, 67
  catabolism 92
lysophosphatidate, biosynthesis 58, 59, 63

McArdle's disease, aetiology 25
MADD see glutaric acidurias
malate
  biosynthesis 48, 50
  decarboxylation (malic enzyme) 50, 51
malate/aspartate shuttle 9, 12, 13
malate dehydrogenase
  catalysis 4, 8, 9
  decarboxylating (malic enzyme) 50, 51

mitochondrial role in gluconeogenesis 36, 37, 104
  in oxaloacetate reduction 8, 9
  plants (glyoxysomes) 41
  metabolic channelling 104
malate synthase, in glyoxylate cycle 41
malic enzyme, malate decarboxylation 50
malonate 7
malonyl-acetyl CoA-ACP transacylase (fatty acid synthase complex) 106
malonyl ACP, biosynthesis 54
malonyl CoA
  biosynthesis 50, 51, 53–5
  fatty acid transport inhibition 70
  and insulin secretion 120, 121
mammals
  amino acid synthesis 88
  fatty acid desaturation 68
  glucose biosynthesis from fatty acids, problems 40–1
mania (bipolar disease), amine hypothesis 100
mannose, insulin secretion stimulation 120
MAO (monoamine oxidase) 89, 99, 100, 101
maple syrup urine disease 96
MARCKS (myristoylated alanine-rich C kinase substrates) 121
maturity-onset diabetes see type 2 diabetes
maturity-onset diabetes of young (MODY), aetiology 120
MCAD (medium-chain acyl CoA dehydrogenase) 70
  deficiency 70, 71
MCPA (methylenecyclopropylalanine) 71
medium-chain acyl CoA dehydrogenase see MCAD (medium-chain acyl CoA dehydrogenase)
melatonin
  biosynthesis 100
  catabolism 100
  metabolism 100, 100
mental illness, and dopamine 98
MEOS (microsomal ethanol-oxidizing system) 48
mercaptopurine, inhibitory activity 108, 110
metabolic acidosis 96, 98
metabolic channelling (substrate channelling)
  enzyme organization 104–5
  evidence for 104
  fatty acid synthase complex 106–7
  isotope dilution studies 104
  urea cycle 104–5
metabolic charts, overview 2–3
metabolic fuel hypothesis, for insulin secretion 120
metabolic pathways
  mutual dependence in Reye's syndrome 116, 117
  subcellular distribution 2–3
metabolites, channelling see metabolic channelling (substrate channelling)
metadrenaline 98
metalloporphyrins 114
metepinephrine 98
N^5,N^{10}-methenyl tetrahydrofolate, biosynthesis 111
methionine, biosynthesis 108
  catabolism 92
  metabolism to fat 67
methionine salvage pathway 108
methotrexate and rheumatoid arthritis 109, 110
  inhibitory activity 109
α-methylacyl CoA racemase (AMACR) 80–3
  deficiency 80, 81
  and disease 82
  known as P504S in oncology (immunohistochemistry) 80
  overexpression in tumours 80
3-methyladipic acid 82
4-methyladipoyl CoA 82, 84
α-methylbutyrate, and maple syrup urine disease 96
N-methyl-D-aspartate (NMDA) receptor, activation by glycine 96
3-O-methyldopa (3-OMD) 98
methylenecyclopropylalanine (MCPA), (hypoglycin) metabolism 71
N^5,N^{10}-methylene tetrahydrofolate 108, 109
  glycine biosynthesis 88
methyl-folate trap, and vitamin B$_{12}$ 108
methylmalonic aciduria 96
methylmalonyl CoA mutase, deficiency 96, 117
N^5-methyl tetrahydrofolate, biosynthesis 109
α-methyl-p-tyrosine (and phaeochromocytoma) 98
mevalonate 85
mevastatin 85
microsomal ethanol-oxidizing system (MEOS), roles, in ethanol metabolism 48
milk, galactose 44
mind's clock see biological clock
mineralocorticoid, biosynthesis 86, 87
Mitchell's chemiosmotic theory 6
mitochondrion 2
  ATP biosynthesis 4, 13
  metabolic pathways in 60, 68, 78, 82, 92
  oxygen transport 14, 16, 17
  PEPCK in mitochondria 66, 67
  respiratory chain 2, 3, 6–7
  swollen in Reye's disease 116

mobilizing lipase *see* hormone-sensitive lipase (HSL)
MODY (maturity-onset diabetes of young) 120
monoacylglycerol lipase, catalysis 60
monoamine oxidase (MAO) 99, 100, 101
monodehydroascorbate reductase 79
monohydroascorbate reductase 41
montanic acid 78
multiple acyl CoA dehydrogenase deficiency (MADD) 70
multiple carboxylase deficiency 117
muscle
  cardiac 32, 33
  Cori cycle 14
  and diabetes mellitus 120, 122
  fructose metabolism 46
  glucose/alanine cycle 90
  glucose metabolism 10, 20, 22
  glycogen metabolism 22, 24–5, 26
  glycogen storage 22
  glycogen storage diseases 25
  glycolysis, regulatory mechanisms 32–5
  insulin resistance 122
  red 14
  white 14
  see also skeletal muscle
muscle AMP deaminase, deficiency 38
muscle cells, glucose transport 10, 94, 118
muscle protein, metabolism and gluconeogenesis 36
myoadenylate deaminase, deficiency 38
myoglobin, roles, in oxygen transport 16
myristic acid 78
myristoylated alanine-rich C kinase substrates (MARCKS) 121
myxothiazol 7

NAD⁺ *see* nicotinamide adenine dinucleotide (NAD⁺)
NADH *see* nicotinamide adenine dinucleotide (NADH)
NADH/NAD⁺ ratio and ethanol metabolism 48
NADP⁺ *see* nicotinamide adenine dinucleotide phosphate (NADP⁺)
NADPH *see* nicotinamide adenine dinucleotide
    phosphate (NADPH)
NAG (*N*-acetylglutamate) 102
neonates
  diabetes 120
  glycine accumulation 96
  insulin receptor defects 120
  jaundice, treatment with Sn-mesoporphyrin 114
neuroblastoma, aetiology 98
neurochemical diseases 100
niacin, deficiency 100
nicotinamide 100
nicotinamide adenine dinucleotide (NAD⁺)
  availability 4, 5
  availability and β-oxidation 70
  biosynthesis 100
  as hydrogen carrier 4
  precursors 66
  reduction 10, 11, 14
nicotinamide adenine dinucleotide (NADH)
  biosynthesis 4, 10
  oxidation 6, 7, 8–9, 13
  P/O ratio 12, 13
  pyruvate dehydrogenase inhibition in diabetes 36
nicotinamide adenine dinucleotide phosphate (NADP⁺), availability and
    pentose phosphate pathway 30, 31
nicotinamide adenine dinucleotide phosphate (NADPH)
  biosynthesis 30–1, 50–7
  NADPH biosynthesis, cytosolic isocitrate dehydrogenase 66, 67
  and pentose phosphate pathway 50
  and pyruvate/malate cycle 50
nicotinic acid 100
  hormone-sensitive lipase, inhibition at pharmacological dose 59
NIDDM *see* type 2 diabetes
nitric oxide, from arginine 88
nitrogen, in urea biosynthesis 102, 103
nitrogen excretion
  Krebs urea cycle 102
  Krebs uric acid cycle 112
2-(2-nitro-4-trifluoro-methylbenzoyl)-1,3-cyclohexanedione (NTBC)
  toxicity 98
  in type 1 tyrosinaemia treatment 96, 97, 98, 99
NMDA (*N*-methyl-ᴅ-aspartate) receptor and glycine 96
nomenclature
  fatty acids 76, 77, 78
  steroids 84
non-essential amino acids 88–9
non-insulin-dependent diabetes mellitus (NIDDM) *see* type 2 diabetes
non-ketotic hyperglycinaemia 96
noradrenaline (norepinephrine)
  S-adenosylmethionine (SAM) methylation 108
  lipolysis stimulation 60
  methylation 99, 108
  in phaeochromocytoma 98
14-norlanosterol 84
normetepinephrine (normetadrenaline) 98

NTBC *see* 2-(2-nitro-4-trifluoro-methylbenzoyl)-1,3-cyclohexanedione (NTBC)
nucleoside diphosphate kinase, catalysis 4, 12
5′-nucleotidase, and adenosine production 34

obesity 65
  and perilipin 60
all *cis*-Δ⁹,¹²-octadecadienoate *see* linoleic acid
all *cis*-Δ⁶,⁹,¹²-octadecadienoic acid 78
all *cis*-Δ⁹,¹²,¹⁵-octadecadienoic acid 78
cis-Δ⁹-octadecenoic acid 78
cis-Δ¹¹-octadecenoic acid 78
octanedioic acid, biosynthesis in MCAD deficiency 71
octanoic acid 78
octanoyl carnitine, biosynthesis in MCAD deficiency 71
octodecanoic acid 78
oculocutaneous tyrosinaemia (tyrosinaemia, type II) 98
oestradiol, biosynthesis 86, 87
oleic acid 78
oligomycin, proton transport inhibition 7
3-OMD (3-*O*-methyldopa) 98
OMP (orotidine monophosphate) 110
'one-carbon pool' 108
ornithine 67, 102
  catabolism 88, 92
  transamination 92
ornithine cycle *see* urea cycle
ornithine transcarbamoylase (OTC), deficiency 102–3
  gene therapy 103
orotate, biosynthesis 103
orotate phosphoribosyl transferase, bifunctional enzyme 110, 111
orotic aciduria 103, 111
orotidine monophosphate (OMP), biosynthesis 110, 111
orotidine monophosphate decarboxylase (bifunctional enzyme) 111
OTC *see* ornithine transcarbamoylase (OTC)
outer mitochondrial membrane, composition 2
ovaries, sex hormone biosynthesis 86
oxaloacetate
  in Krebs cycle 38, 41, 43
  malate/aspartate shuttle 9
  pyruvate/malate cycle 50
  reduction in ethanol metabolism 48
  transamination in urea cycle 102
α-oxidation of fatty acids 80
  phytanic acid 80, 81
β-oxidation of fatty acids 18, 19, 70–3, 76–7, 80
  in ATP biosynthesis 2, 3
  linoleic acid 70, 76, 77
  in mitochondrion 78, 82
  peroxisomal 78–9, 80–3
  in plants 41
  pristanoyl CoA 80
  and Reye's syndrome 116
ω-oxidation of fatty acids 79, 80, 82–3
  phytanic acid 82, 83
  phytanoate 82
oxidative phosphorylation 2, 4, 6, 8, 12, 18, **18**
  not active in red blood cells 16, 17
oxidized glutathione (GSSG) 31
3-oxoacyl CoA thiolases, localization 70
5-oxoprolinuria 30
oxygen debt 14
oxygen transport, in red blood cells 16

palmitic acid (palmitate)
  biosynthesis 52–5, 58, 106, 107
  oxidation 18, **19**, 116
palmitoleic acid 78
palmitoleoyl CoA, biosynthesis 68
palmitoyl CoA
  biosynthesis (mitochondrial chain elongation) 16, 17
  desaturation 68
pancreas
  α-cells and glucagon 36, 122
  β-cells and insulin 10, 28, 32, 60, 61, 120, 121
PAPS (3′-phosphoadenosine-5′-phosphosulphate) 101
Parkinson's disease, aetiology 98
Pasteur effect 14, 15
PBG (porphobilinogen) 114
PBR (peripheral benzodiazepine receptor) and cholesterol uptake 86
PCOS (polycystic ovary syndrome) 87
PDE-3B (cyclic AMP phosphodiesterase-3B) 28, 29
PDH *see* pyruvate dehydrogenase (PDH)
PDK (phosphoinositide-dependent kinase) 123
PDK-1 (phosphoinositide-dependent kinase-1) 123
PDK/PKB hypothesis 123
PDK/PKB pathway 123
PDT (photodynamic therapy) 114
pellagra, aetiology 100
pentose phosphate pathway 30
  enzymes in 2, 3
  in fatty acid biosynthesis 52–5
  lipogenesis 56–7

and NADPH biosynthesis 30–1, 50–7, 66
  in red blood cells 31
  regulatory mechanisms 30
pentosuria, essential 44
PEPCK *see* phosphoenolpyruvate carboxykinase (PEPCK)
PEPCK-C gene 66
perilipin 60
peripheral benzodiazepine receptor (PBR), and cholesterol uptake 86
permanent neonatal diabetes mellitus (PNDM) 121
peroxisomal ATP-binding cassette transporter (ABCD1) and X-ALD 78–9
peroxisomal β-ketothiolase 78
peroxisomal β-oxidation 78–9, 81, 83
peroxisome proliferator activated receptor (PPAR-γ), glitazones and
    diabetes 64
peroxisomes 80
  oxidation of ethanol 48
  proliferation 64, 78
persistent hyperinsulinaemic hypoglycaemic of infancy (PHHI),
    aetiology 120
PFK *see* phosphofructokinase (PFK)
PFK-1 *see* phosphofructokinase (PFK-1)
PFK-2 *see* phosphofructokinase (PFK-2)
phaeochromocytoma, aetiology 98
phenylalanine, inborn errors of metabolism 98, 99
phenylalanine monooxygenase deficiency 96, 99
phenylketonuria (PKU) 96, 97, 98, 99
  aetiology 98
  toxic metabolite hypothesis 98
  transport hypothesis 98
phenylpyruvate, biosynthesis 98
PHHI (persistent hyperinsulinaemic hypoglycaemic of infancy) 120
phlorizin 121
phorbol esters 121
phosphatidate, as intermediate 59, 63, 120
phosphatidylcholine, biosynthesis, role of *S*-adenosylmethionine
    (SAM) 108
phosphatidylethanolamine, methylation, role of *S*-adenosylmethionine
    (SAM) 108
phosphatidylinositol 4,5-bisphosphate, metabolism 123
phosphatidylinositol 3,4,5-trisphosphate, biosynthesis 123
3′-phosphoadenosine-5′-phosphosulphate (PAPS) 100
phosphocreatine, ATP production 4, 34
phosphoenolpyruvate 14
phosphoenolpyruvate carboxykinase (PEPCK) and hepatic
    gluconeogenesis 36
  cytosolic, overexpression in muscle (supermouse) 42–3
  and glyceroneogenesis in adipose tissue 64
  inhibition by insulin 36
  mitochondrial PEPCK 66, 67
  regulatory mechanisms 64
phosphofructokinase (PFK), deficiency in red blood cells 16
phosphofructokinase-1 (PFK-1) 2, 56
  deficiency in muscle 25
  inhibition 36, 54
  metabolic roles 32, 56
  regulation by fructose 2,6-bisphosphate 32, 33
phosphofructokinase-2 (PFK-2), bifunctional enzyme 32, 56
phosphoglucomutase 22
6-phosphogluconate dehydrogenase 30
phosphoglucose isomerase 31
  deficiency in red blood cells 16
2-phosphoglycerate, biosynthesis 14, 94
phosphoglycerate kinase, in glycolysis 4, 12, 28
phosphoinositide-dependent kinase (PDK) 123
phosphoinositide-dependent kinase-1 (PDK-1), functions 123
phosphopantetheine and fatty acid synthase complex 106
phosphoribosyl pyrophosphate (PRPP) and salvage pathway 110
  biosynthesis 108
    in uric acid cycle 112
phosphoribosyl transferases (PRTs), catalysis 110
phosphorylase kinase
  activation 25, 26
  glycogen synthase phosphorylation 26
phosphorylases (glycogen)
  activation 25
  binding and inactivation of glycogen synthesis 123
  catalysis 22, 23, 24
  deficiency 22
  inactivation 26
  inhibition 28
    and hereditary fructose intolerance 47
  properties 22
  regulatory mechanisms 26
phosphorylation
  glycerol 36, 62–4
  oxidative phosphorylation 2, 4, 6, 8, 12, 16, 17, 18, **18**
  protein-serine phosphorylation and regulation of bifunctional
    enzyme 32, 33
  substrate-level phosphorylation 4, 13, 18, **18**
photodynamic therapy (PDT), cancer treatment 114
photosensitivity 114
phytanic acid
  dietary 80

α-oxidation 80, 81, 82
ω-oxidation 82, 83
phytanoate, ω-oxidation 82
phytanoyl CoA 2-hydroxylase 80
   deficiency 80
phytol metabolism 80, 81
picolinic acid (picolinate), biosynthesis 100, 101
piericidin, electron transport inhibition 7
pineal gland 100
pinealocytes 100
PK see pyruvate kinase (PK)
PKA see protein kinase A (PKA)
PKB see protein kinase B (PKB)
PKC see protein kinase C (PKC)
PKG see protein kinase G (PKG)
PKU see phenylketonuria (PKU)
plants
   Krebs–Kornberg glyoxylate cycle 41
   β-oxidation 41
polycystic ovary syndrome (PCOS) 87
polyol osmotic theory for formation of diabetic cataracts 44
P/O ratios 7, 12, 13, 18, **19**, 74, 112
porin, in outer membrane 2
porphobilinogen (PBG), biosynthesis 114
porphobilinogen (PBG) deaminase deficiency (acute intermittent porphyria) 115
porphobilinogen (PBG) synthase, inhibition by succinylacetone in tyrosinaemia I 96, 98
porphyria cutanea tarda, aetiology 115
porphyrias, aetiology 114, 115
porphyrin, metabolism 114–15
potassium channels, adenosine triphosphate-sensitive (KATP channels) 120, 121
potassium inwardly rectifying channel 6.2 (Kir6.2) 120
PP-1 see protein phosphatase-1 (PP-1)
PP-1G see protein phosphatase-1G (PP-1G)
PP-2A see protein phosphatase-2A (PP-2A)
PPAR-γ (peroxisome proliferator activated receptor), glitazones and diabetes 64
PP inhibitor-1 26, 28
pravastatin 85
pregnane 84
pregnenolone, biosynthesis 86
prenylated proteins 85
preproinsulin, metabolism 121
primers, glycogen 22
pristanal 80
pristanic acid 80
pristanoyl CoA, β-oxidation 80
progesterone
   biosynthesis 87
   nomenclature 85
proinsulin, metabolism 121, 122
proline
   biosynthesis 88
   catabolism 92
proline oxygenase, catalysis 92
propionyl CoA, product of ω-oxidation 82
propionyl CoA carboxylase, deficiency 96
14-3-3 protein 101
protein kinase A (PKA)
   activation 24, 26–7, 32–3, 120
   glycogen metabolism 24–7
   inhibition by insulin and A-kinase anchoring protein (AKAP) 26
   melatonin biosynthesis 100
   roles 24–9, 32, 34, 37, 60, 61
protein kinase B (PKB) 123
protein kinase C (PKC) 120
   activation and sorbitol metabolism 45, 120, 121
protein kinase G (PKG), and ANF in exercise-stressed heart muscle 60, 61
protein metabolism
   to acetyl CoA 92
   in diabetes mellitus 118
   during fasting 90
   to fatty acids 66–7
   gluconeogenesis 94–5
protein phosphatase-1 (PP-1) 26–9
   inactivation 26
   regulatory mechanisms in liver 28, 122
protein phosphatase-1G (PP-1G) 26
protein phosphatase-2A (PP-2A) 28
   activation by xyulose 5-phosphate 57
   ChREBP dephosphorylation 56
   PFK-2/F 2,6-bisPase dephosphorylation 57
   phosphorylase kinase dephosphorylation 26, 27, 28
protein phosphatase inhibitor-1, activity 26
proteosomal proteolysis of AANAT 100
proton channels 6, 7
proton extrusion 7
proton transport
   inhibition 7
   processes 6
protoporphyrin IX, biosynthesis 114

protoporphyrinogen IX, biosynthesis 114
Prozac 100
PRPP see phosphoribosyl pyrophosphate (PRPP) and salvage pathway
PRPP amidotransferase 112
PRTs (phosphoribosyl transferases) 110
purine nucleotide cycle 38, 39, 103
   anaplerosis and Krebs cycle 38, 39
purinergic agonists, insulin secretion stimulation 121
purines, biosynthesis 108–9, 110
pyrimidine biosynthesis 110–11
pyroglutamic aciduria (5-oxoprolinuria) 30
pyruvate
   oxidation 10
   pyruvate/malate cycle 50, 51, 66, 67
   reduction 14, 15
      reduction to lactate following ethanol consumption 48
pyruvate carboxylase
   activation 36, 37, **117**
   catalysis 50, 66, 104
   pyruvate/malate cycle 50, 51, 66, 67
   regulatory mechanisms 36
   stimulation 36, 122
   substrate channelling 104
pyruvate carrier, substrate channelling 104
pyruvate dehydrogenase (PDH)
   activation by insulin 66
   catalysis 66
   cofactors 10, 14
   glucose/fatty acid cycle 38, 39
   inhibition 34, 35, 49, 94
   regulatory mechanisms 38, 39
   substrate channelling 104
pyruvate kinase (PK) 56
   activation by protein phosphatase-2A 56
   deficiency in red blood cells 16
   in glycolysis 4, 32
   regulation in supermouse 42, 43
pyruvate/malate cycle, and NADPH biosynthesis 50–1, 66

Q cycle, mechanisms 6, 7
quinolinate , biosynthesis 100

Rabson–Mendenhall syndrome, aetiology, radioisotope dilution and substrate channelling 104
Randle cycle see glucose/fatty acid cycle
Rapoport–Luebering shunt (2,3-BPG) 16–17
reactive depression 100
red blood cells
   Cori cycle 14–15
   enzyme deficiencies 16
   oxygen transport and 2,3-BPG 16, 17
   pentose phosphate pathway and reduced glutathione 30, 31
reductases (fatty acid) 68
re-esterification of fatty acids 60
Refsum's disease 80, 82
rescue pathways 80, 82
respiratory chain 6–7, 12
   ATP biosynthesis 6–7
   in fasting **117**
   in fatty acid oxidation 18, 19, 70, 71
   hydrogen transport 10
   inhibitors of 7
   and Reye's syndrome 116
Reye-like syndrome 116
Reye's syndrome
   aetiology 116, 117
   diagnostic criteria 116
rheumatoid arthritis and methotrexate 110
ribose 1,5-bisphosphate and PFK-1 56
ribose 5-phosphate
   glycogen storage disease I 22
   in purine biosynthesis 31, 108
ribulose 5-phosphate, biosynthesis 30
Richner–Hanhart syndrome (tyrosinaemia type II) 98
Rieske protein 7
RNA, biosynthesis 108
rosiglitazone and glycerol kinase in adipose tissue debate 62
rotenone, electron transport inhibition 7

SAD (seasonal affective disorder) 100
salvage pathways
   methionine 108
   purines/pyrimidines 110
SAM see S-adenosylmethionine (SAM)
sarco(endo)plasmic reticulum CA²⁺ ATPase (SERCA), catalysis 121
SCAD (short-chain acyl CoA dehydrogenase) 70
SCHAD (short-chain hydroxyacyl CoA dehydrogenase) 71
schizophrenia and serine hydroxymethyltransferase deficiency 88
   dopamine hypothesis 98
SCN (suprachiasmatic nuclei) 100
seasonal affective disorder (SAD) 100
sebacic acid in MCAD deficiency 70, 71
seeds, sugar biosynthesis from fat 41

SERCA (sarco(endo)plasmic reticulum CA²⁺ ATPase) 121
serine
   biosynthesis by 'phosphorylated pathway' 88
   catabolism 92
   as glycine precursor 108
   phosphorylation (covalent modification of proteins) 26, 28, 32, 60, 61
   uses 88
serine hydroxymethyltransferase, catalysis 88, 108, 110
serotonin
   biosynthesis 100
   metabolism 100
serotonin reuptake inhibitors 100
sex hormones, biosynthesis 86, 87
short-chain acyl CoA dehydrogenase (SCAD), localization 70
short-chain fatty acids, elongation 68, 69
short-chain hydroxyacyl CoA dehydrogenase (SCHAD), specificity 71
SIDS (sudden infant death syndrome) 70
signal transduction, insulin 29
simvastatin 85
singlet oxygen, photosensitive porphyria 114
skeletal muscle
   Cori cycle 14
   cytosolic PEPCK, overexpression in muscle (supermouse) 42–3
   glycogenolysis 24–5
   GLUTs (glucose transporters) 35
   PFK-2/F 2,6-bisPase isoenzymes 32, 33
skin cancer, treatment 114
Smith–Lemli–Opitz syndrome 84
Sn-mesoporphyrin 114
sorbinil, as aldose reductase inhibitor 44, 45
sorbitol, metabolism 44, 45
sorbitol dehydrogenase, catalysis 44
sport, biochemistry of (see also 'supermouse') 34–5, 42, 43
squalene, biosynthesis 84
squalestatin 85
SREBP, regulation of fatty acid and cholesterol biosynthesis 56
starflower oil, therapeutic benefits 68–9
StAR (steroid acute regulatory) protein 86
starvation
   amino acid metabolism 94–5
   brain energy requirement during 72, 74
   fatty acid mobilization 18, 38
   and gluconeogenesis 36, 94–5
   glucose alanine cycle 90
   glycogen 20–7
   metabolic pathways in liver 116–17, **117**
   muscle protein metabolism during 90
statins (HMG CoA reductase inhibitors) 84, 85
stearic acid 78
stercobilin, biosynthesis 114
steroid acute regulatory (StAR) protein, regulatory mechanisms 86
steroid hormones 84, 86
   biosynthesis 87
steroids, nomenclature 84
sterol response element binding protein see SREBP
stigmatellin 7
Streptococcus mutans, and xylitol 44
suberic acid and MCAD deficiency 70
suberylglycine and MCAD deficiency 70
substrate-level phosphorylation 4, 13
succinate, biosynthesis and glyoxylate cycle 41
succinate dehydrogenase
   catalysis 4, 12
   inhibition by malonate 7
   roles, in respiratory chain 2, 3
succinic acid esters, and insulin secretion 121
succinylacetone
   accumulation, tyrosinaemia type I 98
   porphobilinogen synthase inhibition 98, 115
succinyl CoA
   biosynthesis 4, 35, 92, 93
   catabolism of ketogenic amino acids 91
   condensation 114
   and ketone body utilization 75
succinyl CoA synthetase 12, 13
   catalysis 4, 19
sucrose, average daily intake 46
sudden infant death syndrome (SIDS) 70
sugars, biosynthesis from fats 41
6-sulphatoxymelatonin, biosynthesis 100
sulphonylurea receptor, potassium channel closure 120
sulphonylureas 121
suprachiasmatic nuclei (SCN) 100
synaptotagmin, as calcium sensor for insulin secretion 120

TAGs see triacylglycerols (TAGs)
Tarui's disease, aetiology 25
TDO (tryptophan 2,3-dioxygenase) 100
testes, sex hormone biosynthesis 86
testosterone, biosynthesis 86, 87
tetracosanoic acid 78
tetradecanoic acid 78
trans-Δ²-tetraenoic acid 78

tetrahydrobiopterin, biosynthesis, impaired 96, 98
tetrahydrofolate (THF), biosynthesis 108
tetramethyl-*p*-phenyldiamine (TMPD), in respiratory chain studies 7
thenoyltrifluoroacetone, electron transport inhibition 7
thermogenesis 6, 7, 64
thermogenin 7
THF (tetrahydrofolate) 108
thiamine deficiency, and hyperlactataemia 14
thiazolidinediones (TZDs, glitazones) and PEPCK 64
thioesterase and fatty acid synthase complex 106
threonine
    catabolism by dehydratase pathway in humans 92
        see also chart, back cover
    catabolism by amino acetone pathway in animals *see* chart, back cover
threonine dehydratase pathway for threonine catabolism 92
thymidylate synthase
    catalysis 110, 111
    inhibition 110, 111
thyroid hormones 88, 89
timnodonic acid *see* eicosapentanoic acid (EPA)
tin mesoporphyrin 114
TMPD (tetramethyl-*p*-phenyldiamine) 7
tolcapone 98
toxic metabolite hypothesis (phenylketonuria, PKU) 98
α-toxin (metabolic channelling urea cycle) 104, 105
transamination route, urea biosynthesis 102, 103
transdeamination route, urea biosynthesis 102, 103
transport hypothesis (phenylketonuria, PKU) 98
triacylglycerol/fatty acid cycle, mechanisms 62–5
triacylglycerol lipase *see* hormone-sensitive lipase (HSL)
triacylglycerols (TAGs) 18, 19, 40, 52–65
    biosynthesis (in supermouse) 43
    in diabetes 118
    ketogenesis 72
    lipolysis 60, 61
    metabolism 40
tricarboxylate transporter 54
    metabolic channelling 54
tricarboxylic acid cycle *see* Krebs citric acid cycle
trifunctional enzyme, mitochondrial β-oxidation of fatty acids
    70, 71, 116
triglycerides *see* triacylglycerols (TAGs)
tri-iodothyronine 98
trimethoprim 109
triose kinase, catalysis 46
triose phosphates, biosynthesis 12
tripalmitin, metabolism 50–67
triparanol 85
tryptophan
    catabolism 92
    in depression treatment 100
    and lipogenesis 66
    metabolism 100–1
    oxidation 92
tryptophan 2,3-dioxygenase (TDO), catalysis 100
tryptophan hydroxylase 100, 101
tryptophan pyrrolase *see* tryptophan 2,3-dioxygenase (TDO)
type 1 diabetes, aetiology 120
type 2 diabetes
    aetiology 120

and insulin resistance 120
    in adipose tissue 120
    lifestyle influences 120
    in liver 122–3
    in muscle 120
    risk factors 120
type I glycogen storage disease, aetiology 22
type III glycogen storage disease, aetiology 22
type V glycogen storage disease, aetiology 25
type VI glycogen storage disease, aetiology 22
type VII glycogen storage disease, aetiology 25
type XI glycogen storage disease *see* Fanconi–Bickel syndrome
tyrosinaemia 96, 98, 99
    type I (hepatorenal)
        aetiology 96, 98
        treatment 96, 98
    type II (oculocutaneous) 98
    type III 98
tyrosinase deficiency, albinism 96
tyrosine
    biosynthesis 88
    inborn errors of metabolism 96, 97, 98, 99
    metabolism to fat 66
    uses 88
tyrosine aminotransferase, recessive disorder 98, 99
tyrosine 3-monooxygenase, inhibition by α-methyl-*p*-tyrosine
    98, 99
TZDs (thiazolidinediones, glitazones) and glyceroneogenesis 64, 65

ubiquinol, in respiratory chain 6, 7
ubiquinone
    precursors 84
    in respiratory chain 6, 7, 8
    roles, in fatty acid oxidation 70
UDCA *see* ursodeoxycholic acid (UDCA) and obstetric cholestasis
UDP (uridine diphosphate) 110
UDP-glucose 22
UDP glucuronate *see* uridine diphosphate glucuronate
UDP glucuronyltransferase 44
UMP (uridine monophosphate) 110
uncoupling protein, and thermogenesis 7
unsaturated fatty acids, β-oxidation 76–7
urea, biosynthesis 102
urea cycle
    discovery by Krebs 112
    mechanisms 102–3
    metabolic channelling 104–5
    in Reye's syndrome 116
ureotelism 112
uric acid, and gout 110
uric acid cycle 112
uricotelism 112
uridine diphosphate glucose (UDP-glucose), biosynthesis 22
uridine diphosphate glucuronate 44
uridine diphosphate (UDP) 110
uridine monophosphate (UMP), biosynthesis 110
uridine triphosphate (UTP)
    biosynthesis 110
    reactions, with glucose 1-phosphate 22
urobilin, biosynthesis 114

urobilinogen, biosynthesis 114
uroporphyrinogen I, biosynthesis 114
uroporphyrinogen III, biosynthesis 114
ursodeoxycholic acid (UDCA) and obstetric cholestasis 86
UTP *see* uridine triphosphate (UTP)

vaccenic acid 78
valine
    catabolism 34, 90, 96, 102
    metabolism disorders 96
    oxidation 90
vanillylmandelic acid (VMA) 98
variegate porphyria, aetiology 115
vascular damage, and sorbitol metabolism 44
very-long-chain acyl CoA dehydrogenase (VLCAD), in carnitine
    shuttle 70
very-long-chain acyl CoA synthetase 79
    catalysis 78
very-long-chain fatty acids, chain shortening 78, 79, 80
very-low-density lipoproteins (VLDLs)
    secretion 122
    triacylglycerol transport 58, 59
vitamin B$_6$, and homocysteine catabolism 109
vitamin B$_{12}$ 108
    and homocysteine catabolism 109
    and methyl-folate trap 108
    and methylmalonic aciduria 96
vitamin C, biosynthesis 44
vitamin D, precursors 85, 86
VLCAD (very-long-chain acyl CoA dehydrogenase), in carnitine
    shuttle 70
VLDLs *see* very-low-density lipoproteins (VLDLs)
VMA (vanillylmandelic acid) 98
voltage-dependent calcium channels 120
von Gierke's disease, aetiology 22

white adipose tissue
    fatty acid mobilization from 60–5
    glyceroneogenesis 64, 65

xanthine monophosphate (XMP), amination 108
xanthurenate 101
X-linked adrenoleukodystrophy (X-ALD) 79
XMP (xanthine monophosphate), amination 108
xylitol 44
    biosynthesis 44
    dental decay prevention 44
    metabolism 44, 45
xylulose 44
xylulose 5-phosphate and protein phosphatase-2A activation 56
    biosynthesis 44
L-xylulose reductase, deficiency 44

yeast, alcoholic fermentation 15

Zellweger syndrome, aetiology 80
zona fasciculata, cortisol biosynthesis 86
zona glomerulosa, aldosterone biosynthesis 86
zona reticularis, cortisol biosynthesis 86
zymosterol, biosynthesis 85